GUIDE TO PLANNING AND MANAGING MULTIPLE CLINICAL STUDIES

Guide to Planning and Managing Multiple Clinical Studies

Bert Spilker, Ph.D., M.D.
Head, Department of Project Coordination
Burroughs Wellcome Co.
Research Triangle Park, North Carolina; and
Clinical Assistant Professor of Medicine and
Adjunct Associate Professor of Pharmacology
University of North Carolina at Chapel Hill
Chapel Hill, North Carolina

Raven Press New York

Raven Press, 1185 Avenue of the Americas, New York, New York 10036

Made in the United States of America

Library of Congress Cataloging-in-Publication Data
Spilker, Bert.
Guide to planning and managing multiple clinical studies.

Companion v. to: Guide to clinical interpretation of data, and: Guide to clinical studies and developing protocols.
Bibliography: p.
Includes index.
1. Clinical trials. I. Spilker, Bert. Guide to clinical interpretation of data. II. Spilker, Bert. Guide to clinical studies and developing protocols. III. Title. IV. Title: Multiple clinical studies. [DNLM: 1. Clinical Trials—methods. 2. Drug Evaluation—methods. 3. Research Design. QV 771 S756ga]
R853.C55S653 1987 615.5′8′0724 86-31535
ISBN 0-88167-264-5

9 8 7 6 5 4 3 2

To my children, Adam and Karen.

Preface

Guide to Planning and Managing Multiple Clinical Studies is the third and final volume written as a group of guides to clinical studies.* The first volume deals with a single clinical study, and its three sections describe processes used to (1) choose a study design, (2) write a protocol, and (3) plan and conduct a clinical study. The second volume deals with the clinical interpretation of data that evolve from clinical studies and also describes various aspects of publishing data. The present volume expands consideration from a *single* study (i.e., conducted at either a single site or multiple sites) to consideration of processes involved in planning, conducting, and managing *multiple* (i.e., different) clinical studies. Like the two others, the present volume is intended for a broad range of individuals with industrial, academic, or government affiliations.

This volume continues the practical "nuts and bolts" style established in the first volume by presenting numerous tables of possible interpretations, considerations, and factors to review, as well as including a variety of checklists. Nonetheless, this book is not a "how to" for carrying out multiple clinical studies. Each company, academic group, or government agency differs in critical ways (e.g., standard operating procedures, approaches, ethics, objectives), and it is therefore not possible to present a single meaningful "how to" approach that may be directly used for conducting studies. Each project will also vary, and although the procedures followed may be generally similar, the specific problems and issues to deal with are unique. This book presents many of the options that are available to consider in dealing with issues and problems. The best approach will be achieved by those who are most prepared to solve the novel challenges that arise in all studies.

The chapters in this book are generally autonomous and may be read in any order. There are numerous factors to consider in initiating and carrying out a project that involves multiple studies. Section I presents relevant steps and procedures for (1) choosing a project or drug for evaluation, (2) establishing goals, strategies, and approaches, and (3) designing the project with all of these factors in mind. Specific techniques are presented to integrate efficacy and safety data obtained in multiple studies. Ethical issues involved in both single and multiple clinical studies are also discussed.

---

* *Guide to Clinical Studies and Developing Protocols* (1984) and *Guide to Clinical Interpretation of Data* (1986) are the first two volumes of the group.

Section II describes many considerations that underlie the planning, conduct, and management of special nondrug studies such as those on surgery and medical devices, as well as factors relating to initiating and managing projects in multiple countries. Suggestions are offered for designing single clinical studies in the field of surgery.

Section III presents management techniques that include recommendations for academic or private physicians who are conducting several studies either simultaneously or sequentially. These techniques also apply to sponsors of studies who often develop elaborate systems to allocate resources and plan and monitor clinical studies. Practical details and suggestions are presented to enable the investigator and staff, sponsors, and managers to monitor and review progress in multiple studies relating to drug development and other medical areas.

Acknowledgments

The author sincerely thanks the many people who helped review this manuscript. The major reviewer in this work was Dr. John Schoenfelder, whose perception and logical mind helped clarify numerous vague or questionable passages.

The author also thanks the following people for their review and many valuable suggestions: Mr. J. M. Arnold; Dr. Howard Filstein; Mr. Robin K. Henning; Drs. Allen Lai, Walker Long, and Lloyd G. Millstein; Ms. Erika F. Nissman; Dr. Peter Palmer; Mr. David C. Pressel; Dr. Joel E. Sutton; Mr. Randy Vestal; and Mrs. Cindy F. Wilson.

The author appreciates the technical assistance of Mrs. Joyce Carpunky, Mr. Allen Jones, and Mr. Rolly Simpson, plus the typing skills of Mrs. Judy Appleton and Mrs. Thomasine Cozart.

Thanks are due Manchester University Press of Manchester, England for permission to copy most of my chapter on orphan drugs from the book *Orphan Diseases and Orphan Drugs*, edited by I. H. Scheinberg and J. M. Walshe, 1986.

Contents

Section III: Management of Multiple Clinical Studies

Terminology

RESEARCH (in the Pharmaceutical Industry)

Numerous definitions of research are used both in the literature and among scientists. In the broadest sense, research in the pharmaceutical industry includes all processes of drug discovery, preclinical and clinical evaluation, and technical development. In a more restricted sense, research is used to concentrate on the preclinical discovery phase, where the basic characteristics of a new drug are determined. Once a decision is reached to study a drug in humans, to evaluate its therapeutic potential, the compound passes from the research to the development phase.

RESEARCH AND DEVELOPMENT

When research and development are used together, it refers to the broadest definition given for "research". Some people use the term "research" and others use the term "development" to include most or all of the areas (discovery, evaluation, and development) covered by the single term "research and development". Drug development, in its broadest definition, is exactly the same as the broad definition of research.

DEVELOPMENT OF DRUGS

The term "development" as applied to drugs is used in several different contexts, even within the pharmaceutical industry. This often leads to confusion and misunderstandings. No single definition is preferred, but the particular meaning intended should be made clear by all people using the term. Three operational definitions are presented from the broadest to the narrowest:

1. All stages and processes involved in discovering, evaluating, and formulating a new drug, until it reaches the market (i.e., commercial sale).
2. All stages involving the evaluation and formulation of a new drug (after the drug has been discovered and has gone through preclinical testing), until it reaches the market.
3. Those stages after the preclinical discovery and evaluation which involve technical development. These processes include formulation work, stability testing, scaling-up the compound for larger-scale synthesis, and providing analytical support. Clinical studies are not included in this definition.

List of Tables

Section I

Section II

Section III

Appendix

List of Illustrations

Section I

Section II

Section III

Appendix

Section I

Planning and Conducting Multiple Clinical Studies

1

Choosing a Project or Drug for Evaluation

General Procedures • Criteria to Apply • Preparing Feasibility Reports • Assessing the Feasibility of an Overall Project • Reaching a Decision • Drug Studies Conducted by Physicians in Private Practice

GENERAL PROCEDURES

This chapter is written from the perspective of individuals within a company who have choices to make about which projects to develop. The projects would primarily be oriented toward developing an investigational drug, medical device, or diagnostic test. The same approaches may be used by scientific and clinical investigators in academia who are also choosing a project to develop, which will require multiple clinical studies. A few considerations that specifically apply to academicians will be mentioned. Finally, the chapter concludes with a brief discussion on how physicians in private practice may choose a project or drug for evaluation.

The projects that a company is willing to undertake depend on which other projects the company is pursuing. If there are many other projects under development and limited resources are available, then standards for accepting a new project will be higher than if there are only a few interesting projects or resources are "unlimited." Projects that fall outside the company's usual "comfort zone" usually have a more difficult time gaining resources, unless a strong commitment is made for their development.

In reaching a decision about whether to initiate a new project, the following few steps will usually provide assurance that a reasonable sequence has been followed. These processes may be used to judge each specific criterion as well as the overall project proposed.

1. Specify the objectives to be achieved in making the decision. Do all the relevant people agree on these objectives?
2. Determine and examine each of the available alternatives. Various techniques such as "decision trees" may be useful in creating or looking for additional alternatives.
3. Obtain the necessary information on each alternative.

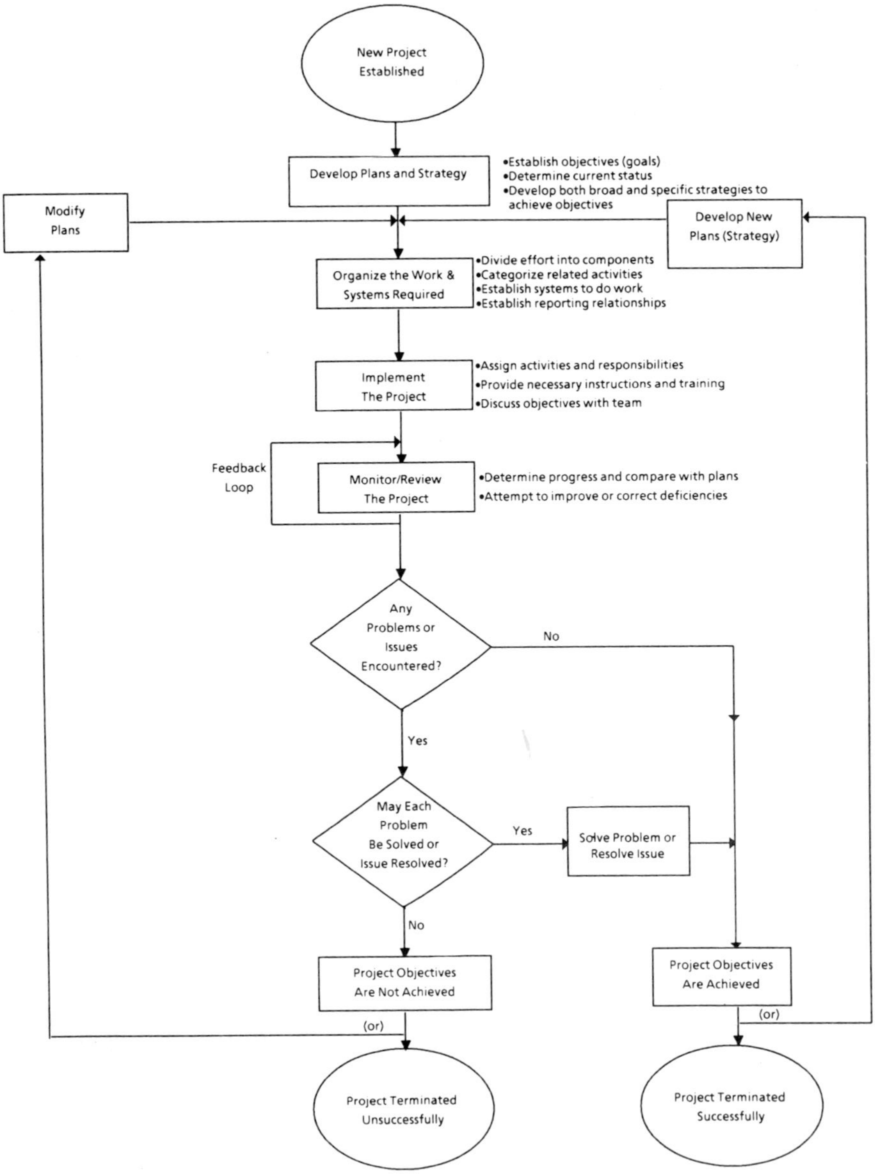

FIG. 1.1. Flow diagram model for establishing and monitoring a project.

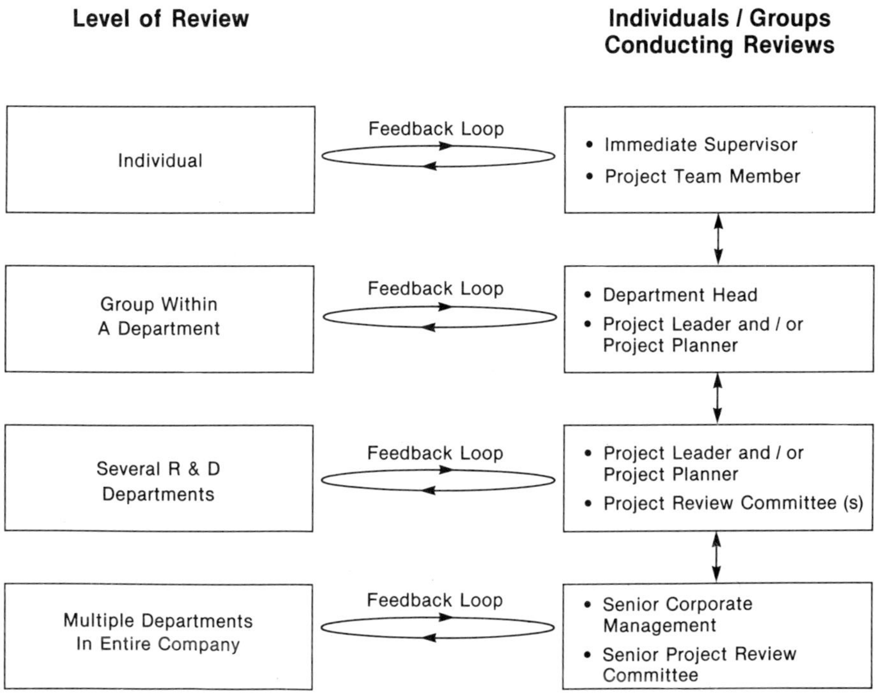

FIG. 1.2. Levels of project reviews within a company.

4. Analyze the uncertainties inherent in each alternative. This may be done qualitatively and/or quantitatively.
5. Evaluate the alternatives and discuss each with relevant people.
6. Based on all of the above information and inputs, reach a decision.

A number of years ago some companies used systems that gave scores to potential projects to determine if they had enough points to enter the project system. The points were based on the types of criteria discussed above and various other considerations. A number of systems that have been used are discussed by Faust (1982). This approach is rarely followed today in the pharmaceutical industry because the elaborate models were found to have numerous shortcomings that were critical factors to consider in selecting projects, but were difficult to include in the models. These factors include (1) personal biases, (2) intuition, (3) risks involved at the time the decision is made, (4) status of other projects, and (5) corporate health. More emphasis is now placed on how the proposed project is perceived to fit into the overall project portfolio, which in turn is defined in terms of medical and commercial objectives plus long-term and short-term goals. The general methods by which a project is established and monitored are shown in Fig. 1.1, and the types of reviews conducted within a company are illustrated in Fig. 1.2.

CRITERIA TO APPLY

There are many criteria to use in selecting a project or drug for evaluation. Although some criteria are highly specific and are related to the specific attributes and characteristics of the potential project or drug, there are many guidelines and criteria that are considered in most situations. The primary categories of criteria to be discussed are (1) scientific merit, (2) medical utility and uniqueness, (3) commercial value, (4) practical considerations, and (5) organizational factors.

Scientific merit includes consideration of how scientifically interesting the project or drug's preclinical, biological and/or chemical profile is assessed to be. Scientific interest, in turn, is often based on the differences and similarities between the new drug and known agents, how well the drug's profile meets the minimal and ideal goals set for the drug, and the nature of how the drug works. In addition, the project may have special attributes of interest to the developers and/or scientists.

Medical utility and uniqueness are often clear when discussing major breakthroughs in new drug development, but are less clear when discussing drugs that may have a more minor role for patient therapy, prevention, or diagnosis. One gauge of assessing medical uniqueness is to determine the number of patients who would be expected to be treated per year if the drug is shown to have the expected clinical profile. If this criterion is used to make a choice among multiple drugs it will favor that drug (or drugs) which will be used most often.

A more humanistic approach to choosing among multiple drugs with different indications is to also consider the percent of patients with the disease who will be treated and helped with each drug, and not solely the numbers of patients treated. Thus, a novel drug for a rare disease that has no current therapy should acquire 100% of that small market (e.g., 1,000 patients) and may represent a more important project to develop (in terms of medical interest and humanitarian concerns) than one that will only attain a 10% share of a larger market (e.g., 1,000,000 patients) where adequate therapy exists. It is also possible to consider both aspects (i.e., number of probable patients to be treated and market share) when determining which project to develop.

If there are new compounds that may become breakthrough drugs which are not being developed because of financial limitations, then the potential drug may be licensed to another developer such as the federal government, independent foundation, institute, or to another company. Another possibility is to establish a collaborative approach or joint venture to pursue the new drug's development. Joint development may make consideration of selected orphan drugs more attractive.

Commercial value is usually an important factor to consider in choosing a project and may be assessed in many ways. Marketing considerations include (1) projections of sales and profits, (2) fit of the potential project with marketed products and other projects, (3) commercial need for a new drug with the characteristics anticipated in the potential project, and (4) status of the competition in terms of existing and investigational drugs.

For academicians who do not envision a commercial product resulting from their project, the commercial aspects usually relate to relative costs in terms of staff, equipment, and time required to pursue a particular project and also the likelihood that a given project will be funded through competitive grants or other mechanisms.

The fourth and fifth major types of criteria used to choose projects are practical considerations and organizational factors. The term "practical considerations" refers to how easily and conveniently the project fits into the particular investigator's plans or sponsor's organization. Timing is an important consideration since the ability to pursue a project depends to a large degree on which other projects are ongoing and what potential each of those projects has in medical and commercial terms. The situation is actually more complex for many companies that wish to maintain a balance of short-, medium-, and long-term projects, in terms of the anticipated duration of their premarketing clinical studies. In addition, companies often have short-, medium-, and long-term objectives in terms of therapeutic areas or types of products they wish to emphasize.

The impact of the proposed project and ability to pursue it expeditiously in terms of resource requirements and availability (e.g., number of staff, expertise, equipment, facilities, money) must be considered, as well as the likelihood of success. A resource-intensive project that will have a major impact on other projects in terms of staff requirements for a protracted period must be considered differently than a project that has only a negligible or temporary effect on the others. Another resource issue is whether the appropriate expertise is available to carry out and complete the project.

One particular aspect of the resource issue which is often relevant to consider relates to short-, medium-, and long-term financial commitments in taking on a new project. Some companies consider this issue through brief informal conversations among research managers using as a theme the questions "Can we afford to take this project on?" and "Can we afford not to take this project on?" Other companies resort to detailed business analyses of what the market for the therapeutic class is expected to be like in 10 or another number of years and the expected market share for the proposed drug, based on established and projected new competitive products. Common analyses and estimates include consideration of specific advantages of the new drug, date of launch, and strength of the patent(s). These companies then determine anticipated sales and profits considering the above factors plus manufacturing, marketing, promotion, and other costs.

Another criterion to consider in choosing which drugs to develop is the public exposure one receives by deciding to develop a given project or drug.

There are clearly diseases for which drug development will enhance the image of the sponsor, either because the development may be viewed as an altruistic effort (such as for rare diseases where the sponsor may actually lose money) or as a valuable service in an area of great societal need (e.g., a major advance in chemotherapy for lung or colon cancer).

Thus, the desire of medical and commercial personnel to choose new projects that will fit the overall portfolio must be carefully assessed in conjunction with numerous additional practical and organizational factors that relate to the entire company.

The manner by which the criteria used to choose a project are applied depend in a large measure on the nature of the group that must choose a project to develop. If there is a preponderance of either medical, scientific, or marketing personnel involved in the final decision, then that particular aspect will likely have a major influence on the decision reached.

Some groups apply these criteria in an overall subjective approach, whereas others resort to sophisticated scales that delve into many details (Mazzoni, 1972). There is a wide spectrum between simple and complex approaches to this discussion and the drug industry appears to be moving away from complex approaches.

Role of Marketing Input in Choosing Research Directions and Projects

Many pharmaceutical corporations attempt to avoid placing a heavy emphasis on short-term marketing considerations in choosing corporate goals. One danger of this marketing approach is that the organization may focus too closely on what appears to be profitable in the short term (e.g., line extensions of marketed products) at the expense of important medical opportunities and long-term commercial success.

A traditional marketing approach to choosing future areas for new drug discoveries and innovations is based on examining the past performance of drugs in various therapeutic areas. A previously successful therapeutic field from the perspective of drug sales is usually viewed as having great potential to be taken over by a more therapeutically valuable drug. Therapeutic areas where current sales are small or are actually declining are often viewed with skepticism. On the other hand, a creative individual will view a number of these "unpromising" therapeutic areas as providing great opportunities to make important medical breakthroughs, while also reaping large commercial success. For example, prior to the introduction of cimetidine (Tagamet), drug therapy of ulcers was a small market primarily limited to the use of antacids, but cimetidine markedly enhanced total drug sales in the entire therapeutic area. Cimetidine paved the way for other antiulcer drugs to become both scientifically acceptable on a rational basis and commercially attractive. Unless unexpected adverse effects are reported, or other toxicities develop, cimetidine will continue to be both commercially and medically successful for many years. Similar situations have occurred in other therapeutic fields influenced by breakthrough drugs. If a new safe and effective drug were discovered for weight reduction or dementia it would stimulate an enormous demand and a huge new commercial market would be created overnight.

It is not suggested that well-worked therapeutic areas (e.g., cephalosporins, β-receptor antagonists) should either be specifically avoided or pursued in the search for new drugs. The consideration of developing novel approaches to patient treatment in certain important therapeutic areas where some therapy already exists is a worthwhile concept to explore, especially when there are significant limitations in the safety and/or efficacy of current therapy. This situation can be illustrated through the use of propranolol in hypertension. At the time of its development there were many drug treatments available for patients with hypertension, but none of them were ideal. Although propranolol, too, is not a totally ideal drug, it offered greater benefit to many patients with hypertension than previous therapy and spawned the discovery and development of a large number of other β-receptor blocking drugs. Propranolol was not the ultimate antihypertensive drug, and both calcium channel blockers and angiotensin I converting enzyme (ACE) inhibitors have made further advances in this field.

There are many appropriate stages of drug development at which to consider commercial information. The first such time is during the early stages of research when targets are sought for new chemical compounds. Many compounds, however, are often found to affect targets other than those for which they were originally intended. This occurs either early on in the research process during screening and testing in animal models, or later during the clinical development or marketing phases. Nonetheless, it is relevant for commercial influences to have some input in the decisions made about the original targets that the scientist and/or scientific management chooses. As a drug moves through a variety of tests, hurdles, and problems, its profile becomes progressively better defined, especially in terms of relative benefits and risks. The estimates of the drug's potential commercial return becomes more accurate, especially toward the end of Phase II studies. Usually the best marketing estimates may be made of the drug's commercial value at the time of launch, after many years and many millions of dollars have been spent. But, even these estimates are based on many unknown factors and may prove to be highly inaccurate.

It is generally well accepted that approximately 1 in 10,000 newly synthesized compounds becomes a marketed drug, so that the rate of attrition is extremely high for newly synthesized compounds. Most compounds are synthesized with hopes for their success, whereas others are made for improved patent protection or for different reasons. The ratio of drugs that become marketed to those compounds tested in humans varies from approximately 1 in 4 to 1 in 10, depending on the source of information and also what standards are used to choose those drug that are tested clinically.

As the costs of taking new compounds with clinical studies increases in the United States, fewer sponsors are willing or able to simultaneously progress two or more compounds from the same chemical series to initial clinical tests in humans. Instead, they select the best compound from a single chemical series for clinical evaluation based on animal and other data. This has meant that the ratio of marketed drugs to those tested in humans has increased over the last two decades and a greater percentage of apparent success has been achieved. The increased cost of the entire drug development process has also put pressure on sponsors to increase the standards used for choosing drugs to test in humans.

Licensing of Drugs or Products

There are few major pharmaceutical companies that rely entirely on discovering new drugs within their own research and development departments and are not proactively seeking to license drugs from other companies. Other companies have adopted a reactive posture and respond to offers received. When sponsors are considering either licensing-in compounds from other companies or licensing-out compounds to other sponsors to develop and/or market, the importance and influence of commercial input is often paramount to the decisions made. In licensing drugs the company must strongly consider commercial potential for the compound, drug, or product being discussed, as well as commercial aspects of the proposed business arrangements (e.g., royalties, fees, countries involved).

Drugs may be licensed in (or out) at any stage of development. The further along the development track the product is at the time of licensing, the more accurately its potential value may be estimated. A newly synthesized compound that is found to have activity in an initial screen may have enormous long-term commercial potential but relatively little value for licensing. As the compound survives additional rounds of biological testing its real value steadily increases. Each stage in the drug development process usually represents a difficult hurdle and culls out many drugs, usually for reasons of toxicity or insufficient therapeutic activity.

In addition to the licensing of drugs from other companies, drugs may be licensed from the academic community, which often has the chemical and biochemical means to synthesize drugs, but lacks adequate resources for testing or developing drugs through formulation development, toxicology, and clinical trials. There are also instances of commercial or research groups outside academic centers or corporations who synthesize drugs that eventually are tested by companies.

Although licensing drugs from other sponsors may seem to be a means of avoiding the high costs of research, many of the major clinical, toxicological, and technical development costs usually remain. These latter costs are almost always much more than those spent on the discovery and early animal studies of the compound that is being developed.

Drugs may also be licensed (in or out) after they have been approved for marketing. A major reason why a sponsor might license a drug to another company *after* it has been approved for marketing would be because the original sponsor could not market the drug as effectively as the company to which it was licensed. For example, a relatively small company with a limited number of marketing representatives usually can not generate as much revenue with a specific drug as a sponsor with a much larger number of sales representatives. A company may also wish to expand its sales in regions of the world where its presence is currently small or nonexistent.

Cross-Licensing

Another reason for licensing a marketed drug might result as part of a cross-licensing agreement. If two companies develop drugs that are outside their usual zones of marketing, then swapping products (with appropriate financial, legal, and other safeguards) may be a sound business arrangement for both companies. For example, if one company's products are primarily concentrated in the cardiovascular area and those of another company are concentrated in the surgical area, then each of their sales forces will normally direct their promotional campaigns and efforts toward different types of specialists and practitioners. A new product in a different therapeutic area might be difficult for them to promote and a cross-licensing agreement could be a mutually beneficial solution. Two companies that sell drugs in different regions of the world could also benefit in some cases from a cross-licensing arrangement.

Joint Development and/or Marketing

The original developer of a drug might wish to retain the rights to sell it as well as license it or obtain expertise or funds for its development. Thus, there could be an agreement between two sponsors to jointly develop and/or market a drug.

The types of arrangements for jointly developing a drug vary enormously. Some situations exist where one company does all of the technical and clinical work and the other company provides financial support. In other situations, the two companies either divide the work equally between them or work jointly on all tasks.

Under confidentiality agreements many companies are willing to openly discuss most of their ongoing efforts on hot leads and new drugs with a competitor if a cross-licensing or joint-marketing arrangement is considered likely. By initially discussing results in general terms there is little chance of divulging information that is unprotected.

Licensing Agreements

The licensing patterns and product "mix" of large and medium-size drug companies reveal an amazing variety of business arrangements. Many research-based companies have a few products that they have licensed-out to other companies, whereas other products may have been licensed-in, and certain other drugs are being jointly developed.

This discussion has so far omitted one of the most important factors—that each agreement covers certain countries but not others. Therefore a company may license a single drug to several different companies, but each company will get the rights to sell the drug in a different country. Another complicating factor occurs when a drug is available in multiple dosage forms such as an oral capsule, intravenous solution, and eye drops. Each of these dosage forms may be licensed-out separately to different companies for development and/or marketing in the same country.

PREPARING FEASIBILITY REPORTS

Before making a firm commitment to conduct clinical or preclinical research in a therapeutic area, initiate a new biological project, or develop an interesting chemical lead as a new drug, it is usually important to prepare a feasibility report. In the academic community, a feasibility evaluation or report may assist in the preparation of a grant application, whereas in the drug industry a feasibility report is usually related to the development or licensing of a new drug. Feasibility reports vary in scope and magnitude, ranging from a superficial review of the proposed project, drug, or area for investigation to a thorough evaluation and analysis of the project requiring a major commitment of time, effort, and money.

The feasibility report usually presents a global view of the proposed strategy that has been designed to achieve the project's objectives. For the purposes of this discussion it is considered that the feasibility report is prepared either shortly prior to or shortly after the decision is made to initiate a project. In the former case the document is created to assist in the decision-making process, whereas in the latter case it is used as one of the initial steps to assist in the planning of a project's development. Other possible uses of a feasibility report are to (1) define the goals and objectives of the project, (2) identify the most efficient and rapid route(s) for reaching the goals, and (3) show that the steps in this route are possible to conduct.

The major purpose of a feasibility report is to examine the factors that may affect whether the project or clinical development can be conducted successfully. If certain factors are uncovered which will probably or definitely play a critical role and affect the success of the project, then additional attention can be placed on those factors as the strategy for the project is developed. A detailed strategy to achieve or fulfill the goals of the project should not be developed until after it has been determined that an overall strategy is feasible. There is usually some overlap in the content of both the feasibility of a project and the specific strategies to be used. For the purpose of this discussion, however, these two processes will be separated, and the development of strategies is discussed in Chapter 2.

One of the most important reasons for preparing a feasibility report is to identify both actual and potential problems that may be encountered in pursuing a project. If significant problems are uncovered it may be necessary to (1) terminate the project, (2) establish a new goal that will avoid the anticipated problem(s), or (3) develop a strategy that will overcome the anticipated problem(s). The unstated axiom in this situation is that the better one is able to anticipate problems, the better one is able to deal with them. Although this is not always correct it is usually in the interests of the leaders of a project to have a clear view of the path they are traveling and the obstacles that may block their route.

Another objective of the feasibility report is to convince others of the project's value. For instance, in preparing a grant application in the area of

TABLE 1.1. *Sample table of contents for a clinical feasibility report—I*

Section headings	Section contents
1. What?	What is proposed?
2. Why?	Why is it proposed? How does the study fit the overall strategy?
3. Where?	Where are the proposed studies to take place?
4. How?	How will the project be organized, monitored, and reviewed?
5. Who?	Who will run the project, manage the project, design the protocols, conduct the studies, monitor the studies, analyze the data, and interpret the analyses?
6. When?	When will the studies be started, reach various milestones, and be completed?
7. How much?	How much will the studies cost individually and for the entire project? What are the other costs?
8. Verification?	Has it been verified (insofar as possible) that the studies can be conducted as planned within estimated times and budgets? What steps were conducted to verify these factors?
9. Success?	What are the chances of success (i.e., achieving the objectives)?
10. Recommendation?	What are the recommendations for the project?

TABLE 1.2. *Sample table of contents for a clinical feasibility report—II*

A. Abstract
B. Background
C. Summary information on the drug
  1. Chemical structures of pertinent compounds or drugs
  2. Pharmacological synopsis of the primary compound or drug
  3. Clinical pharmacology synopsis on the project drug and standard drugs
D. Pharmacology and other preclinical data (e.g., biochemical, physiological)
  1. Summary of pharmacological and other tests related to primary activity
  2. Summary of any other biological tests
  3. Suspected or known mechanism of action
  4. Additional nonclinical studies that will be (or may be) performed
  5. Toxicological results
E. Clinical data available
  1. Activity of the project drug and/or of standard drugs
  2. Clinical conditions that cause, result from, or are associated with the target disease
  3. Physiological and biochemical mechanisms underlying or associated with the target disease
  4. Currently available drug and nondrug therapy for treating the target disease—advantages and disadvantages
  5. Drug–drug interactions
  6. Other available data
F. Patent status
G. Regulatory considerations
H. Formulation and other aspects of technical development considerations
I. Marketing considerations
  1. Present market size
  2. Future trends in market growth
  3. Present drugs available
  4. Limitations of currently available drugs
  5. Competitive drugs currently under investigation (e.g., indications, pros and cons, pharmacological characteristics, current status)
  6. Estimated ranges of future sales plus caveats
J. Financial considerations (e.g., development costs, payback time, projected profit)
K. Rationale for human investigation
  1. Summary of primary clinical objectives
  2. Clinical data available
  3. Animal data and extrapolatability of those data to humans
  4. Potential advantages of the project drug versus currently available drugs and other therapies
  5. Potential disadvantages of the project drug versus currently available drugs and other therapies
  6. Overall strategies for clinical development
L. Clinical studies to be considered
  1. Overview of clinical studies proposed[a]
  2. Protocol for initial study (or studies)
  3. Estimated costs and time of initial study and for entire program
  4. Clinical personnel required
    a. At drug company (sponsor)
    b. At academic institutions
    c. At private clinics or other facilities
M. Summary
N. Recommendations
O. Bibliography
P. Appendixes
  1. Details of drugs currently marketed for the proposed indication
  2. Details of drugs chemically related to the study drug
  3. Additional chemical, pharmacological, clinical, or other information

[a] This list may not be complete and may only cover Phase I or Phases I and II.

TABLE 1.3. *Sample table of contents for a clinical feasibility report—III*

1. Rationale for clinical development
2. Comparison of the proposed drug with an ideal drug
3. Comparison of the proposed drug with presently available drugs and drugs under development
4. Current clinical data available (if any)
5. Proposed strategy for clinical development
6. Proposed clinical studies to be conducted
7. Proposed development of a core package of clinical studies
8. Coordination with drug development in other countries
9. Timetable of regulatory submissions
10. Work-force requirements
11. Financial costs
12. Summary
13. Recommendations

clinical research, one attempts to convince the group that is deciding how to dispense funds that the goals indicated within the grant are both worthwhile and attainable. Thus, the feasibility report will help the investigator define the objectives or goals, describe the path to follow, to reach, or to approach the goals; and identify potential problems that are likely to arise.

There are many different styles for preparing a feasibility report. Three styles are shown in Tables 1.1 to 1.3. The first is intended as a more informal approach that addresses the basic questions about most projects. The second is a more structured and detailed approach, better suited for situations where a formal review of the report will be conducted. The third emphasizes strategies and international development of a project. These tables indicate major areas that should be included (or at least considered) in most feasibility reports.

After a feasibility report has been prepared it may be used in many different ways. One common use is for the supervisors or managers who control the decision making to evaluate the report and to reach a decision as to whether the author(s) have demonstrated that the project is feasible. It should be mentioned that a feasibility report does not necessarily have to be a positive report in favor of conducting a project. There are many situations in which a negative report that presents reasons for not conducting a project is far more valuable. For instance, a well thought out and logically developed feasibility report that strongly criticizes the proposal may save the sponsor many millions of dollars on a project with flawed logic or undesirable goals, or one that has an extremely small chance of meeting its objectives.

ASSESSING THE FEASIBILITY OF AN OVERALL PROJECT

In an ideal drug development scenario, the individual who is planning the clinical program of a new drug will develop a list of the types of clinical

TABLE 1.4. *Multiple clinical studies are generally required for the projects listed*

1. Phase I, II, III, or IV clinical evaluation of a new drug
2. Postmarketing surveillance studies of a newly approved or marketed drug
3. Pharmacokinetic profile of an investigational or marketed drug
4. Comparison of a test drug, treatment, or procedure with a standard drug, treatment, or procedure
5. Evaluation of a theory, hypothesis, or mathematical model of a biological effect
6. Evaluation of a new or modified medical device
7. Evaluation of a new indication of a marketed or investigational drug
8. Evaluation of a new formulation, dosage form, or dosing schedule
9. Evaluation of a new therapy in a specific patient population (e.g., geriatrics, infants)
10. Evaluation of a drug's general safety profile and/or a specific question about a drug's toxicity
11. Marketing-oriented studies designed to compare a test drug and a competitor's drug. Evaluations may focus on the drug, formulation, indication, dosage form, dosing regimen, route of administration, or other factor
12. Evaluation of a new methodology for assessing safety or efficacy of a drug or other modality
13. Evaluation of known or potential drug interactions

studies that should be conducted in all four phases of drug development. Questions of what will need to be known about a new drug in 10 or more years, relating to postmarketing surveillance, will often influence the direction that is taken at the outset of the initial clinical studies. If the general planning and strategy of a clinical study program is haphazard and random, then errors in the project's direction will undoubtedly occur. These errors may become part of that drug's history and reputation and may affect the entire medical and commercial life of the drug, even years after it is eventually marketed. For example, if an inappropriate indication is initially chosen to be pursued and the drug performs badly, then a stigma will probably be created, which may take a long time to overcome even after the drug is developed for a more appropriate indication. Moreover, valuable time will be lost in the drug's development when such tangents are pursued.

Various types of projects which usually require multiple studies are listed in Table 1.4, and factors to consider in determining whether to initiate a new project are shown in Table 1.5. With any of the types of projects shown in Table 1.4, one must assess or consider all information available before deciding to undertake the project. This information should be examined for hints of potential problems to avoid at different stages [e.g., avoid including patients in Phase II studies who are receiving concomitant drugs (if possible) or who have renal disease with compromised renal function]. Also examine preclinical and clinical data available for potential toxicities that should be carefully monitored in future studies with special tests (e.g., ophthalmological examinations) and determine whether more frequent use of commonly used tests (e.g., electrocardiograms, blood tests) is advisable to monitor

TABLE 1.5. *Selected factors to consider in determining whether to initiate a new project*

1. Determine how worthwhile the project is from a scientific, medical, and commercial viewpoints
2. Determine whether adequately trained personnel are available for all aspects of the project. If not, estimate the probability that they can be recruited and hired by the time they are needed or may be recruited as consultants
3. Determine whether adequate financial resources are available to conduct the entire program. If not, estimate the likelihood that they will be obtained
4. Determine whether some or all of the financial and other resources necessary for the project have to be taken from other projects. If so, determine which projects have a greater priority
5. Determine the adequacy of the facilities and equipment that are presently available
6. Determine how much time the project will require to complete. Estimate the probability that the project will be completed by a given date if the drug or treatment has the desired properties
7. Estimate the likelihood that most (or all) technical, ethical, patent, legal, and regulatory problems that will be encountered during the project are presently known and can be effectively addressed and solved
8. Determine the activities that are currently being conducted at other academic centers, institutes, and drug companies that might influence the project (e.g., compete for a limited patient population, compete for a limited number of investigators, solve the same medical problem, evaluate the same issue, reach the market sooner) and decrease its value or affect the overall objectives
9. Determine the potential impact that the project will have on publicity

patients. In some situations it is useful to evaluate data available on close chemical analogs of the study drug for hints of potential value. Careful review of the data will minimize the chance of obtaining either false-positive or false-negative results with the drug being evaluated.

Three questions one usually desires to answer in formulating an approach to developing a new drug in the most rapid and efficient manner are:

1. Which appears to be the best or most nearly optimal dosage form, formulation, patient population, indication, and/or dosage regimen to *initially* utilize in clinical studies?
2. What is (or are) the *ultimate* dosage form(s), formulation(s), patient population(s), indication(s), and/or dosage regimen(s) desired?
3. At what phase of development will other dosage forms, formulations, patient populations, indications, and/or dosage regimens be added or evaluated in the clinical program as a transition is made from the initial to hopefully final goals?

Once these questions have been considered and a decision is reached to proceed with a drug's development, then additional strategies and plans may be developed that will assist progress in reaching the goals identified.

Whether a drug is developed successfully primarily depends on the nature of the drug and the individual people who are collectively developing it. The type of organization and systems used by the company or sponsor are usually secondary considerations. Well-developed plans are important, but they can only cover a limited number of possibilities and often have limited usefulness when problems arise. The individuals running and managing the development must have "prepared minds" as well as a sense of readiness to effectively deal with any uncertainty and unanticipated problems that arise.

REACHING A DECISION

A series of steps is described to assist in choosing a single potential drug candidate when several or many compounds are available for consideration.

1. Determine the relevant criteria to be used in evaluating the compound. Include both criteria (objectives) of activities the compound should possess and not possess. Generally, limit the number of criteria to about six.
2. Establish minimum standards that a compound must meet to be selected for development.
3. Rank order the objectives. Assign approximate weights to each objective (if possible), depending on its relative importance.
4. Rank order the potential candidates according to how well they achieve each objective.
5. List important caveats about each compound which may affect the decision.
6. Determine which additional tests, if any, should be conducted on the lead compound(s).
7. Determine which compounds, if any, meet the minimum criteria needed to choose a compound for development.
8. Determine which non-compound-related factors (e.g., financial resources, work force) will affect the decision, and list how they will affect it.
9. Consider all of the above factors and choose the best compound.
10. If the best compound to choose is not obvious, consider and critique each compound in turn. Then compare the evaluations.

Everyone would like to work for an organization where the drug or medical device chosen for development is the one that has the best chance for success and offers the best medical and commercial opportunities. Unfortunately, this scenario does not always occur. When multiple compounds (or sometimes even a single compound) are being considered for development the quality of the presentation where the proposal is made may influence or even determine which drug is chosen. The specific people who serve as backers of a compound are sometimes a critically important influence in the choice that is reached. One means of controlling for these factors is to arrange for an independent person or group to review the decision. This group could consist of consultants or scientists who do not report to the group that made the decision. This independent person (or group) should be able to reach a decision based on scientific and business criteria only.

DRUG STUDIES CONDUCTED BY PHYSICIANS IN PRIVATE PRACTICE

Most of the foregoing discussion centered on studies that an academic or industrial group or individual scientist might choose to pursue. There are also studies that might be pursued by physicians in private practice. These require a number of special considerations that will be described.

The term *drug studies* is used in a more broad context in this section than in the rest of this book. It includes participation in any type of medical research, including presenting posters at medical conventions and reporting cases in the medical literature, as well as participating in formal drug studies using prepared protocols.

Which Studies to Conduct

Possibly the most simple approach for many physicians who are interested in research is to analyze and write a report of unusual case(s) that provide important lessons or information. Another approach is to contact the manufacturer of a drug whose safety or efficacy profile is of particular interest. Many companies are willing to help private practitioners conduct small studies on topics of mutual interest.

Physicians who have little training in conducting drug studies would find it easier in most cases to begin with a Phase III or Phase IV study. Such a study would generally be performed in outpatients and would not be as demanding for either patients or the investigator as Phase II studies. Phase III and IV studies usually have fewer demands in terms of patient visits and tests that must be evaluated or performed at each visit; these studies may generally be integrated more easily into an outpatient clinic setting in a hospital or private clinic than Phase II studies.

Sponsored Studies

There are numerous practical factors for a physician in private practice to consider in deciding whether to conduct sponsored studies. These include the (1) number of staff members and time required to fill out and maintain the sponsor's data collection forms, which are often quite extensive, (2) amount of resources required to process and analyze data adequately (this step is usually performed by the sponsor or by a statistical collaborator), (3) liability insurance to protect oneself against unforeseen problems with a new drug or treatment, (4) monitoring resources if several private practitioners are collaborating on a project, and (5) sufficient motivational drive and desire to withstand the demands of conducting a study throughout its duration. It is clearly better to conduct a simple study and do it well than to attempt a more ambitious one and not succeed.

There are many questions than an investigator will desire to ask a sponsor or their representatives. These are so extensive and are in so many areas that they are not listed. The reader is advised to consider all of the issues discussed in *Guide to Clinical Studies and Developing Protocols* (Spilker, 1984) and in this book, but from their own perspective. Issues involve all aspects of the study, from initiation to data analysis to publication, and from protocol design to study conduct and to terms of financial payment.

Independently Conducted Studies

One of the major areas in which private practitioners may contribute to medical research, apart from conducting drug studies, is to publish case reports of adverse experiences observed with new drugs. It is important when describing adverse reactions to indicate the number of patients with the problem and the number of patients with the same treatment who did *not* have the problem. It is only through such incidence data that a realistic perspective of the clinical importance of the reported event may be established. Details on severity, duration, outcome, rechallenge with drug, and other factors are also important to include. These are more completely described in Chapter 8 of *Guide to Clinical Interpretation of Data* (Spilker, 1986).

Private practitioners are sometimes recruited by sponsors to treat some of their patients with a drug and to monitor prospectively for adverse reactions (Drury and Hull, 1981). One of the common traps of this type of observation is that it is easy to overreport and to speculate that an adverse reaction is a result of a particular drug the patient is receiving. It is usually a difficult, time-consuming, and sometimes expensive task to prove that this association is real and not a chance association or a result of a spurious relationship based on a bias of the patient or investigator. The consequences of false associations of drugs with adverse reactions may be far-reaching and extensive. Significant medical resources and efforts may be unnecessarily spent evaluating nonexistent relationships. Patients may be unnecessarily deprived of a useful treatment that was withheld or withdrawn from the market. Patients may needlessly suffer psychologically or develop sequelae through stress created, or they may experience physical complications during studies conducted to evaluate the issue.

The result of underreporting adverse reactions is equally undesirable. If physicians are either unfamiliar or uncomfortable with the FDA 1639 forms or UK "Yellow Card" (see Chapter 21), then they will be less likely to use these systems for reporting potentially important adverse reactions. There are numerous other means for potentially important adverse reactions to be reported (e.g., through publications, directly to the manufacturer), but for this to occur the physician must (1) recognize the event as an adverse reaction, (2) recognize the potential value of reporting the adverse reaction, (3) have the knowledge of how to report it, and (4) have the interest and time to follow through his/her good intentions.

Other types of nonsponsored studies that may be conducted by private practitioners include (1) those where a small number of patients are required, (2) those with single straightforward objectives, and (3) various types of multicenter studies. If and when problems arise the private practitioner may obtain advice or assistance from peers, nearby hospital staff, academic center staff, drug companies, and individuals who have published related articles.

The rules a potential investigator should follow in conducting a study are identical to those applicable to a group of experienced academicians who are conducting a large study. These are described in this and the other volumes of this group of guides. Perhaps the most important suggestion would be to enlist the aid of a statistician who is knowledgeable about clinical studies, before getting too deeply involved in a project.

Studies may be conducted in even a single patient under certain circumstances. A few of the designs that may be used are mentioned in Chapter 5 of *Guide to Clinical Interpretation of Data* (Spilker, 1986). See also Guyatt et al. (1986) and McLeod et al. (1986).

Investigator's (IND) Notice of Claimed Investigational Exemption for a New Drug

There are often situations where an investigator approaches a sponsor with a request to study one of the sponsor's marketed (or nonmarketed) products for a new indication or in a new group of patients. Nonsponsored studies may require the investigator to obtain regulatory approval. If so, it may be necessary to obtain an IND. Some companies prefer not to have investigators conduct this type of investigational study under the company's IND. One reason for this decision might be that the company does not wish to dedicate the resources necessary to help design as well as monitor the study. The company may be willing, however, to supply drug to an investigator who has obtained his own IND. An investigator who wishes to obtain his own IND to conduct clinical studies should communicate directly with the company that manufactures the drug of interest and discuss the various possibilities for obtaining regulatory approval. If an investigator's IND is chosen as the most desirable approach, then the investigator must submit the information listed in Figs. A1 to A3 (Appendix) to the Food and Drug Administration (FDA). The company must provide a letter to the FDA allowing cross-reference of the investigator's IND to all previously submitted preclinical data.

2

Establishing Project Strategies and Goals

Definition and Description of Strategies • Definitions and Types of Objectives and Goals • Types of Strategies • Developing a Strategy

DEFINITION AND DESCRIPTION OF STRATEGIES

There are many uses of the word "strategy" and many types of strategies that may be developed. Strategies are operationally defined as dynamic concepts, plans, or principles (written or unwritten) that describe the means or approach to be used to move a project from its present or current position and to achieve the goals that have been established. Strategy is a dynamic term that describes how a project (or other well defined entity) will move from its current status to achieve its goals. The three major elements of a strategy are (1) the current position, (2) the goals, and (3) the means of moving from the current position to the goals. The term "tactics" denotes the specific details and methods that are used to initiate, implement, and complete the strategy.

In developing strategies, it is necessary to consider four major factors:

1. *Duration* of time that the strategy will cover (e.g., 1 week, 1–3 years, indefinite).
2. *Level* at which the strategy will operate (e.g., within a specific department, corporation, drug or nondrug project, single-drug study, or single activity within the study).
3. Whether the strategy will emphasize *general or specific details*. A research and development strategy may be created along general or specific lines. A general research strategy may describe how a specific therapeutic area will be explored to search for new drugs. A less general strategy may describe how both targeted (e.g., disease oriented) and nontargeted research within that therapeutic area will be pursued to achieve specified goals. Specific aspects of a research strategy used for each target might include: (1) the nature of activities to be followed, methods to be used, and how resources will be allocated for targeted

and nontargeted research; (2) how the balance of research efforts in targeted and nontargeted areas will be monitored and reviewed; and (3) how short-, mid-, and long-term research programs for each target fit into the general strategy. At a certain level of detail one ceases to describe strategies and enters the area of tactics (specific mechanisms and details followed to implement a strategy).

4. *Description of the present position and the goal.* In formulating a strategy it is possible to consider either one aspect of the present position and goals or else to consider the total complexity of each. Each of these two focal points may be considered in general terms and attention may be concentrated on the in-between area (i.e., the strategy for achieving the goals). It is also possible to define and describe the present position in too much detail or to overly describe one's goals. Detailed documents or reports that focus too strongly on either current status or goals are not describing strategies. Moreover, it is not always necessary to define current status or final objectives if only general strategies are derived. These factors, however, are essential for developing strategies for specific projects or activities.

DEFINITIONS AND TYPES OF OBJECTIVES AND GOALS

As with strategies, the definitions of objectives and goals depend to some degree on the level within the company or organization that is being considered. At the overall institutional level (e.g., agency, company, university) level, the objectives are general statements about future direction of the entire organization. These statements are neither quantified nor tied to specific completion dates. They are often related to values and philosophies on both a personal and business level and may describe a desired state of being. It is not necessary for an organization to have clearly established objectives.

Goals are more specific targets than objectives. Goals may be quantified and time limits may be associated with them. Organization-wide goals are usually developed after objectives and are intended to help achieve the objectives. Goals usually are established to include measures of performance. Goals usually answer the question of "What" a group wants to get or be.

At lower levels in an organization the distinction between objectives and goals tends at first to blur and then to disappear altogether. One reason is that a general business philosophy and values, which are critically essential at the overall organizational level, are not necessarily important for each individual department. The department's overall mission tends to be seen in this context as a manifestation of their contribution toward the organization's objectives. Department goals that may be quantitated may be viewed as indistinguishable from their objectives.

In the rest of this chapter and book no distinction is made between ob-

TABLE 2.1. *Example of general project goals*[a]

1. Submission of an IND, NDA, or other regulatory application
2. Solve a current issue or problem
3. Support (or challenge) a current view, theory, hypothesis, or scientific model
4. Develop the characteristics and profile of a new drug, medical device, or surgical procedure either in various populations or under various conditions
5. Evaluate the mechanism of action of a drug
6. Evaluate the incidence of adverse reactions in a large patient population
7. Compare a new or established drug with other standard drugs or other treatment modalities

[a] Two or more of these goals may exist for any project.

jectives and goals. It is clear that such distinctions may be made, but they are not generally considered useful except as they relate to an overall organization.

In the most broad context, development of a new drug involves several types of goals. These include humanitarian (including medical), scientific, and commercial goals. In addition, goals may include discovery of a drug, conduct of preclinical studies, and development of a drug to the market. Within each of those general goals of the drug discovery and development process, other goals are established [e.g., develop a clinical plan, prepare a New Drug Application (NDA) in an efficient manner and with a minimal amount of time]. Examples of general project goals are listed in Table 2.1, and a few specific goals that could be sought for a drug that would provide delivery of a constant dose are listed in Table 2.2.

TYPES OF STRATEGIES

Deriving a useful strategy to achieve a goal requires knowledge of both the current status of the project and its therapeutic area, as well as the goal.

TABLE 2.2. *Establishing specific scientific and/or clinical goals of a project*[a]

Goals may be to:

1. Improve patient compliance
2. Decrease dosing frequency
3. Increase duration of the therapeutic effect, especially with drugs having short half-lives
4. Avoid plasma peak concentrations and hopefully decrease toxicity
5. Avoid plasma trough levels that may lie below minimal therapeutic concentrations
6. Avoid first-pass effects

[a] The example used is that of a drug delivery system which provides constant blood levels.

Goals are generally more ambiguous and speculative than one's current position. If only the current status is considered, then the strategy created may lead in numerous directions, many of which would be tangents and not lead to the desired goals. If one focuses on only the past and the present status of a project, a direction may be created that will lead forward. But, without establishing a clear goal, the place one is headed toward may be uncertain or unknown.

Three examples of the type of information included in a research and development unit's general strategy are presented to illustrate the wide diversity possible in establishing even a single type of strategy:

1. Principles, philosophy, and values with which the unit operates to achieve its goals.
2. General and specific approaches to develop drugs that result from the principles, philosophy, and values of the group. These approaches will theoretically be the same in future years as they are today. This definition does not depend heavily on the specific characteristics of current products and activities, but is a reflection of underlying approaches and methods to be followed.
3. To achieve corporate and research and development goals it may have been decided to concentrate efforts in certain therapeutic areas. There are other therapeutic areas that may be considered for development if certain circumstances (e.g., chemical leads) are present. There is a third group of therapeutic areas that are not to be considered as targets for various reasons (e.g., they lie outside the corporate "comfort zone"). Research efforts and projects must be targeted to the first two groups of therapeutic areas.

Examples of Overall Strategies for Specific Projects

It is important to have an overall strategy for each individual project. Agreement on an overall strategy for pursuing each individual project usually precedes discussion and agreement on the specific project strategies and tactics which enable the overall strategy to be achieved. Individual projects have a variety of overall strategies associated with them. Some specific examples of overall strategies for individual projects of new chemical entities (NCEs) include (1) focusing all efforts on the single indication and dosage form for which an NDA may be achieved most rapidly, (2) conducting Phase I and early Phase II studies only and then licensing the drug to another company, (3) choosing the most commercially rewarding indication as the initial target for the drug's first NDA, (4) developing a combination product prior to the single entity, (5) initially developing the drug for a specific patient population, and (6) screening many potential indications in early Phase II before targeting one (or more) for further development. The initial overall

TABLE 2.3. *General purposes, durations, and levels of various types of strategies*

A. Purpose
  1. Global strategies[a] may be used to:
     - Establish general types of mechanisms and procedures to be used
     - Develop the values, philosophy, and approaches to be used
     - Determine the specific projects to be pursued
  2. Operational strategies[b] may be used to:
     - Solve a specific problem
     - Address a specific issue
     - Guide a specific project or multiple projects
     - Conduct a single activity or multiple activities

B. Duration of an established strategy[c]
  1. Definite
     - No revisions are anticipated
     - Revisions required at fixed time intervals (e.g., monthly, yearly)
     - Revisions required at variable times[d]
  2. Indefinite
     - No revisions are anticipated
     - Revisions required at fixed time intervals (e.g., monthly, yearly)
     - Revisions required at variable times[d]

C. Line management level within the organization at which the strategy will operate
  1. Top managerial level (e.g., corporate-wide, university-wide)
  2. Multidepartmental within the same division or unit
  3. Single department
  4. Group or section within a department
  5. Single individual

D. Matrix level within the organization at which the strategy will operate
  1. Across different functional groups at the top of the corporation or university
  2. Across different departments within one or multiple divisions
  3. Across different groups or sections within a department or departments
  4. Among different individuals from different groups but working as a team

E. Level of activity[e]
  1. Activity within a department on one part of a drug's development
  2. Activity within a department on an entire drug's development
  3. Activity within multiple departments on a single drug
  4. Activity within multiple departments on multiple drugs

[a] Global strategies provide a general approach that will be used to achieve the goals.
[b] Operational strategies provide the specific details required to achieve the goals.
[c] For both operational and global strategies.
[d] Criteria may or may not be established for determining when revisions are required.
[e] Selected examples only.

goal for these projects would generally be similar, namely, to reach the market in the shortest possible time with the best labeling possible and in the most cost effective manner.

To carry out development of a new drug that is to enter Phase I studies and to adhere to an overall strategy, an entire series of other strategies must be created. Many of these will be oriented toward enabling the individual departments or groups to complete their part of the effort. A number of types of strategies are shown in Table 2.3.

Overall NDA Strategy

This is often initially articulated in a clinical feasibility report prepared by medical personnel, which is reviewed and accepted by senior managers. This report may indicate, for instance, (1) that the most rapid way to achieve an NDA is to develop indication A before indications B or C and to not explore indications D and E until after an NDA for indication A is submitted, (2) that patients who have certain disease characteristics (e.g., anatomical locations, severity, or classification) would be easier to enroll in studies than other patients with the same disease, (3) that a specific formulation or dosage form might be preferable to develop first, or (4) that certain investigators should (or should not) be contacted for any of a variety of reasons. Numerous other factors could be explored that would be part of the detailed strategy to reach a successful NDA in the shortest possible time and still obtain acceptable drug labeling.

Specific Strategy to Develop Each Indication and Dosage Form

This type of strategy could be prepared either for the entire period from IND (or pre-IND) through NDA approval, or could be limited to the period between two project milestones. Alternatively, this type of strategy could focus on a specific time period, such as a few months, a year, or some other fixed period. Short-term strategies must be periodically updated, because they rapidly become outdated and obsolete. General purposes, durations, and levels of various types of strategies that may be used for projects are presented in Table 2.3.

Production and Marketing Strategies on a Project

Specific production and marketing strategies may be developed for relevant projects. Although production considerations usually become relevant only when a drug reaches Phase III there may be specific production issues that should be discussed when a compound is first considered for project status, or even before this time, so that optimal input into a drug's development may be achieved. Relevant production issues might relate to the lack of equipment or technology, the hazardous nature of the chemical synthesis, or problems associated with certain types of production. In practice, many drug companies only seek production input during late Phase II or during Phase III after efficacy has been demonstrated, and an NDA is being planned or assembled.

The research-and-development-oriented strategies described in this chapter are generally intended for a project on an investigational drug. Analogous overall and/or specific marketing and production strategies will also be developed for each investigational drug. There are (or should be) clearly delineated marketing and production strategies for each marketed drug. Marketing strategies may also be developed for early preclinical research programs or projects. A discussion of marketing strategies is presented in Chapter 22.

DEVELOPING A STRATEGY

Once the feasibility report is reviewed and accepted by management, the information included may generally be converted into a global operating strategy. The feasibility report usually includes information on the current status of knowledge in a field or on a known chemical compound and describes goals of the project. The means (i.e., strategy) of achieving these goals may be presented in general or specific terms. A number of formats that may be used to delineate and present strategies are shown in Table 2.4.

Overall Approach

The traditional means of developing a strategy starts with goals and then develops one or more alternative ways (i.e., strategies) to achieve those goals. If the goals relate to an entire corporation or large organization, rather than to a specific project or activity, then it may be relevant to start with the resources available and develop a strategy before establishing the goals. This approach was advocated by Hayes (1985). The author believes that this approach may be relevant for a large organization but is inappropriate for developing the strategy for a particular project.

TABLE 2.4. *Potential formats to delineate and present strategies*[a]

1. Algorithms
2. Flow charts
3. PERT[b] network, critical path method, precedence charts
4. Activity schedules of descriptions by department or group
5. Preset forms of questions to complete
6. Tables of activities to conduct
7. Grid charts
8. Prose—from short terse statements to expanded discussions
9. Gantt charts
10. Milestone charts
11. Critical path method

[a] See Chapter 18 for a discussion of most of these formats.
[b] PERT, Program Evaluation and Review Technique.

Initial Steps

The initial step in developing a strategy is to produce a clear statement and description of both current status and goals for the project or activity. It is sometimes impossible to define goals clearly. A general description of the area in which the goals exist or a clear direction to be followed may be used in such cases, and specific goals may be identified later. There may also be occasions when the current status of a project is not clear and cannot be well defined. In such situations a broad description of this area may suffice.

It is usually impossible to develop a single strategy to meet all of a project's needs. This is partly because of the great differences that exist in approaching short-term and long-term goals within a project. For example, one cannot develop a global strategy using the long-term ultimate goals to be achieved in several years and incorporate all short-term specific goals one hopes to achieve on a month-to-month (or other) basis. Multiple strategies are also necessary because many types of workers and managers at various hierarchical and functional levels will need different strategies to plan their work and to judge completed efforts.

When multiple goals exist it is important to determine whether they will be approached simultaneously through one strategy or whether each will require a separate strategy. It is usually possible to establish and clarify goals that can be pursued simultaneously. When there are also a series of goals to be approached sequentially, it may only initially be possible to develop a strategy that addresses the first or first few goals to be pursued.

Strategies exist at many hierarchical levels in an organization, and in many projects multiple strategies are operating at the same time. Some are general strategies, whereas others are extremely specific. Some relate to complex coordinating activities among many departments or groups, and others refer to activities conducted by a small cadre of people. Some strategies require a few days or weeks to complete, whereas others require years or are indefinite in length. Therefore, there are many "current positions" and "goals" to consider within any given project and these differ greatly from each other, depending on the nature of the particular strategy that is being developed.

How to Develop an Overall Project Strategy

If an overall strategy is to be developed for all projects, it may evolve through "bottom-up" or "top-down" techniques. In the bottom-up approach, consideration is given to combining the desirable aspects and principles of individual project strategies. An attempt is made to discern what is common to most or all projects and to bring those aspects together. The top-down approach starts from an overall view of research and development goals and seeks to identify the specific project strategies that would best fit that overall approach. This overall strategy concept is then used as a model from which the individual strategies are derived. Certain elements of this overall strategy might be (1) to concentrate activities on a few (e.g., three to six) selected projects to reach the NDA submission stage most rapidly, (2) to spread resources thinly across many projects to increase the chances that some will reach an NDA stage, or (3) to focus attention on a single indication for each project so that the NDA may be attained most rapidly.

Approaches to Developing Strategies

The person or group responsible for developing strategies must initially determine:

1. The level(s) in the organization to be included in the activities or plans created.
2. The duration of the strategy or strategies.
3. The number and purpose of each of the strategies to be developed.
4. The degree of specific details to be used.

After these aspects are established the following approaches may be considered from the perspective of identifying specific strategies that will best address their objectives. Five types of approaches to developing strategies are briefly described (in no particular order):

1. *Backward Approach.* In this approach it is necessary to initially focus on the goals and then develop strategies on the basis of their likelihood of achieving these goals. Activities may combine both intergroup (i.e., matrix) and intragroup (i.e., line management) aspects.
2. *Forward Approach.* This approach focuses on the resources, current status, and interests of the group and creates strategies that allow those factors to be developed in the manner determined by the decision makers. This approach is more suited for some large companies than it is for a research department or other group that usually has clear-cut goals.
3. *Line-Function Approach.* This approach limits strategies to those that lie within the purview of a specific function, department, or other group. This approach avoids considerations of matrix strategies.
4. *Matrix Approach.* Developing a matrix strategy (or strategies) cuts across multiple units or groups within a company or research and development group.
5. *Key Question Approach.* Strategies are developed on the basis of how they fit key questions that are identified as focus points. A person or group assigned to each question could develop the specific strategies

TABLE 2.5. *Selected elements that may be included in a brief document summarizing a project's strategy*

A. Identification material
   1. Project name and/or drug name
   2. Date of report
   3. Project code number
   4. Project leader or manager

B. Clinical synopsis[a]
   1. Specific indication or disease studied or to be studied
   2. Dosage form
   3. Status of each indication and dosage form (e.g., 1, U, P, F)[b]
   4. Next decision point for each type of study (e.g., efficacy, safety pharmacokinetic)[c]
   5. Date next decision point is expected for each study being conducted. Identify protocol numbers and nature of the decision
   6. Other present or future activities of importance and estimated dates of completion

C. Operational strategies for each clinical indication[c]

D. Technical development issues and activities
   1. Present activities
      - Analytical development
      - Chemical development
      - Pharmaceutical development
      - Final formulation
      - Stability studies
   2. Issues and/or problems
      - Analytical development
      - Chemical development
      - Pharmaceutical development
      - Final formulation
      - Stability studies
   3. Comments

E. Toxicology
   1. Studies in progress
   2. Studies planned to start within 1 year
   3. Issues and problems
   4. Comments

F. Other relevant activities and issues

[a] The first five points may be used as headings for a table, to present the data.
[b] 1, Primary indications or dosage form studied; U, study (or studies) underway, P, study (or studies) planned to start within 1 year; F, future study (or studies) planned to start after 1 year.
[c] A one- to three-sentence synopsis is given for each indication listed.

to answer or pursue that question. Examples of relevant questions could be:

a. What therapeutic areas should be emphasized?
b. What types of projects should the portfolio contain?
c. How may projects be developed more efficiently?

Different types of project, department, or even institutional strategies will require different approaches. These approaches are not mutually exclusive as either the forward or backward approaches may be combined with either line-function or matrix approaches. After the strategies are created they must be tied in with other strategies that already exist. Selected elements that may be used to summarize a project's strategies are listed in Table 2.5.

While strategies are being developed (or after a draft is completed) it is necessary to insure that they make sense. This is achieved through various analyses. The analyses should demonstrate that the proposed strategies are both realistic and have a reasonable probability of achieving the intended goals. Either before or after the strategies and analyses are accepted by managers, the means to implement the strategies must be established. The proposed means may include simple or highly complex methods whereby everyone necessary is informed about the strategies and understands their roles in the implementation process.

A Few Pitfalls

One potential danger in developing strategies is when one strategy document attempts to accomplish too many different functions. If several types of strategies are mixed together in one document, there is a danger of creating confusion in the minds of those who must use these documents to plan their activities. Consideration of multiple levels or multiple time frames within a single document may lead to confusion. Mixing principles, values, current status, and goals with strategies is common and often hinders, rather than facilitates, communications. Another common problem is to identify a goal that is not the most appropriate one and thus to initiate activities in pursuit of secondary or inappropriate goals.

Reviewing and Monitoring a Strategy

It is important to have a mechanism to periodically review and update strategies. This process may be conducted at fixed intervals or on an as-needed basis. Although neither approach is *a priori* preferable, it is useful to consider the question of periodic reviews and revisions at the outset of a project. It is also important to determine the number and nature of different strategies that will be helpful to use in a project. These strategies should be developed in the early stages of a project's life to facilitate their acceptance and increase their usefulness.

In critiquing a proposed strategy the first step is to insure that both the current status and goals are clearly defined. Their appropriateness must be ascertained relative to the purposes for which the strategy was created. Then the strategy must be evaluated as to how effectively and efficiently it will allow and facilitate progress toward the goals. Next, evaluate whether any relevant problems or issues have been overlooked and determine if there are unanswered questions. Several different strategies should usually be developed on any one project to (1) expedite decision making by project leaders, (2) allow for delegation of responsibilities, (3) facilitate management review, and (4) achieve an overall uniformity in approach.

One of the major purposes of a strategy is as a monitoring tool to assist an individual, group, department, or larger unit to adhere to a preset course. When the person or group deviates from the agreed-on course, the strategy should serve to raise a warning flag. Alternatively, the deviation may indicate that the strategy itself has to be modified to incorporate the implications of the new information that has made the departure necessary.

3

Designing the Overall Project

Types of Projects • Initial Steps • Choosing the Approach • Visual Models of Drug Development • Considerations for a Clinical Program in Phases I, II, and III • Choosing Efficacy Parameters to Measure • "Catch-22" and Other Issues

TYPES OF PROJECTS

In designing an overall project the initial step is to establish the type of project to be created. Common types of new projects include:

1. Development of a new chemical entity (NCE) from discovery of its biological activity to its marketing as a new drug.
2. Development of a line extension for an already-marketed drug.
3. Development of a new indication for a marketed prescription drug.
4. Conversion of a marketed drug from prescription to nonprescription [i.e., over-the-counter (OTC)] status.
5. Development of a combination drug.

There are many similarities among these five types of projects in the approaches followed to design, monitor, and manage the studies. The similarities will be discussed in this chapter rather than concentrating on the many differences that also exist. Some considerations that apply to the different phases of drug development will also be discussed. Combination drugs are specifically discussed in Chapter 15.

INITIAL STEPS

For projects involving drugs it is usually mandatory to identify the clinical indication and dosage form that will be the initial focus of activity. Once this goal is agreed on, a detailed clinical plan may often be drawn. If the project involves a therapeutic area where the nature of most Phase I, II, and III clinical studies are well worked out and accepted, developing a clinical plan will be a relatively straightforward exercise. Even in this situation,

TABLE 3.1. *Initial activities conducted to establish a new project*

A. Establish an overview for the project
   1. Determine overall objectives
   2. Determine how strategies to accomplish overall objectives will be established, reviewed, and reestablished
   3. Develop an overall plan using networks and charts to document how the overall objectives will be accomplished
B. Activities related to project management
   1. Assess the relative priority of the project
   2. Assess the resources needed to accomplish the project's objectives
   3. Assess the resources available to the project
   4. Determine the major milestones and decision points
   5. Determine how progress will be monitored and status reported
C. Activities related to project personnel
   1. Choose the leader or manager of the project
   2. Determine which disciplines/departments should be involved
   3. Choose the members of the project team
   4. Determine workloads and responsibilities for each member
   5. Establish reporting methods to be followed
D. Activities related to progressing the drug toward human studies
   1. Determine the preclinical studies that must be conducted
   2. Determine all reports that must be prepared prior to testing the drug in humans
   3. Identify and evaluate actual or potential problems
   4. Determine quantities of drug needed for the initial phases of development
E. Activities related to testing the drug in humans
   1. Choose the indication(s) to pursue
   2. Choose the initial route(s) of administration to be developed
   3. Choose the initial dosage form to be developed
   4. Identify the initial clinical studies to be conducted
   5. Determine the type(s) of patients to include in the initial studies

however, various modifications will be required throughout the drug's development. If the drug is intended for use in a new therapeutic field or in a field that does not have clear guidelines and well-established clinical endpoints for drug development (e.g., irritable bowel syndrome, senile dementia), it may be impossible to develop a detailed clinical plan for the entire development process. Nonetheless, plans for a few initial studies and a general direction must be established.

There is no single best order of steps to follow in initiating and designing a project. Many steps are necessary to consider and initiate. A selected list of these steps is given in Table 3.1. Establishing a project plan generally follows the steps shown in Fig. 3.1. Individual tasks may be illustrated with the type of bar chart shown in Fig. 3.2 or with charts that show the interactions between various activities (see Chapter 18). Individual studies planned may also be illustrated with bar charts (Fig. 3.3). Concomitantly with the development of the project's plans it will be necessary to hold meetings at which the choice of specific steps and tasks are discussed.

Establishing the overall goals of a project is an essential part of the initial

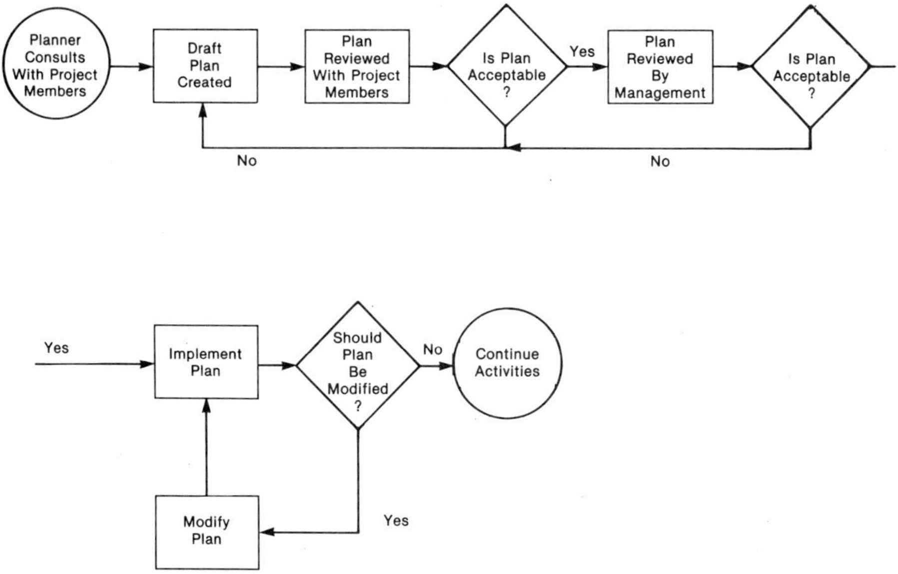

FIG. 3.1. Establishing a project plan to achieve certain objectives. General procedures for reviewing and approving a project plan. The modified plan may have to be reviewed by management prior to implementation.

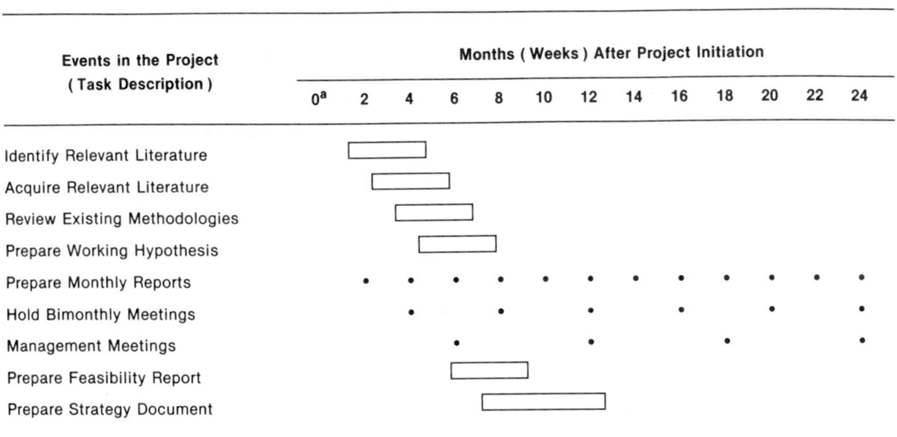

[a]0 date is set at the initiation of the project (e.g., January 15, 198__).

FIG. 3.2. Selected tasks in a hypothetical project illustrated by a Gantt chart.

FIG. 3.3. A hypothetical bar chart illustrating the initiation and completion dates for numerous clinical studies on a single drug. The hatched lines indicate the time required to process the data on the study. Times required to prepare statistical and medical reports could also be illustrated with other types of hatches or marks. N/A, study number not yet assigned.

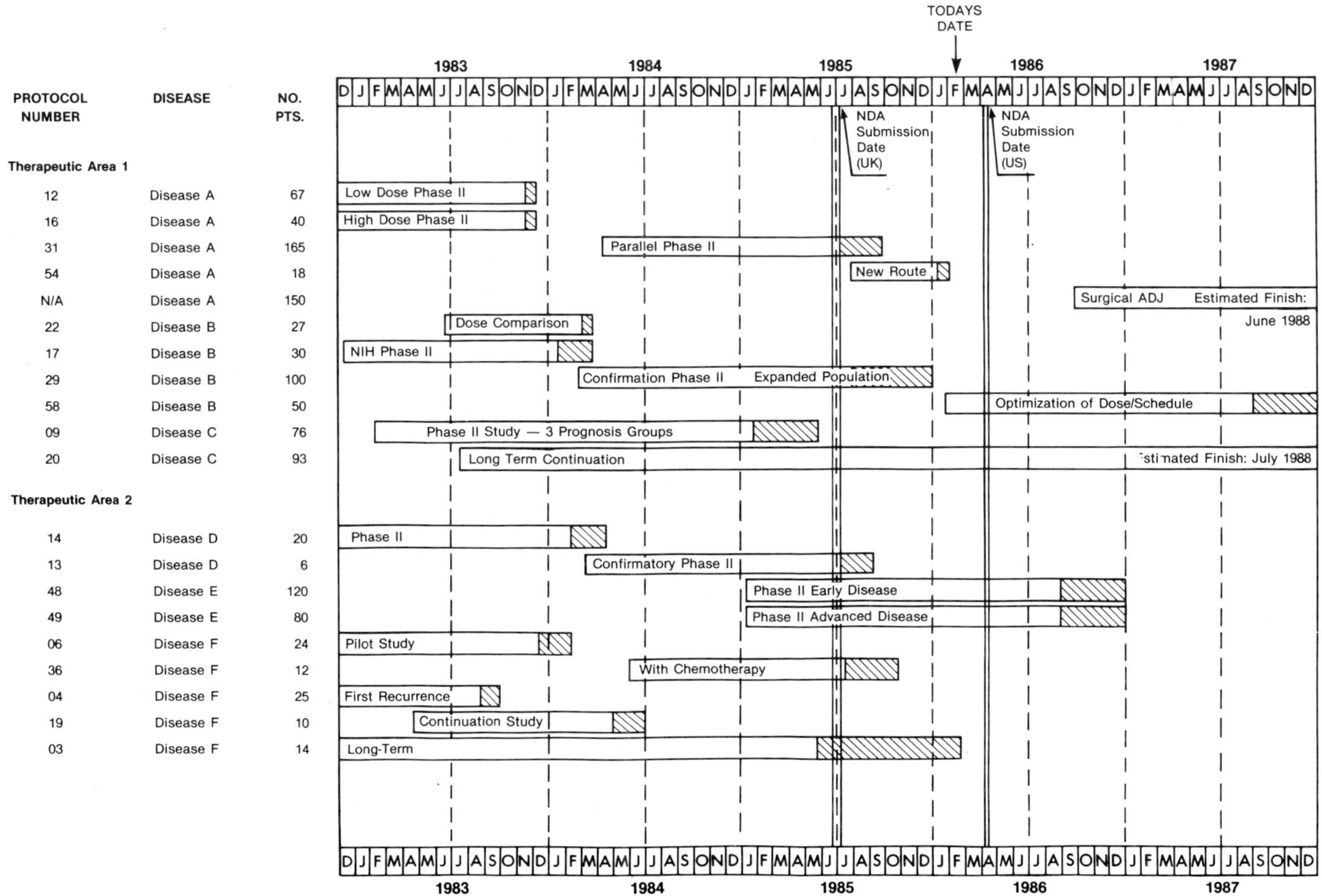
TODAYS DATE
1983
1984
1985
1986
1987
D J F M A M J J A S O N D
PROTOCOL NUMBER
DISEASE
NO. PTS.
NDA Submission Date (UK)
NDA Submission Date (US)
Therapeutic Area 1
12 Disease A 67 Low Dose Phase II
16 Disease A 40 High Dose Phase II
31 Disease A 165 Parallel Phase II
54 Disease A 18 New Route
N/A Disease A 150 Surgical ADJ Estimated Finish: June 1988
22 Disease B 27 Dose Comparison
17 Disease B 30 NIH Phase II
29 Disease B 100 Confirmation Phase II Expanded Population
58 Disease B 50 Optimization of Dose/Schedule
09 Disease C 76 Phase II Study — 3 Prognosis Groups
20 Disease C 93 Long Term Continuation Estimated Finish: July 1988
Therapeutic Area 2
14 Disease D 20 Phase II
13 Disease D 6 Confirmatory Phase II
48 Disease E 120 Phase II Early Disease
49 Disease E 80 Phase II Advanced Disease
06 Disease F 24 Pilot Study
36 Disease F 12 With Chemotherapy
04 Disease F 25 First Recurrence
19 Disease F 10 Continuation Study
03 Disease F 14 Long-Term

TABLE 3.2. *Sample table of contents for an investigator's brochure*

1. Summary
2. Introduction (e.g., proprietary name, generic name, chemical name, salt, empirical formula, structural formula, type of drug)
3. Chemistry (e.g., physical characteristics, pK_a, solubility in different solvents, stability under different conditions, assay method)
4. Pharmacology
   - Primary activities (e.g., animal tests used, results)
   - Secondary activities (e.g., animal tests used, results)
   - Mechanism of action studies
   - Effective dose range and duration of action
   - Biochemical effects
   - *In vitro* effects
   - Other studies
5. Toxicology and experimental pathology[a]
   - Acute studies (e.g., species, routes, results)
   - Subacute studies (e.g., species, routes, doses, duration, results)
   - Chronic studies (e.g., species, routes, doses, duration, results)
   - Special studies (e.g., teratology, mutagenicity, reproduction)
6. Metabolism and pharmacokinetic studies[a]
   - Animal data (e.g., absorption, distribution, metabolism, excretion)
   - Human data (e.g., absorption, distribution, metabolism, excretion)
7. Clinical data[a]
   - Diseases in which the drug is being studied
   - Rationale
   - Safety profile
   - Efficacy profile
8. Pharmaceutical results (e.g., pH, physicochemical compatibilities, stability, expiration date, packaging and storage requirements, dissolution data)
9. Regulatory history and status
10. Marketing status of other dosage forms
11. Basic information for clinical investigators[b]
12. Published literature and unpublished references

[a] Each section may be subdivided depending on type and amount of data available.
[b] May be written in the form of a package insert. This should include information on manifestations and treatment of overdosage.

processes. The specific nature of the initial steps conducted must lie within the general framework of the organization sponsoring the project's development. There will be numerous organizational constraints within which the project leader or manager must operate to initiate and develop activities. Depending on the nature of the organization there may be more or less flexibility in approach or style that is permitted. Individual approaches to project activities are not permitted in some organizations and would probably not flourish, whereas in other institutions, individual solutions to designing and conducting project activities are actively sought and encouraged.

After the clinical direction of a project is established, certain aspects of technical development may be determined. The most basic aspect of technical development concerns the choice of dosage form(s) to be developed (e.g., parenteral, enteral). If the drug is to be given orally, then the amount

TABLE 3.3. *Selected aspects to modify or consider as one progresses from study to study within the same project*

1. Patient inclusion criteria
2. Duration of drug exposure
3. Dosing regimens
4. Indications
5. Formulations
6. Initiate continuation protocols
7. Compassionate plea protocols
8. New types of patient populations
9. Revise estimates of patient entry rates

of drug in each capsule (or other dosage form) must be determined. This determination is usually based on anticipated human doses to be used in the initial clinical studies. The fewest number of separate dosage strengths should be prepared because of the large amount of work and quantity of drug required for each size. Based on the numbers of volunteers and patients in the first few studies, plus drug requirements for toxicology and other preclinical studies, one or more orders for additional chemical synthesis will probably be necessary. Formulation development and stability testing will be initiated. Analytical development work to develop assays will be initiated based on known compounds, analogs, early chemical studies, and other data. Additional activities required to file a Notice of Claimed Investigational Exemption for a New Drug (IND) or to achieve the initial milestone in the project are similarly planned and scheduled. One important activity involves the creation of an investigator's brochure. A sample table of contents is shown in Table 3.2. This brochure should be updated periodically with new data. Between revisions the new data may be indicated in the clinical protocol so that it may be reviewed by the investigator and his Institutional Review Board (IRB).

Various activities required to assemble an IND are scheduled in a way that prioritizes certain steps which take place before others. If an individual is assigned the role of planner for the project, he or she helps organize and coordinate various activities with the project leader or manager. These activities are described further in Chapter 18.

As one progresses from study to study there are numerous clinical aspects to modify. Some of these are shown in Table 3.3. A number of selected pitfalls to avoid in conducting studies are listed in Table 3.4. Possibly the single most important point to consider in designing the clinical development of a drug is that it is better to have fewer studies of higher quality than many studies of lesser quality.

TABLE 3.4. *Selected pitfalls to avoid in conducting clinical studies*

1. Overestimating the number of suitable patients that are currently available or will in future be available to enter the study
2. Overestimating the rapidity with which patients can be entered
3. Underestimating the demands of the study in terms of time requirements for (1) evaluating patients, (2) discussing patient's clinical status and requirements with staff, (3) completing data collection forms, and/or (4) performing other necessary administrative activities
4. Applying the inclusion criteria inappropriately and entering unsuitable patients, or entering patients before all of their laboratory data are returned
5. Failing to notify the sponsor and/or the Institutional Review Board (IRB) within 24 hours after a serious adverse reaction has occurred
6. Failing to notify the sponsor and/or the IRB about serious clinical events that are not believed by the investigator to be drug related, but which could be study related (e.g., suicide of a patient who was receiving placebo)
7. Paying inadequate attention to important details in the protocol for conducting the study (e.g., how to modify doses after adverse reactions occur)
8. Failing to adequately complete data collection forms
9. Handing out bottles of medication or assigning patient numbers haphazardly, instead of following the randomization code. Patients are therefore not entered and randomized to treatment in the appropriate predetermined sequence

CHOOSING THE APPROACH

In choosing an approach to be used in developing a drug there are two major influences. They are the nature of the drug and the specific situation and/or conditions of the institution that will develop the drug. The major choices of an approach are visually illustrated later in this chapter.

The nature of the drug has to do with whether objective clinical criteria or endpoints may be used to evaluate the drug and reach a go/no-go decision during Phase II. Drugs such as diuretics or weight-reducing agents have clear clinical endpoints. If this type of endpoint is present then a highly focused approach may be initially followed. If the drug is an anticancer agent or in a therapeutic area where many disease targets may be affected, then it will often be advisable to evaluate the drug in several different areas during Phase II studies. Even during Phase I studies numerous approaches may be used to identify the maximally tolerated dose using various dosing regimens and schedules. If the endpoints are generally nonobjective, such as for antipsychotic drugs, then a different type of approach must be used which emphasizes well-controlled studies. If criteria on which to base a go/no-go decision with regard to developing the drug to a new drug application (NDA) status are not established before studies begin, then there is more of a chance for personalities and nonscientific influences to affect this decision.

Choosing Sites at Which to Conduct Studies

Pharmaceutical companies pursue Phase I to III evaluations of drugs at various types of sites and in a variety of ways. These can be generally summarized as utilizing a mixture of the following types of options:

1. Clinical facilities, owned and operated by the sponsor, that conduct clinical studies. These facilities are primarily, but not exclusively, used for Phase I studies.
2. Clinical facilities established by the sponsor in a hospital that may be part of a medical school. The hospital is often located near the sponsor, but some notable exceptions exist.
3. Some academic institutions have established clinical facilities that are used to conduct clinical studies. These study sites are sometimes physically separated from the hospital wards. These facilities may be reserved for faculty members to use and may be primarily oriented toward sponsored clinical studies.
4. Some departments within a medical school have established facilities that solicit sponsored studies as a source of training for the staff and students; these facilities also act as a source of revenue for the department, staff, and institution. These funds are sometimes directly applied to support other clinical studies that are of particular interest to the unit's staff or recipients of the funds.
5. Some contract organizations have established independent clinical facilities that pursue clinical studies as a business enterprise. The physicians who are part of these groups may or may not be associated with a nearby hospital to which patients may be brought if an emergency develops.
6. Some contract organizations have organized a network of hospitals in which clinical studies are conducted.
7. Some contract organizations have organized a network of private practitioners and/or group practices who are able to conduct clinical studies. The physicians may be located in one city, a particular region, or throughout the country.
8. Some contract organizations do not conduct any clinical studies themselves, but act as intermediaries to find a solution for the sponsor's needs, and attempt to place each study where it may be successfully conducted.

In choosing among these options (and others), sponsors usually balance (1) consideration of expected quality of the study, (2) control of the study retained by the sponsor, (3) turnaround time to initiate and complete the study, (4) costs, (5) reputation of the site(s), and (6) numerous other factors.

Phase I Studies

In Phase I studies the major factors in most sponsors' deliberations on whether to establish an independent facility are control, cost, and anticipated turnaround time. When Phase I studies are conducted by physicians who are employees of the company the sponsor has more control on the timing of the study and ordering of priority than for studies conducted by outside investigators. The costs and maintenance of the physical facilities, plus salaries of the staff and anticipated degree of use must be balanced against the expected convenience, added control, ease of utilizing other Phase I facilities, and costs of those studies.

It is a significant step for a company to establish an independent Phase I unit. This unit must have excellent staff and should be close to a population of potential volunteers. A local college or university will not necessarily provide a reliable source of volunteers, because (1) the school may have rules that prohibit certain types of activities, (2) the unit may not be able to advertise in the school paper or post notices on bulletin boards, (3) there may be difficulty gaining access to students, or (4) students may have religious or philosophical views that do not allow them to volunteer for drug studies. Moreover, students usually take long summer and midsemester breaks that may adversely affect scheduling student participation of some important studies.

Phase II and III Studies

Phase II and III studies are generally conducted through a variety of mechanisms at various types of institutions and with both narrow and broad patient populations. Although the majority of studies on most new drugs are conducted at teaching institutions, Phase III studies are often conducted at community hospitals (Begg et al., 1982) and at other facilities (e.g., nursing homes, private clinics).

Clinical Facilities Established by Sponsors

Clinical facilities that are established by sponsors at hospitals have certain advantages over an independent unit that is entirely owned and operated by the sponsor. A unit at a hospital would especially be useful to a sponsor who did not have the volume of studies to keep an independent unit operating at or near full capacity. Arrangements with the hospital could be established to allow studies by other sponsors or the hospital faculty to be conducted during slack periods. Whether this unit would be better to locate in a private community hospital or in a hospital that is part of a medical school would depend on the terms and conditions of the relationship established, the availability and suitability of the facilities, and various other factors.

Contract Organizations

Conducting Clinical Studies

Contract organizations vary widely in their structure and in their approach to conducting clinical studies. Basically, they either conduct the clinical studies themselves or place them at other sites where they are conducted. Many sponsors use such groups during all phases of drug development. In Phase I studies, most contract organizations do the clinical studies themselves. There are a relatively large number of such groups, as well as numerous academic institutions that are able to conduct this type of study.

In Phase II studies most contract groups place a sponsor's studies at centers where they will be conducted. Since these studies may require a relatively large number of homogeneous patients with the disease being evaluated, few contract groups will have direct access to such patients. On the other hand, certain outpatient Phase II studies and many Phase III studies are able to be conducted directly by some contract groups. Whether these studies are conducted by the contract group or by investigators at other sites depends on the contractor's facilities, patient availability, and the relative ease or difficulty of the study.

In detailing arrangements between sponsors and contractors who will not conduct studies themselves it is important to clarify all important areas, including:

1. How will investigators be chosen?
    - The contractor may make the final decision.
    - The contractor may choose the investigator, but the sponsor has the right of refusal.
    - The sponsor must evaluate each proposed investigator and choose those who will conduct the study.
2. Who will be responsible for monitoring the studies?
    - Only monitors from the sponsor.
    - Monitors from the sponsor always accompanied by a monitor from the contractor.
    - Monitors from the sponsor with or without a monitor from the contractor.
    - Monitors from the contractor with or without a monitor from the sponsor.
    - Only monitors from the contractor.
3. How many monitoring visits will be made by the contractor?
    - Number to be determined solely by contractor.

- Number to be determined solely by sponsor.
- Number to be determined through joint discussions.

4. How will drug supplies be handled and shipped to the study site?
   - Various possibilities will be explored and agreement will be reached.

Conducting Nonclinical Activities

Contract organizations have broadened the services they offer in recent years to include numerous other nonclinical activities related to clinical drug studies. These services include laboratory evaluations of biological samples, processing of data collection forms, analyzing data statistically, writing final medical reports, and preparing regulatory submissions.

VISUAL MODELS OF DRUG DEVELOPMENT

A few simple models are described as a means of establishing a frame of reference for considering how drug development changes within a project during the years it takes to proceed to an NDA. These approaches do not illustrate the quantity of work involved in moving from the project's initiation to NDA. The magnitude of work required is almost always believed to multiply manyfold as a compound progresses toward an NDA. In some cases there appears to be more of a logarithmic, rather than an arithmetic, increase in the amount of work. Some people have described the increasing quantity of work as an inverted pyramid or a mushrooming effect.

The models refer primarily to the number of (1) different dosage forms (e.g., solution, capsule, tablet) that are studied, (2) different indications pursued, (3) different routes of administration being tested, and, to a lesser degree, (4) different formulations, (5) patient populations, and (6) dosing regimens. These models are illustrated in Fig. 3.4 and refer primarily to Phases II and III of clinical development, but also include technical development, toxicological, and other nonclinical activities. Consideration of Phase I clinical activities may sometimes be included in these figures. Hybrid and other models also exist.

Some companies generally adopt one or more of these approaches. No company will entirely be representative of a single approach. Ideally, the approach chosen should fit the drug. Two of the major influences on the approach chosen relate to the nature of the drug being developed and the personality of the individual who has the major "say" or makes the final decision regarding the approach taken. At most drug companies, this individual is usually the head of research and development.

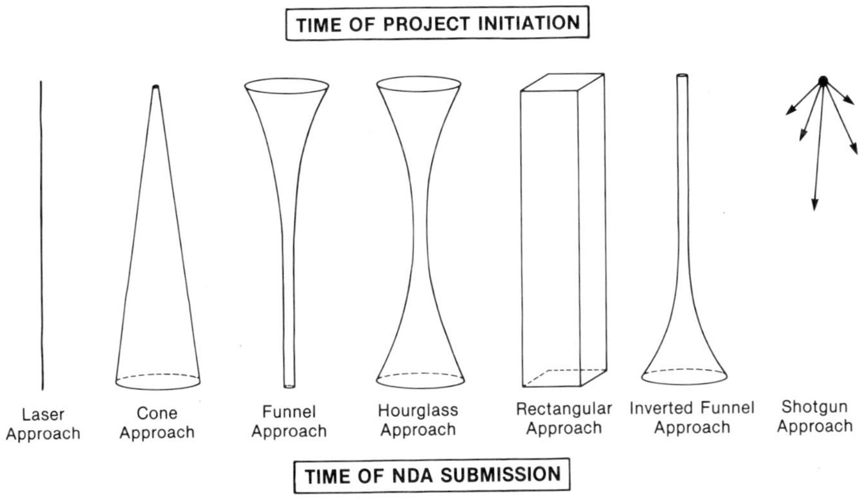

FIG. 3.4. Visual models of drug development illustrating different types of approaches followed. See text for details.

Laser Approach

A single dosage form and single disease indication are targeted at the initiation of the project. This target is pursued without expanding the studies to other indications, formulations, or dosage forms until after the NDA is filed (or approved). In the most pure form of the laser approach, a wide variety of dose schedules and patient populations are not necessary to evaluate. This type of project moves along a highly focused path.

Cone Approach

A single dosage form, formulation, and target disease are initially evaluated. Gradually, as the compound progresses toward an NDA, more and more dosage forms, formulations, routes of administration, and/or indications are pursued. This is the most common approach followed in new drug development.

Funnel Approach

After initial Phase I studies demonstrate that a drug should enter Phase II, multiple indications are evaluated. From the results of numerous studies, a single or small number of the more promising indications are chosen to be pursued. These are followed in well-controlled Phase II studies and Phase

III evaluations. The size of the funnel's stem will vary, depending on how focused the activities are during later Phase II and Phase III.

Hourglass Approach

As in the situation above, multiple indications are focused to a small number. The number of activities are then gradually expanded in terms of additional dosage forms, formulations, dosage regimens, and patient populations as the project nears the NDA. The top part of the hourglass usually illustrates a focusing of indications, and the expanding lower part illustrates an increase of other aspects of the project (e.g., multiple dosing regimens, multiple dosage forms).

Rectangular Approach

This is the "broad-front" approach where multiple dosage forms, indications, and routes of administration are followed throughout the life of a project. Whereas some of these will probably drop out, others may be added. A comparable image would be that of a cylinder.

Inverted Funnel Approach

A narrow focused approach is followed for most of a project's life. Shortly before (or after) the NDA is submitted, the number of activities greatly increase. Other possible indications are pursued and other dosage forms or routes of administration may be studied.

Shotgun Approach

To proceed from project initiation to an NDA requires planning, vision, persistence, and many other desirable attributes. When some of these characteristics are missing from a project team or management, the project may proceed in different directions either simultaneously or sequentially. When this occurs the project rarely succeeds. The difference between this approach and the funnel, hourglass, and rectangular approaches is that the latter three represent an organized approach to pursuing a project and build continually in an effort to reach a goal. If the project's efforts are not continually directed toward the goal, it is easy for a project's direction to wander.

It is often only in hindsight that a shotgun approach may be diagnosed. At the time that studies are in progress the project may be presented to others on the team, or to management, in the guise of funnel, hourglass, or rectangular approach.

Tangents

A tangent is defined as activities on a project which are not adhering to the general approach being followed. They may be purposely initiated to explore specific issues, questions, or therapeutic areas. As such, they may represent or lead to modifications in the approach being followed. Thus, a project that starts out following one of the diagrams shown in Fig. 3.4 may change and become one of the other approaches, or a hybrid approach may result.

Tangents may also develop inadvertently or purposely, but without appropriate sanction. In either case it is the responsibility and one of the major roles of management to prevent or minimize the number and extent of tangents. Many individuals associated with a project will present "good reasons" for exploring an area or a question that is later diagnosed as going off on a tangent. The most effective means of preventing tangents is to question how the proposed study or activity will help achieve the project's goals. Hopefully, this question will be asked at the stage when the work is proposed and not after it has been initiated or completed.

It is rare for most projects to reach their goals without having explored a number of unplanned tangents. Many tangents offer the potential of valuable benefits which may improve the project. Nonetheless, if tangents become too commonplace in number or too extensive in size they may threaten progress on a project. Tangents require company resources and will diminish productive work that will help move a project toward its goals. There is clearly a balance that must be achieved among the interest, excitement, and creativity often associated with exploring tangents and work on the main thrust of a project. Management must determine which tangents to allow because most will not be successful and there are usually insufficient time and resources to try all possible tangents. Tangents that occur within a single clinical study often represent protocol violations and are not discussed in this section.

CONSIDERATIONS FOR A CLINICAL PROGRAM IN PHASES I, II, and III

Most of the general approaches and specific considerations relating to this topic have been discussed widely throughout the three books of this series. This section will indicate some of the general aspects to be considered in each clinical phase of development.

Various factors that may decrease the time to proceed from IND to NDA are listed in Table 3.5. A number of suggested approaches to increasing the efficiency of clinical studies are presented in Table 3.6, and typical types of studies conducted in each phase of study are listed in Table 3.7. Situations

TABLE 3.5. *Factors relating to clinical studies to consider in minimizing the interval between submitting IND and NDA applications*

1. Adopting a feasible clinical strategy
2. Developing a regulatory strategy and core clinical package where each study serves an important purpose for the indication(s) that will be requested
3. Reviewing each strategy periodically and revising them appropriately
4. Utilizing appropriate staff and resources to carry out the clinical strategy
5. Utilizing appropriate study designs to achieve study objectives and overall objectives
6. Utilizing well-developed protocols that have a high likelihood of being successfully completed
7. Utilizing efficient investigators and staff who are highly motivated and have demonstrated their abilities
8. Insuring rapid patient entry—insofar as possible
9. Utilizing a sufficient number of study sites to achieve objectives
10. Conducting studies with adherence to high standards
11. Monitoring studies both at the study site and sponsoring institution on an appropriate periodic basis, paying close attention to effective monitoring
12. Utilizing reasonable and effective project management systems to insure efficient allocation and use of resources
13. Processing and analyzing data according to a plan developed prior to study initiation
14. Conducting meetings with regulatory authorities to present data and plans and to solicit feedback on their responses to the clinical plan for drug development
15. Developing a realistic and efficient plan to write and assemble the various parts of the NDA

in which various study blinds are used are listed in Table 3.8. Finally, sources of scientific information to help in planning projects are given in Table 3.9.

The definitions of the three phases of clinical development given in *Guide to Clinical Studies and Developing Protocols* (Spilker, 1984) are not absolute. Different individuals or groups sometimes use other definitions, such

TABLE 3.6. *Means to increase efficient conduct of drug studies*

1. Incorporate elements of proven value from earlier protocols
2. Eliminate problem areas encountered in conducting earlier protocols
3. Choose collaborators (or investigators) who have proven their reliability, dependability, cooperativeness, and overall ability
4. Include a research coordinator at the study site, especially for complex studies, whose primary or sole responsibility is to help conduct the study
5. Establish both formal and informal systems that have been proven to be useful in initiating, conducting, and monitoring studies
6. Periodically review how different aspects of conducting a study can be improved (e.g., follow-up of missed appointments can be handled with telephone calls and reminder cards)
7. Discuss problem areas with staff and colleagues to reach acceptable solutions
8. Discuss issues or problems with a consultant or panel of consultants
9. Determine which individuals have specific responsibilities

as ones based entirely on the chronological order in which clinical studies are conducted. Using that approach, Phase I studies are the first clinical studies conducted on a new drug. This is often an unsatisfactory definition, because later in a drug's development program during Phases II or III it may be necessary to conduct additional Phase-I-type studies (e.g., to explore a higher drug dose in normal volunteers), which should be referred to as Phase I. Another reason against using a chronological definition is that pharmacokinetic studies are often referred to as Phase I studies, although they are conducted throughout a project's three phases.

Phase I Studies

The types of studies conducted during Phase I are listed in Table 3.7. These studies usually progress from single-dose studies to multiple-dose

TABLE 3.7. *Typical types of clinical studies conducted on investigational drugs*[a]

A. Phase I
   1. Single-dose tolerance study of volunteers and/or patients who are exposed to a single dose of the drug[b]
   2. Multiple-dose study (for *X* days) of volunteers or patients. The subjects usually receive a fixed dose of drug, although dose titration is sometimes permitted
   3. Initial pharmacokinetic evaluations. These are often combined with, and conducted as part of, the above studies
   4. Increasing the dose range of a new investigational drug to define the upper limit of safety or to insure safety when lower doses have failed to demonstrate activity in Phase II studies
   5. Interactions of the drug with food or other interventions in normal volunteers
   6. Pharmacokinetic studies in normal or various patient populations (e.g., elderly, hepatic impaired) using unlabeled or radiolabeled drug

B. Phase IIA[c]
   1. Pilot study (or studies) of a drug in patients. These studies may be conducted in either an open-label or a single- or double-blind manner[d]
   2. Pilot study (or studies) of a drug in normal volunteers challenged to determine the efficacy of a drug (e.g., castor oil may be used to cause diarrhea, citric acid may be used to produce cough, syrup of ipecac may be used to produce emesis)
   3. Dose–response study of patients to identify the range of active doses
   4. Studies evaluating variations in dose level and/or dosing schedule
   5. Initial pharmacokinetic studies of patients as opposed to volunteers, who are enrolled in most Phase I studies[e]

C. Phase IIB[f]
   1. Placebo-controlled double-blind study (or studies) conducted at one or at multiple sites
   2. Placebo-controlled and active-drug-controlled, double-blind study (or studies) conducted at one or at multiple sites
   3. Active-drug-controlled, double-blind study (or studies) conducted at one or at multiple sites
   4. Dose–response-controlled, double-blind study (or studies) conducted at one or at multiple sites

(*continued*)

TABLE 3.7. *(Continued)*

D. Phase III
   1. Open-label and both single- and double-blind studies of larger numbers of patients with fewer protocol exclusions than in Phase II
   2. Humanitarian studies conducted in severely ill patients
   3. Evaluation of potential new indications
   4. Evaluation of new dosage forms
   5. Evaluation of new formulations
   6. Evaluation of new dosing regimens
   7. Pharmacokinetic studies required for characterizing a drug's activity
   8. Specialized studies dictated by the specific profile of the drug
   9. Evaluation of specific patient populations (e.g., geriatrics)
   10. Large-scale open-label studies to obtain broad exposure in a wide variety of patients
   11. Drug interaction studies
   12. Comparison with known therapies
   13. Premarket surveillance studies to better characterize the safety profile

[a] The actual studies utilized to evaluate an investigational drug depend on many factors, including the pharmacological nature and characteristics of the drug, disease, and patients, plus ethical and commercial considerations.

[b] In some studies a second (or third, etc.) dose is given to the same volunteer a number of days or weeks later.

[c] Studies in Phases II and III may evaluate the drug either as monotherapy or as add-on therapy.

[d] See *Guide to Clinical Studies and Developing Protocols* (Spilker, 1984) for a discussion of this point.

[e] Pharmacokinetic studies are always considered as Phase I studies by some individuals.

[f] Single-blind or open-label studies may be conducted under certain circumstances when double-blind studies are either impractical or impossible for ethical or other reasons.

studies and include as much pharmacokinetic evaluation as appropriate. The philosophy of attempting to identify a maximum tolerated dose is stressed, because it provides an upper limit to use in planning Phase II and III studies. Some individuals have questioned the ethics of this approach because it doses normal volunteers until at least moderately severe adverse reactions occur, and this may be at doses higher than those considered necessary to test for efficacy in Phase II studies. The counterargument is that an adequate degree of efficacy may not be observed at the expected doses in Phase II studies and it may be necessary to evaluate higher doses, which will not have been tested in normal volunteers. If that has to be done, then additional Phase I studies in normal volunteers must be considered. Moreover, Phase I testing is relatively safe and few volunteers who provided an honest medical history have ever been seriously injured (see Chapter 7 for references).

The pharmacokinetic program should be developed by experts in the area, but most specialized studies are generally not conducted until after the drug has demonstrated sufficient activity to warrant full clinical development. Many pharmacokinetic studies are thus conducted during late Phase II and throughout Phase III.

TABLE 3.8. *Situations and uses for various types of study blinds*

A. Open-label
   1. Pilot studies conducted prior to a more definitive study, when endpoints measured are objective and less subject to investigator and patient bias
   2. Case studies in life-threatening situations
   3. Unusual situations where definitive data may be obtained in (e.g., patients in a coma)
   4. Exposure of drug to a broad patient population to gain information of efficacy and safety for situations in which the drug will be used (e.g., premarketing surveillance)[a]
   5. Postmarketing surveillance studies to obtain data on drug safety and general tolerance
   6. Studies where ethical considerations do not permit blinding

B. Single-blind
   1. Provides a degree of control when a double-blind study is impossible or impractical to conduct
   2. Provides a degree of assurance of the data's validity as compared with open-label studies

C. Double-blind
   1. Best-controlled study design in most situations. Allows strongest interpretation of data if:
      a. all other aspects of the study were properly designed and conducted
      b. the blind remained intact
      c. the protocol was not seriously breached
      d. the power of the study was adequate
      e. the patients were compliant
      f. all appropriate, relevant, and useful factors and data were considered

[a] Definitive efficacy data are rarely obtained from open-label studies.

Phase I studies may enroll patients in addition to volunteers (although in separate studies) if it is believed that patients may metabolize the drug differently than normal volunteers. This is often the case in epileptic patient populations, because these patients are often receiving drugs that affect hepatic microsomal enzymes.

Phase II Studies

Pilot efficacy studies should almost always be double-blind, because open-label studies in all therapeutic areas studied yield far more false-positive results than do double-blind studies. This topic is discussed at length in Chapter 32 of *Guide to Clinical Interpretation of Data* (Spilker, 1986). A drug's entire dose–response range should be evaluated. This issue refers back to the discussion about identifying the maximum tolerated dose in Phase I. Unless this is done, it often creates problems in deciding about the maximum dose that may be used in Phase II studies. If this maximum tolerated dose is known, then Phase II dose-ranging studies may titrate patients up to this level, while evaluating both safety and efficacy. Because the maxi-

TABLE 3.9. *Sources of scientific information available to clinicians, scientists, and the public*

1. Computerized data bases of clinical and scientific data (e.g., Medlars, Medline, Toxline)
2. Computerized data bases of clinical and scientific reports
3. Computerized collections of data bases (e.g., Dialog)
4. Drug information services (e.g., hospital based)
5. Poison control centers
6. Pharmaceutical companies
7. Trade associations (e.g., Pharmaceutical Manufacturer's Association, Association of the British Pharmaceutical Industry)
8. Professional associations
9. Disease-oriented societies (e.g., American Cancer Society, American Heart Association)
10. Medical societies (e.g., State Medical Society)
11. Under the Freedom of Information Act (e.g., companies such as FOI in Rockville, MD)
12. Foundations[a]
13. Professional colleagues, friends, and peers
14. Well-known experts in the area
15. Medical libraries at universities, institutions, and the National Library of Medicine
16. Various government agencies [e.g., National Institutes of Health (NIH), Food and Drug Administration (FDA), and the United States Department of Agriculture]

[a] See the *Foundation Directory* (10th edition, Foundation Center, New York, 1985) for an extensive listing of foundations.

mum dose is known it is easier to identify the dose that achieves maximum efficacy with minimum adverse reactions. If Phase I dosing has only explored the range of doses predicted to be effective in Phase II, it is generally only possible in Phase II to evaluate those doses that were studied in Phase I. The major drawback of this approach is that an effective dose may be found and subsequently evaluated in many new studies, but that dose may be substantially lower than one which yields a greater degree of efficacy with minimal or no loss of safety. Thus, using a limited approach to exploring doses in Phase I may not lead to evaluating an important part of the dose–response relationship in Phase II. It is important in Phase II studies to evaluate the entire range of doses that may be used to treat patients. If a company has two research locations that approach this drug development issue from different perspectives, then a different dosing regimen may eventually be recommended for marketing in different countries. This will not arise because of relevant differences (e.g., weights of patients, cultures, genetic differences), but because the two research groups each explored different parts of the dose–response relationship.

In choosing the patient population to evaluate it is essential to consider whether the risks of treatment are justifiable on the basis of the benefit-to-risk ratio, for all patients with the disease. It may be necessary to limit drug exposure to those patients with either mild or severe forms of the disease.

Phase III Studies

Major issues include (1) identifying the specific patient populations to evaluate, (2) whether to expand studies to new indications, formulations, and routes of administration, (3) the numbers of patients to be included in a regulatory submission, (4) whether to initiate marketing studies and when they may be initiated, and (5) when to decrease the number of studies and increase the efforts spent on preparing a regulatory submission(s).

At some point during clinical development of a new drug (or of a marketed drug for a new indication) it should be considered as to whether the drug affects the natural history of the disease. If this has not been considered and/or evaluated in Phase II studies, then it should be considered during Phase III. Unfortunately, little is known about the natural history of many diseases.

There has been a general trend away from conducting many Phase III studies in the offices of private practitioners over the last twenty or so years. Nonetheless, many Phase III studies are still performed by practitioners working in solo or group practices. Some contract companies have established networks of private offices/clinics to conduct drug studies. Sponsors should be cautious about the quality of the laboratories in private offices used for hematology, clinical chemistry, microbiology, or urinalysis testing. There is no federal regulation of office laboratories and only three states (Idaho, Pennsylvania, and Wyoming) have comprehensive regulations (Crawley et al., 1986). These authors report that many problems in office laboratories that existed in Idaho before their regulations were greatly improved when the offices were assessed after the regulations. These problems included (1) lack of quality control in testing procedures, (2) lack of knowledge about quality control, (3) lack of adequate procedure manuals, (4) lack of preventive maintenance, (5) lack of knowledge about laboratory safety, (6) errors in proficiency testing conducted during onsite visits, and (7) inability to understand and retain information about quality assurance guidelines.

Unfortunately, problems in laboratory quality are not localized to laboratories in physician's private offices. The Centers for Disease Control (CDC) reported on an evaluation of the quality of 13 laboratories which serve 262 methadone treatment facilities. Ten drug-spiked urine samples were sent quarterly (i.e., 40 samples per year) to each laboratory for identification. Their study covered data obtained between 1973 and 1981. They found that the percent of laboratories with an acceptable performance was 9% for barbiturates, 0% for amphetamines, 50% for methadone, 9% for cocaine, 15% for codeine, and 8% for morphine (Hansen et al., 1985).

Phase IV studies are discussed in sections on postmarketing surveillance studies in the first two books of this series.

CHOOSING EFFICACY PARAMETERS TO MEASURE

In choosing efficacy parameters to evaluate in a clinical program it is especially beneficial if the parameters chosen can demonstrate endpoints related to:

1. Objective measurements that are validated and accepted to represent appropriate criteria of efficacy. Some subjective measurements may also be relevant to include as parameters.
2. Reduced progression or even reversal of the disease process (e.g., reduction of the number, area, or severity of lesions; reduction of the number, severity, or other manifestations of disease episodes; increased number of cured lesions; decreased duration of disease).
3. Improved quality of life. This aspect is becoming increasingly important to measure. Both quantitative and nonquantitative parameters are available to evaluate this endpoint. Some are more objective (e.g., number of days worked in a given period) while others are more subjective. It is possible to use standard questionnaires for some diseases being studied, standard measures of daily living and functioning interviews, or even just a few questions that assess those aspects that are of primary importance to the patient.
4. Reduced mortality in those studies in which this parameter has relevance.
5. Clinical global impression of both the physician and patient.
6. Reduced number or severity of risk factors.
7. Improved symptomatology of the patient.
8. Biochemical measures which assess the underlying state of the disease.
9. Direct visualization and measure of the lesion (e.g., in ulcer disease, in arterial blockage).

Some parameters require a long period to illustrate changes (e.g., wall thickness in congestive heart failure). One must examine more rapidly changing parameters in shorter-term studies. Parameters for acute studies must be able to demonstrate effects of the drug within the time period studied. Other types of parameters are listed in Table 10.4 of *Guide to Clinical Interpretation of Data* (Spilker, 1986).

Utilizing multiple approaches usually is able to provide the most convincing data of a drug's efficacy, assuming that the most accepted parameters of efficacy are included. By including parameters at different levels of organization (e.g., biochemical, pathological, pharmacological, physiological, symptomatic, objective clinical), it assists the process of extrapolating data to other patients. The relative importance of the various parameters should be established prior to the study and indicated in the protocol. In some situations, what is measured is not the true endpoint of the drug [see Table 23.1 in *Guide to Clinical Interpretation of Data* (Spilker, 1986)].

To identify the parameters that are best able to measure these attributes it may be desirable to convene a panel of experts and/or general practitioners. Debating the pros and cons of available parameters will indicate:

1. The parameters that are most important for influencing physician's decisions to switch to a new drug therapy. How do the physicians rank these in importance?
2. The combination of parameters that is most practical and makes the most sense to measure in a study.
3. The hard objective (i.e., quantitative) parameters that provide less information than soft-objective or subjective parameters. For example, the erythrocyte sedimentation rate is a precisely quantitated laboratory value measured in many studies conducted in arthritis patients, although it is subject to daily variation within a single patient. It provides less information on patient response than does the "softer" measure of morning stiffness.
4. How much of a change in the parameters would be clinically important. Also, how much of a change in the parameters would be sufficient for these physicians to switch therapy in some (or most) of their patients?

In some diseases the major efficacy parameter to measure is clear. For example, in patients with essential hypertension, blood pressure is measured. But even in this disease with an objective endpoint there are multiple means of presenting the data (e.g., initial fall of blood pressure over *X* weeks, maintained blood pressure loss for *Y* months, maintained normal pressure for *Z* months). The choice of one of these or other formats for presenting data depends on the study's objectives and should be determined prior to the study. For post myocardial infarction patients who are to be treated with a drug to prevent reinfarction and/or sudden death the choice of parameters to measure is much more complex. One may measure the number of deaths at one year, ventricular function either invasively with dyes or noninvasively, clinical endpoints relating to quality of life, or others.

Establishing Efficacy of a New Drug

To demonstrate that a new drug (drug A) has improved efficacy over standard drug therapy used to treat a disease, there are several areas that may be explored. Clear-cut advantages of drug A over available drugs could be in terms of (1) time to onset of effect, (2) magnitude of effect, or (3) duration of effect. There are also other means by which greater efficacy may be objectively and/or subjectively demonstrated. A few of these include: (1) different and more relevant parameters may be studied; (2) reduction in the number, severity, and/or duration of subsequent episodes of the disease; (3) improved quality of life; and (4) a decreased rate of relapse after therapy is discontinued.

There are numerous aspects of the profile of a new drug that may indirectly contribute to its efficacy but are not efficacy measures per se. Examples of this would be any characteristic of the drug that leads to increased patient compliance (e.g., lower cost, better taste, decreased number of tablets per dose, decreased number of doses per day).

It is important to evaluate efficacy data for a new drug to critically assess whether or not efficacy has been demonstrated and full-scale drug development should continue or be initiated. This usually occurs sometime during Phase II. The methods used to establish efficacy must be the most relevant ones or a mistaken conclusion may be drawn. If individual patient histories are used there must be adequate controls. If measurements are compared with baseline (or other approaches used) then statisticians must confirm that the conclusions reached are appropriate. If different forms of the drug are being developed then a different risk to benefit assessment must be made for each.

Dose-Response Relationships

In interpreting data where two drugs are being compared to determine which has the greater efficacy, the data may be relatively clear-cut, but still yield a mistaken view. For example, dose–response curves are often expressed using percent values of the effect measured (to 100%) on the ordinate. Two drugs will each reach 100% regardless of the response they cause. Figure 3.5 shows that drug A is less potent than drug B, but its effect (i.e., activity) is greater. In some cases a misleading interpretation of clinical efficacy is obtained, when information on only relative potency is presented without information on relative activity.

Relapse Rates

The measurement of relapse rates is especially relevant for drugs that are not intended to be used permanently. Relapse rates are also relevant for measuring effects of drugs in diseases marked by discrete episodes. One therapeutic area where relapse rates have been evaluated is in peptic ulcer disease. It is important to note that objective observations through endoscopes and not patient symptoms were used as a clinical endpoint in establishing whether a patient had relapsed. Endoscopic examinations were scheduled to occur at periodic times after drug treatment was discontinued.

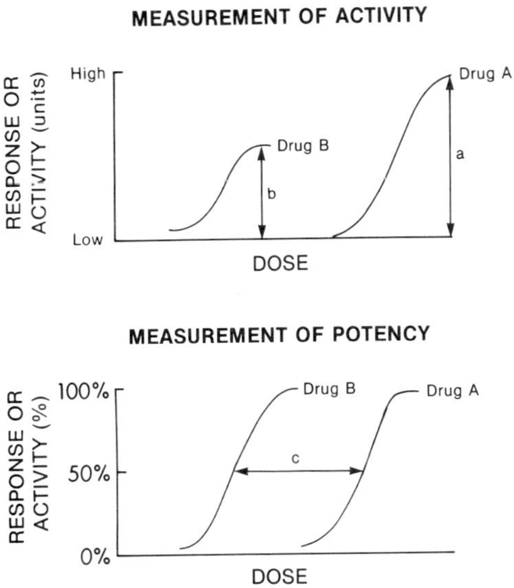

FIG. 3.5. Measuring activity and potency of drugs through use of dose–response curves. In the **upper graph** the activity of each drug is noted by the *vertical arrow*. In the **lower graph** the comparative potency is shown by the *horizontal arrow*, such that at 50% response drug B is more potent than drug A by the magnitude c.

The basic study design used in these evaluations is to initially administer to patients drugs that heal their ulcers. A healing rate (percent of patients whose ulcers heal within a certain time) is then determined. At that point, drug treatment is discontinued and the recurrence rate of endoscopically proven ulcers is determined over a fixed time interval (see Fig. 3.6).

This evaluation of both ulcer healing and recurrence yields several inter-

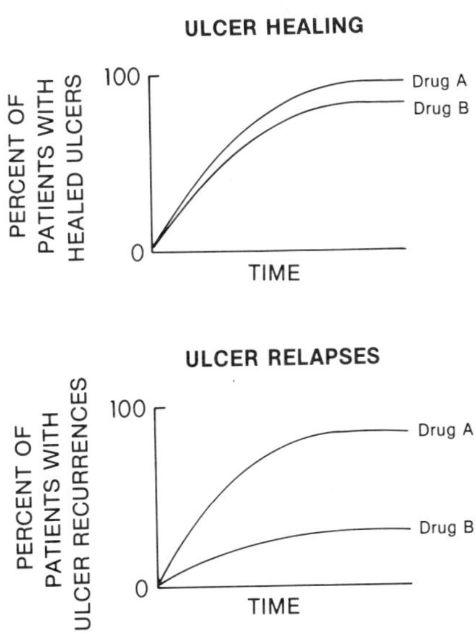

FIG. 3.6. Hypothetical rates of ulcer healing for two drugs (**upper graph**) and recurrence of disease (i.e., relapses) after drug treatment is discontinued for the same two drugs (**lower graph**).

esting possibilities. The drug with the highest rate of cure may also have a high rate of ulcer recurrence. Thus, the percent of patients who can be successfully treated for a given period and then remain disease free may be greater for a drug with a smaller initial cure rate. If the safety and pharmacokinetic profiles of drugs A and B are identical, then the "most effective" drug would be drug B for most patients.

A relevant comparison is to subtract the number of patients who relapsed from the number of patients cured to determine the number of patients with long-term cures, presumably resulting from the initial treatment. The numbers can be converted to percent of initial patients treated and two or more drugs may be compared. This comparison can become highly complex if retreatment of patients with these drugs yields different types of curves or if the safety or pharmacokinetic profiles of the drugs differ to a degree that is clinically important.

"CATCH-22" AND OTHER ISSUES

"Catch-22" (Circular, Paradoxical, or No-Win) Issues in Planning Multiple Studies

"Catch-22" situations often arise when many activities of drug development are attempted simultaneously. It is not advisable to conduct all development on a drug sequentially nor is it possible to do it simultaneously. Neither approach on its own is satisfactory, and judgment should be applied in each separate case in arriving at a reasonable balance. This balance will vary during the stages of drug development.

If the metabolism of a drug is studied in animals before human studies are initiated and a number of metabolites are identified, then it is easier to look for active metabolites in humans. If a parent drug is found to be acting as a prodrug, then there might be advantages in developing the active metabolite instead of the parent drug (e.g., to minimize adverse reactions, to reduce dosing variability). To develop this degree of knowledge at an early stage of drug development, however, usually requires additional time to conduct metabolism studies, which would be obtained at the expense (in part) of conducting clinical studies (as rapidly as possible) to learn whether the drug possesses efficacy. If efficacy is not found, then the drug will be dropped and there is usually no reason to evaluate and/or consider the development of a metabolite. Resources spent on identifying metabolites could have been used to develop metabolic profiles on other drugs that had demonstrated efficacy. This is clearly a circular argument.

Another example of a "Catch-22" situation is that the most important well-controlled Phase II clinical study should ideally be conducted with the final drug formulation, but it often takes significant time and experience to identify and produce the final formulation, shape, and color of a solid (or liquid) dosage form. If a company waits to finalize each of these (and other) characteristics before the major Phase II studies are initiated, too much lost time will occur. The alternative that is usually followed is to use a temporary dosage form (e.g., capsule) and to conduct a bioequivalence study at a later time with the final dosage form (e.g., tablet). It is assumed that the data for the temporary and final dosage forms will be comparable. If not, then additional clinical data with the final dosage form will be required.

In a model of mild pain (e.g., dental pain from tooth extraction) the degree of patients' pain may be adequate to allow a statistically significant separation between pain relief from a standard analgesic drug and placebo to be observed. There may not, however, be adequate residual pain (below the ceiling effect) to show that a new drug relieves more pain than the standard drug. Therefore, it would be necessary to study a new versus old analgesic using a different pain model, which could be used to evaluate drug responses to more severe pain. In this model there would be adequate residual pain to demonstrate a significant pain-relieving effect of the test drug if it were more active than the standard drug. But, mild analgesics are not expected to be active in models of severe pain, and therefore the study would not be worthwhile to perform.

Another example of a "Catch-22" situation concerns the aggressiveness and enthusiasm of project champions. If they are too cautious or even negative about their project in reports and verbal presentations, then management will be reluctant to commit significant resources to their project. It is also possible, of course, that management will replace the project champion with a more forceful and dynamic individual. Champions who are enthusiastic beyond what the data justify may acquire large quantities of resources too early in the projects' life, before it is even known whether the drug has demonstrated activity. If a company encourages and rewards this type of over-optimistic reporting of a drug's progress, then it has a negative effect on the other champions who attempt to present a balanced view of their projects and who do not seek resources before it is appropriate. In addition, resources inappropriately allocated to one project are unavailable to others.

Compassionate Plea Protocols

At some stage of developing a new drug the question may arise of whether to treat patients using a compassionate plea protocol. This type of protocol is for individual patients who are unable to enter formal studies because they do not qualify, live too far from a study site, and so on. These studies are also referred to as humanitarian studies. There are also situations when it is advantageous to enter relatively large numbers of patients in compassionate plea protocols to gain additional safety data shortly before a drug is to be marketed. Some important considerations in deciding whether to utilize compassionate plea protocols are: (1) availability of alternative therapy, (2) efficacy and safety of alternative therapy, (3) seriousness of the disease, (4) relative safety of the new therapy, (5) difficulty involved in using the new drug correctly and appropriately, (6) medical benefits available to patients, (7) propensity for the drug to be misused, (8) stage of the drug's development, (9) views of the relevant regulatory agency, and (10) ability to monitor the sites of physicians who are given the drug to dispense. The study may include all or most patients that physicians have who are available or are in need of treatment. It is not always necessary for patients to meet specific entry criteria to enter a compassionate plea study. Physicians may be required to submit periodic data on all patients to insure patient safety and to check on physician compliance with the protocol. A simple data collection form may be used for this purpose. Physicians who are noncompliant may be deleted from continued participation in the study.

Humanitarian studies should be designed and conducted to meet the highest standards of science rather than current regulations or personal ideas of regulatory reviewers. Reviewers and even regulations will change, but aiming at high scientific and ethical standards are the best guidelines to use. Even though patients may be treated as individual cases and no actual protocol may exist, a form to collect relevant safety and efficacy data should be designed and sent to the physician along with the drug. In some situations a formal protocol will be prepared to assist (and control to some degree) the treatment of individuals or groups of patients. Utilizing a written protocol for compassionate plea studies is the preferable approach.

Blinding Two, Three, Four, or More Groups of Individuals in a Study

Many publications glibly state that their study was conducted in a double-blind manner and do not provide information on (1) how well the blind was maintained, (2) whether it was verified, and (3) whether other individuals associated with the study were kept blind. Insofar as a double-blind study is defined as one in which neither the patient nor the investigator *knows* what treatment the patient was randomized to receive, most studies remain truly double-blind. Nonetheless, many investigators and patients have a good to excellent idea of the specific treatment received by that patient.

The treatment's identity is usually guessed on the basis of clues provided by the treatment itself, relating to adverse reactions, efficacy, laboratory measures, or drug interactions. For example, many drugs cause specific adverse reactions that are difficult or impossible to mask, especially if the patient has been given information about them in the informed consent. A second means of identifying active treatment (as opposed to placebo) is on the basis of clinical improvement. Drugs that are tested in diseases where it is ethical to give a placebo may yield clear evidence of efficacy, although a number of false-positive responses will usually be obtained in a clinical study. A third category is through alterations in laboratory parameters which may yield a clear indication of the patients' treatment. Methods to avoid these or other tip-offs (e.g., drug interactions in add-on studies) may be used in some studies, especially when considered in advance of the study.

Few studies have systematically attempted to evaluate how well patient or physician blinds have been maintained and what influence this may have had on the data obtained. This topic is discussed more fully in Chapters 3 and 37 of *Guide to Clinical Studies and Developing Protocols* (Spilker, 1984).

Blinding of Other Individuals Involved in a Study

In addition to blinding patients and investigators there are other individuals connected with clinical studies who are sometimes kept blind with regard to patient treatment. There are as yet no standards as to whether this practice is desirable, essential, or unimportant in most double-blind studies. The author considers it desirable. Clinical publications rarely specify these details, usually of course because they are not followed.

Outside of patients and investigators the most important people to blind in a study are the monitors who interact with investigators and study personnel. When an investigator notifies the sponsor of a patients' adverse reaction, the decision to unblind that patient's treatment to the investigator should not be made on the basis of the monitor's knowledge of the patient's true treatment. If the monitor has this information and somehow conveys it or an impression to physicians, then patients receiving placebo will tend to be kept in a study more than will patients who are receiving active treatment. Once a decision is made to remove a patient from a study, then their treatment should be unblinded to assist in the treatment plan.

Some monitors may remain blind to individual patient treatment throughout a study but be privy to information on how well the overall study is progressing in terms of efficacy through interim analyses. The wisdom of this partial unblinding must be questioned because of the possibility that the monitor may influence investigators either consciously or not.

Professionals who interpret data within a study (e.g., pathologists who review tissue slides, radiologists who interpret X-rays) should generally remain blind to the treatment and/or diagnosis of the patient. Pharmacists who dispense drugs may remain blind by having the prescription filled by another pharmacist. Statisticians who analyze data may deal with treatments labeled as A, B, and so on, rather than with the name of the drug or the term placebo. They could remain blind until they have chosen all of the statistical methods that will be used to analyze the data. Finally, clinicians who interpret data should in some instances be unaware of which result was from the drug group and which was from the placebo group.

There are extremely few, if any, studies blinded to this degree and it is not the author's contention that such blinding is either necessary or desirable in all cases. Nonetheless, it is certain that strong biases enter many studies because one or more of these groups were not blinded or were inadequately blinded. It is hoped that future studies will pay greater attention to this issue and will more completely document the types of blinds used, as well as indicating how the effectiveness of the blind was ascertained.

4

Recording, Coding, Processing, and Analyzing Data from Multiple Studies

Flow of Clinical Data • Classification of Diseases • Dictionaries of Adverse Reactions • Designing Data Collection Forms • Systems for Coding Data • Analyzing Data

FLOW OF CLINICAL DATA

Clinical data obtained in a study usually flow from investigator to monitors to data processors to statisticians to medical monitors and back to the investigator. Numerous variations in this pattern exist and depend on factors such as whether the study is sponsored, whether data are entered directly in computers, and the nature of the sponsor's organization. The flow of clinical data after a study is completed is shown in Fig. 4.1. Some means of improving data flow are listed in Table 4.1, and sample headings of tables used to monitor this flow are shown in Table 4.2.

TABLE 4.1. *Means of improving the efficiency of clinical data flow*

1. Design standard operating procedures that make sense and are simple to use
2. Design standard data collection forms for use in multiple studies on a project
3. Use data collection forms with responses that can be completed with a check mark or cross rather than requiring a fill-in
4. Design data collection forms to minimize write-in comments
5. Implement standard easy-to-use systems that take data step by step, from data editing to data entry to statistical analysis to clinical interpretation to report writing
6. Coordinate the procedures involved in data flow to allow integration of relevant systems and information with other divisions (e.g., marketing, production, technical development) and other countries
7. Explore automation of various steps (e.g., transfer of clinical laboratory data in machine readable form, use of optical scanners to "read" data collection forms, remote data entry)

TABLE 4.2. *Sample table heading formats used to monitor activities on multiple clinical studies during data processing, analysis, and report-writing periods*

A

Category of study	Study number	Principal investigator	Number of completed patients	Projected[a] date of last DCF to sponsor (* = actual date)	Projected date of last DCF to data processor (* = actual date)	Projected date of draft statistical report (* = actual date)	Projected date of final statistical report (* = actual date)	Projected date of draft medical report (* = actual date)	Projected date of final medical report (* = actual date)

B

Study number	Estimated[a] date of study completion	Estimated date of last DCF to data processing	Estimated date of data-base release	Estimated date of statistical report completion	Author of statistical report	Estimated date of medical report completion	Author of medical report

[a] The term "Projected" or "Estimated" may be changed in the heading to "Actual" when all items in that column are completed. Alternatively, an asterisk or other symbol may be used to indicate that the task has been completed.

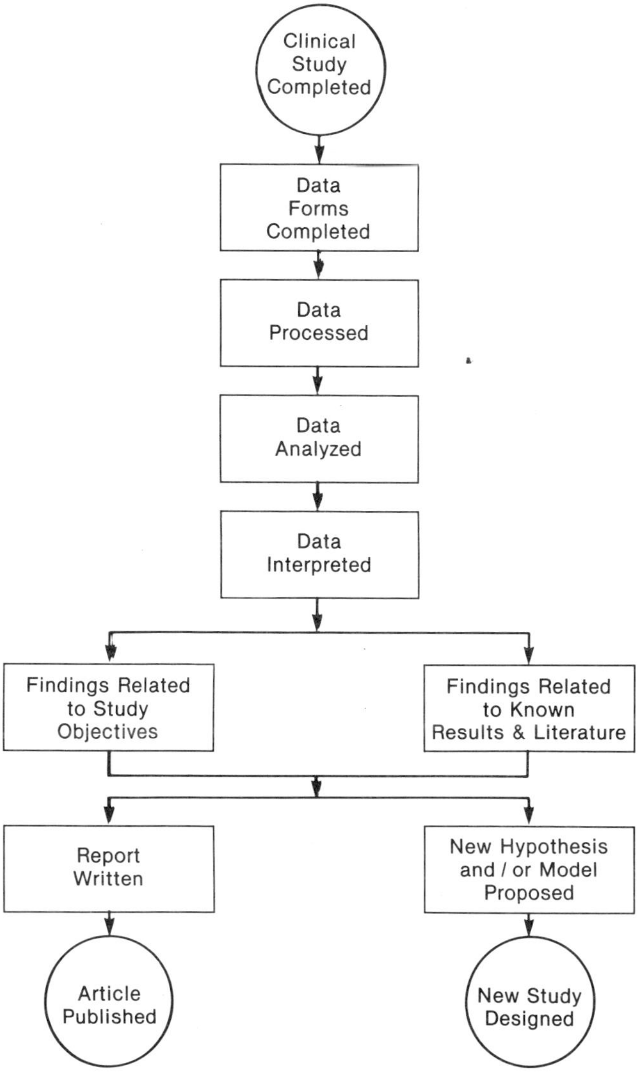

FIG. 4.1. Poststudy flow of clinical information and data. General flow of data after they are collected.

CLASSIFICATION OF DISEASES

There has been an increased use of dictionaries and systems in recent years to define diseases by code numbers, especially for patients entering hospitals. The spread of Diagnosis-Related Groups (DRGs) in hospitals will undoubtedly increase the use of these standardized categories. Some of these systems or dictionaries are created by professional societies (e.g., DSM-III in psychiatry was created by the American Psychiatric Society), and others (e.g., ICD-9) have resulted from international interest in this area. In some clinical studies the enrollment of patients with a standard diagnosis such as one listed in DSM-III is highly pertinent to obtaining the desired patient population. Nonetheless, in most clinical studies patient entry requirements are not tied to standardized diagnoses.

In certain therapeutic areas (e.g., epilepsy) most clinical researchers and many private practitioners adhere to a standard international classification for diagnosing patients. In other fields, however, there have been differences in the classifications used between countries. For instance, DSM-III is used in the United States to classify patients with various psychoses, but ICD-9, which is a morbidity and mortality coding system developed by the World Health Organization, is used (partially or completely) in many other countries for this purpose. In addition, numerous professional societies have prepared glossaries and/or classifications to assist in diagnosis of disease and treatment of patients.

A brief history of the classification of diseases is given by Côté and Robboy (1980). This article concentrates on Systematized Nomenclature of Medicine (SNOMED) and describes some of the problems with the International Classification of Disease (ICD) system. These authors propose that a merger of the two systems, using SNOMED as the starting point, would provide the most useful system of medical nomenclature. Various other coding systems and thesauri have been proposed for disease classification, including "Medical Subject Headings" of the National Library of Medicine in the United States.

DICTIONARIES OF ADVERSE REACTIONS

Dictionaries of adverse reactions are created by individual companies, large professional societies, health agencies, and regulatory agencies. Those created by sponsors are developed for all clinical studies on a particular drug or for all studies of the sponsor. Presently there are no universally accepted dictionaries of adverse reactions, although there have been and still are attempts to achieve this goal. One important reason for creating an adverse reaction dictionary is to allow different investigators (at different sites or at the same site) to identify the same adverse reaction with the same term and to identify different adverse reactions with different terms. Even one investigator may use different terms for the same reaction in different patients or for the same reaction in the same patient at different times. An investigator may label an adverse reaction as "drowsiness" at one visit and as "sleepiness" at a later visit if the patient is still complaining of the same problem. The investigator may not have the patient's data collection form from the previous visit readily available for reference and thus may write a different term in the medical record. This may be later transcribed as "sleepiness" on the data collection form, and without using a dictionary that rates these two adverse reactions as identical, a potential issue may be created.

Although the particular problem in this example is minor, the problem becomes much greater when magnified by 1,000 patients, by 10 visits per patient, and by other synonyms that may be used by other investigators for the same symptom (e.g., fatigue, somnolence, tiredness). In addition, there are other terms that differ slightly in meaning but may actually represent the same symptom (e.g., restlessness, irritability).

One counterargument to standardizing adverse reaction terminology prior to a study is that supplying even brief dictionaries to investigators or precoding data collection forms provides a stimulus that may increase the frequency of adverse reactions. Many clinical monitors prefer to assign the correct term to adverse reactions after all of the data have been collected.

A standard dictionary to be used in a clinical study does not have to be many pages long, and it is generally easier for investigators and their staff to use if it is short. The most important and frequently observed adverse reactions observed with the same drug in previous studies should be defined, synonyms should be presented, and a preferred term should be selected. If this practice is established, then when data are entered in a computer (or even written on a sheet) undesired terms may be removed and the appropriate synonym may be inserted. At a more sophisticated level, this process may be programmed into a computer.

When dictionaries of adverse reactions were first developed, each drug under investigation or even each clinical study had a home-grown list of preferred terms along with anticipated synonyms. In subsequent years some pharmaceutical companies (e.g., Eli Lilly) developed their own dictionaries or thesaurus of adverse reaction terms and synonyms. Some companies use the World Health Organization (WHO) Adverse Reaction Terminology (e.g., Schering-Plough: see Saltzman, 1985), or variations of the COSTART (*C*oding *S*ymbols for a *T*hesaurus of *A*dverse *R*eaction *T*erms) system (e.g., McNeil: see Teal and Dimmig, 1985). These lists are often divided by body system and certain terms carry an asterisk with the notation "Caution, other classification terms may be better suited." Other companies utilize standard systems such as COSTART.

COSTART System

COSTART provides a basis for vocabulary control of adverse reaction reports that emanate from a variety of sources. In that sense it is actually much more like a thesaurus than a dictionary. The orientation of COSTART is primarily anatomic. It has a hierarchical arrangement of terms, from the broadest (body-system categories) to narrowest (specific preferred terms or even special search categories). The COSTART dictionary is used and maintained by the Center for Drugs and Biologics at the FDA for marketed drug surveillance and has been endorsed by many senior managers in the various reviewing sections.

There are four indexes in COSTART:

Index A. Consists of three lists of search categories: (1) body-system search categories, (2) special search categories (e.g., neoplasia, superinfection), and (3) special search categories for fetal–neonatal disorders.

Index B. Consists of an alphabetical listing of all the coding symbols, plus preferred terms and primary search categories (optional categories).

Index C. Consists of a listing of coding symbols by body-system categories.

Index D. Consists of an alphabetical list of terms commonly used by physicians to report adverse reactions to drugs, plus numerous related terms and the coding symbol to be used. This index is extensively cross-indexed.

WHO Adverse Reaction Terminology

The WHO terminology system of adverse reactions is relatively short, containing approximately 1,100 terms. A code number is assigned to each of these terms. This provides the advantage that the same code is retained when the term is translated into different languages, although between countries there are some differences in definitions of specific terms. The WHO system uses a hierarchy of "preferred terms" to describe adverse reactions. Other commonly used terms are called "included terms." These are listed with their preferred term.

FDA Adverse Reaction Drug Dictionary

The FDA and many drug companies have gone through an evolution of systems in how they obtain, collect, process, and define adverse reactions. The drug dictionary currently used by the FDA (*The Center for Drugs and Biologics Ingredient Dictionary*) is described by Forbes et al. (1986), and the processing of adverse reaction reports by the FDA is described by Turner et al. (1986).

Advantages and disadvantages of COSTART, ICD-9, Medical Subject Headings, SNOMED (2nd edition), and WHO Adverse Reaction Terminology are succinctly listed by Stephens (1985).

DESIGNING DATA COLLECTION FORMS

Data collection forms contain raw data generated in a clinical study. Study data must be taken from these forms, entered onto other tabulation forms or directly into a computer, and eventually tabulated and analyzed statistically. The data are then interpreted and utilized to prepare medical reports or articles for publication, as well as for planning additional clinical studies, modifying plans, and adjusting strategies. When data collection forms are well designed they allow efficacy (and safety) data to be integrated from multiple studies most easily.

Some of the more common approaches to designing data collection forms for a single clinical study are presented in Chapter 27 of *Guide to Clinical Studies and Developing Protocols* (Spilker, 1984). It was also stated in that book that when multiple clinical studies are being conducted with one drug, consideration should be given to designing generic data collection forms to improve the ease of combining data from different studies. Types of generic data collection forms are listed in Table 4.3. Various pitfalls to avoid are listed in Table 4.4. The remainder of this chapter considers issues raised when data from multiple clinical studies are combined.

In planning and designing data collection forms for multiple clinical studies a number of basic approaches may be followed. Both a "backward" and "forward" approach will be described. In the backward approach, one starts with an idea of what type of information and format one desires in the statistical reports or synopsis of data. This information is then tracked backward to the data collection form, which is designed to capture data in a manner that allows it to be easily converted or directly placed in the desired tables or figures.

The forward approach starts by considering the type and quantity of raw data that are to be collected and then designing the data collection forms to collect these data. The analyses of the data to be done determine the statistical tables and figures that may be generated. If the statistical tables (or figures) that may be generated are not considered optimal to use in integrating data from multiple studies (or from a single study) then the protocol and design of the data collection form should be modified to allow collection of more appropriate data.

One result of using either one or both of these approaches for designing data collection forms is that a group of generic forms are eventually established. These forms are presumably available in some type of "library" and may be modified as required for a particular study. The significant efforts that are generally expended in creating data collection forms for a specific study become lessened as more clinical studies are conducted. The potential danger in not considering this issue at the outset of a project is that similar

TABLE 4.3. *Types of generic data collection forms that may be prepared*[a]

1. Patient demographics[b] (initials or name, address, birthdate, social security number, sex, marital status, race, education)
2. General medical history
3. Specific medical history focusing on the therapeutic problem being evaluated
4. Clinical chemistry
5. Blood sample: profile of time after drug administration versus drug and/or metabolite concentration
6. Hematology and urinalysis
7. Urinary, fecal, or other sample: profile of time after drug administration versus drug concentration
8. Urine screen for illegal drugs
9. Radiology reports
10. Electrocardiogram
11. Other laboratory examinations (e.g., pathology reports, biological samples, physiological examinations)
12. Physical examination. Forms for both complete and abbreviated examinations may be prepared
13. Vital signs, height, and weight
14. Neurological examination and/or other specialized physical examinations. Forms for both complete and abbreviated examinations may be prepared
15. Disability tests
16. Psychological and/or psychiatric tests to be used
17. Quality of life measurements
18. Concomitant medications
19. Drug dosing record for chronic study—prescribed and actual daily, weekly, or monthly dose
20. Drug dosing record for acute study—precise amount and time of each dose given, plus amount prescribed
21. Drug dispensing record
22. Compliance check—such as pill count
23. Adverse reactions—summary form for study
24. Adverse reactions—general form for times of onset and cessation plus number of occurrences
25. Adverse reactions—specific form for exact times of onset and cessation
26. Clinical global impression (to be completed by the investigator)
27. Clinical global impression (to be completed by the patient)
28. Premature discontinuation of patient
29. Efficacy measurements that are constant or similar between studies
30. Termination record
31. Posttermination record for patient follow-up after the study would have normally stopped
32. Investigator's comment log

[a] Some of these topics may be combined on a single page of the data collection forms. For many of these categories several generic data collection forms may be prepared. These would include abbreviated and full reports. Different formats could be prepared for each form, which would allow for either one or multiple patient visits on a single sheet.

[b] Patient confidentiality must be maintained in sponsored studies or if the data will be made public. Therefore, the patient's name should not appear on data collection forms that will be given to a sponsor or made public, nor on correspondence with the sponsor. Indicating the patient's birthdate is preferable to listing the patient's age.

TABLE 4.4. *Pitfalls to avoid in designing data collection forms or in determining the amount of data to collect at different time points*

A. Designing data collection forms
   1. Requesting information without providing adequate instructions on the data collection forms (or elsewhere) regarding how to complete the forms
   2. Using multiple pages for a single category of information that could easily fit on one page
   3. Requesting an excessive amount of information to be put on a single page, which makes monitoring, editing, and data entry difficult
   4. Using jargon unfamiliar to the person filling out the form. Some individuals advocate eliminating all jargon
   5. Using a check-off system to obtain responses to a question, but not including all possibilities or an "other" category, where different responses may be listed
   6. Collecting all or almost all data in the form of write-ins, so that data obtained from multiple patients are difficult or impossible to rapidly combine and/or condense
   7. Using codes on the form that are only relevant to data processors and make the forms difficult to complete by investigators or their staff
   8. Not combining or attaching all of the pages of the data collection forms for each patient in a manner that is easy to use, store, and retrieve

B. Determining the amount of data to collect at different time points in one or multiple studies
   1. Not collecting sufficient data at baseline or posttreatment
   2. Not collecting any data at the most relevant time points (e.g., taking an electrocardiogram before a drug is given and after the effects have worn off, but not during the period of clinical activity while the drug is in the plasma or the plasma levels are at or near their peak)
   3. Not collecting adequate data at the relevant time points
   4. Collecting unnecessary data

data from separate studies collected on different forms may become difficult or even impossible to combine in an integrated manner.

SYSTEMS FOR CODING DATA

As data flows from the data collection forms to final medical reports (see Fig. 4.2) the flow is made easier when data are easier to handle. One means of accomplishing this is to code selected data either before or after the study.

Precoding Data

In some clinical studies all or almost all of the possible responses to questions or examinations are presented on the data collection forms. The investigator or research coordinator merely has to check off the box with the appropriate response (see Fig. 4.3, part A). In other studies, the investigator is asked to write the code of the correct answer (Fig. 4.3, part B). If each question is precoded, it becomes even easier to subsequently process and

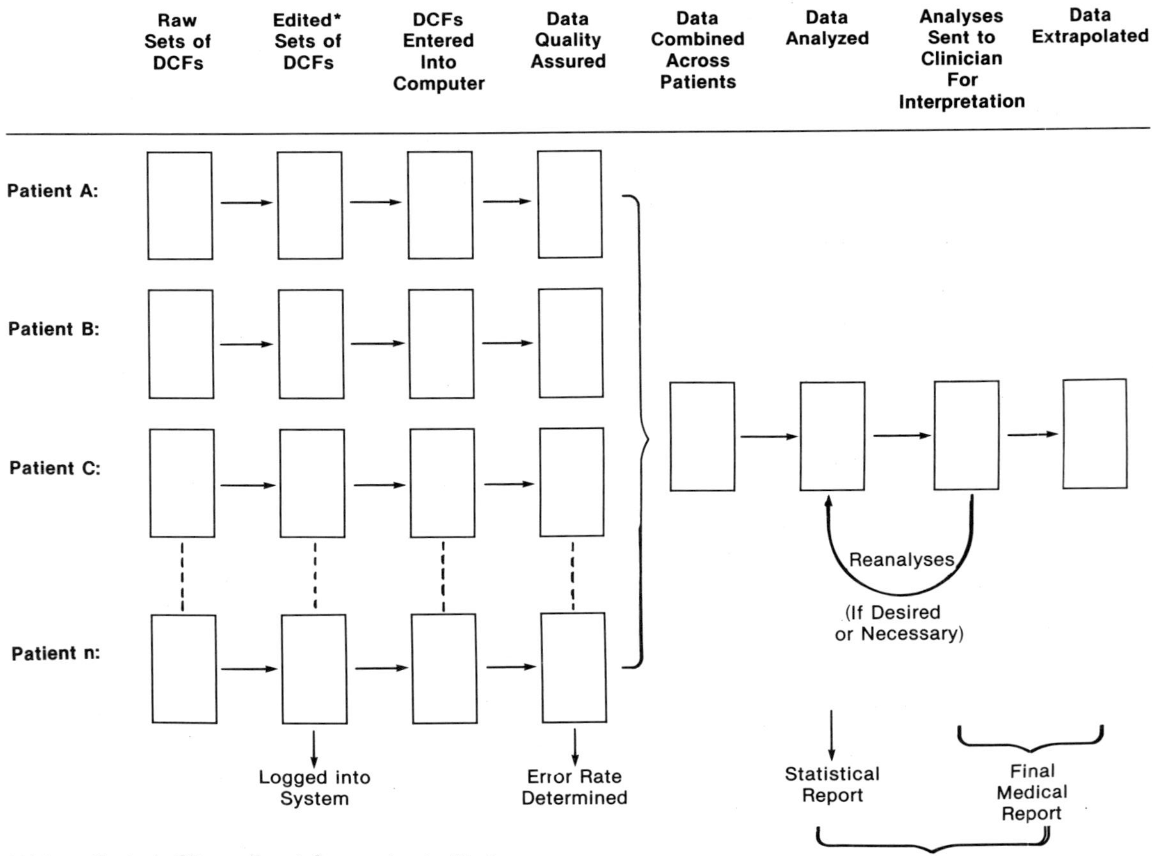

*At Investigator's Site and/or at Sponsoring Institution.

FIG. 4.2. Flow of data from data collection forms. General procedures conducted on data as they move from forms to a final medical report.

A. During the last month, how many episodes has the patient experienced?

Check one:

0	☐
1	☐
2 to 5	☐
6 to 10	☐
11 or more	☐

B. During the last month, how many episodes has the patient experienced?

Place the code for the correct number inside the box. ☐

a	=	0
b	=	1
c	=	2 to 5
d	=	6 to 10
e	=	11 or more

C. During the last month, how many episodes has the patient experienced?

Write the appropriate number inside the box. ☐

FIG. 4.3. Options in designing data collection forms. Various means of collecting data are shown in response to the question "How many episodes has the patient experienced?" The box for the answer may also be labeled with the question number to assist data entry.

validate the data collected in a computer preprogrammed to associate question number *X* on page *Y* with the specific question posed.

If one assumes that the distribution of responses to the hypothetical question posed in Fig. 4.3 would elicit only a few "e's" in part B and little information is lost by not subdividing the "11 or more" category, then there would be little benefit to posing the question in the manner that used to be commonly asked on most data collection forms (Fig. 4.3, part C). In the particular example given; however, the responses to part C would be more amenable to determination of specific means, medians, and error measurements than would the data from parts A or B.

Postcoding Data

In many clinical studies it is possible to go through the data collection forms after the study is complete and to assign codes as was done in the above precoded examples. There are several advantages to doing this coding after the study is complete. One possible advantage would be in a situation

A. Location of Pain? ______________________________

____

____

B. Location of Pain? Shade all affected areas on the drawings of the figure (front and back)

C. Location of Pain? Check All That are Appropriate:

					Do Not Complete or Mark
Head	_____				a
Neck	_____				b
Chest	_____				c
Back	_____				d
Abdomen	_____				e
Groin	_____	Right	_____	Left	f, g
Arm	_____	Right	_____	Left	h, i
Leg	_____	Right	_____	Left	j, k
Foot	_____	Right	_____	Left	l, m
Hand	_____	Right	_____	Left	n, o

D. Location of Pain? Check All That are Appropriate:

Head	_____	a
Neck	_____	b
Chest	_____	c
Back	_____	d
Abdomen	_____	e
Arm (s)	_____	f
Leg (s)	_____	g
Hand (s)	_____	h
Foot (Feet)	_____	i

FIG. 4.4. Options in designing data collection forms. Various means of collecting data are shown in response to the question "Where is the pain located?" The outline drawings of the front and back of a human for answering questions in part B would be attached.

where confusion might arise if a long list of medical terms and associated codes were put on a data collection form and it was not clear which code or codes were to go in which places on the data collection forms. Under these circumstances, placing a blank line next to each term with instructions to "check those answers or categories that are appropriate" would be clear to the investigator and a code (either printed or not printed) on the data collection form could be entered into a space or box at a later time. An example of this approach is illustrated in Fig. 4.4. Part A shows a simple response that will be extremely time consuming to enter in a computer and difficult to integrate with responses about other patients. Part B provides visual information, which is often useful as a supplement but is also difficult to integrate across patients. Part C is a postcoding example where staff assign letter codes to items checked by the investigator. A more simple version is shown in part D.

ANALYZING DATA

It is impossible to discuss data analysis without reference to, and consideration of, statistical methodology. This section is limited to presenting a few general principles and practical points. Individuals should refer to standard statistical texts and/or consult a statistician for details and specific methodologies appropriate to their particular issues.

Academicians who conduct clinical studies often become associated with a statistician who they trust and find to be either knowledgeable about their specific area of research or willing to collaborate in their activities. Statistical input is important (or essential) throughout the course of a study but is almost always mandatory before a study is initiated and after a study is completed. There appears to be a growing trend to have statisticians kept blind to the identity of treatment groups and to analyze data from groups A, B, etc., rather than from groups labeled study drug or placebo. Some statisticians consider this approach preferable for interim analyses rather than for final analyses. This approach may also be followed by committees who are deciding whether to stop a study prematurely.

Prior to the study it is important to identify the major statistical evaluations that will be conducted on the data. Data must be collected in a manner that will allow those methods to be used. During a study there are often unforeseen issues that arise, thus preventing the desired statistical tests from being used and requiring significant modifications of the statistical methods. A number of practical pitfalls in the statistical approach to study design and data analysis are discussed by Pocock (1985). He illustrates that even a single patient's outcome in a large study may markedly affect overall results and the interpretation reached.

It is critical that the statistician not initiate and conduct analyses on data sets that are believed complete (i.e., have data from all patients to be analyzed) but are really incomplete (i.e., data of some or all patients are missing). A system of communications between the clinical monitor, data processor, statistician, and possibly others is important to prevent this problem from occurring. One element of this system should include a means of identifying

Clinical Data Collection Form Reconciliation

Statistician to Complete Top Portion and Send to Clinical Monitor.

Drug Number / Name ______________________________

Protocol Number ______________ Study Number ______________

Investigator ______________ Investigator's Site ______________

Name of Statistician ______________ Date of Form Initiation ______________

....

Clinical Monitor to Complete Rest of Form and Return to Statistician.

Name of Person Completing This Form ______________________

Number of Patients: **Total Number and Patient Numbers if Available:**

Scheduled (at this time) for Completion of Study ______________

Who Have Actually Completed the Study ______________

Complete DCFs Received From Site ______________

Incomplete DCFs Received From Site ______________

Complete DCFs Sent for Data Entry ______________

Incomplete DCFs Sent for Data Entry ______________

Data Entry Performed On ______________

On Whom Data Should Have Been Received by Statistician ______________

Comments, Qualifications, Modifications: ______________________

____

____

____

____

____

____

FIG. 4.5. Clinical data collection form reconciliation. Sample methoa to confirm that data entry and statistical analyses are being conducted on the correct number of patients.

which data are in which data set and how complete each data set is at all points in the data flow. Figure 4.5 illustrates a simple form of this type.

If several similar statistical reports are to be prepared on different (but related) studies, then the initial statistical report may be used as a model. The approach used in this model may have input from the medical personnel who are involved with the studies, as well as the principal investigator in some cases. These medical personnel will help insure that the study analyses are presented in a format that can be clinically interpreted most effectively.

TABLE 4.5. *Selected pitfalls to avoid in analyzing clinical data*

1. Analyzing data without a full consultation and/or association with a professional statistician
2. Using statistical techniques that fail to meet currently acceptable standards (unless there is a strong rationale for the choice of techniques used)
3. Analyzing incomplete data sets
4. Performing an unplanned interim analysis, which will compromise the analysis of the final data
5. Prematurely unblinding the study
6. Inadequately quality-assuring the data
7. Inadequately documenting the analyses conducted (e.g., the rationale for excluding specific data or patients from the analysis)

Sophisticated analyses that are not meaningful to the investigator will generally not be meaningful to most clinically oriented individuals who read the medical report or a clinical article prepared for publication. If statistical details are important to the audience of the report, then they should be included as a footnote or appendix to the clinical report or article. Statisticians should present data in a way that clinicians can readily comprehend the results, even if the clinicians are not statistically sophisticated. If multiple clinical studies are being conducted using a similar or related study design, then each statistical report should be as similar as possible to the original model. Approaches used to analyze efficacy data are described in statistical texts. A few selected pitfalls to avoid in analyzing clinical data are listed in Table 4.5.

The specific patients who are eliminated from data analysis must be determined through nonbiased criteria, which should be enumerated before the study begins. This issue is extremely controversial because inclusion of inappropriate patients in a study analysis may bias data or create more "noise" in the results, which could mask true effects. On the other hand, if patients were treated with the study drug it is usually not considered acceptable to eliminate their data from analysis. An excellent example of this was reported by Sackett et al. (1985) in their Table 7-9.

Analyzing Data From Patients Who Do Not Meet Entry Criteria or Do Not Complete the Study

How does one deal with data from patients who did not meet entry criteria for a study? There are various situations when it is uncertain at the time of enrollment if a patient will eventually be found to meet entry criteria. These situations include studies where all data are not available on entry. For example, in a study where patients must be treated within a few hours of a myocardial infarction, patients with suspected myocardial infarctions may be enrolled but later found not to meet entry criteria. Another example is of patients with various types of infections who are of necessity treated with a study drug before microbiological culture results are available. These results are necessary to provide the evidence of whether their infections met entry criteria. Another complicating factor is that many patients are either mistaken or less than totally honest about their past medical history and are later found not to meet entry criteria.

There are numerous ways to deal with data from patients who either do not meet entry criteria or do not complete the study. The author agrees with those statisticians who advocate performing multiple analyses of the data. Multiple analyses have the advantage that all major views of the data are conducted and interpreted. Analyzing data from all patients treated in a study is important since (1) the patients were treated in the study, (2) in other situations similar patients will likely be treated, and (3) the ability to extrapolate data could be compromised if some treated patients were excluded from analysis. This analysis includes patients studied because of the investigator's "intention to treat."

There are different categories of patients who do not meet entry criteria. These categories include (1) patients entered legitimately who were later found to be in violation of criteria designed to preserve the integrity of the efficacy evaluation, (2) patients who did not meet entry criteria because of minor differences in age or another relatively inconsequential parameter, (3) patients who lied about their previous medical or nonmedical history, but met other criteria, and (4) patients who did not meet criteria designed to insure patient safety.

In all analyses, it is possible to consider either those patients who completed the study or all patients who entered the study regardless of whether they completed it. For those who entered the study but did not complete it, it is possible to carry their last observed efficacy values forward to each of the times when no values were obtained or to simply ignore their missing values in the analysis from the time when they dropped out (of their volition) or were discontinued by the investigator. Patients who drop out and do not complete a study because of adverse reactions are often considered as a separate group. Their data are often treated differently than data from patients who drop out of their own volition for reasons unrelated to the study.

These considerations indicate that there are various categories of patients to review when data are being assembled for analysis. These categories include

1. All patients entered in a study (i.e., those who signed an informed consent) regardless of whether they received any drug treatment.
2. Patients who received at least one dose of a drug.
3. Patients who completed at least a prespecified portion of the study.
4. Patients who completed the entire study.

5. Patients who dropped out of the study on their own volition, because of lack of efficacy.
6. Patients who dropped out of the study on their own volition, because of clinical improvement.
7. Patients who dropped out of the study on their own volition, because of adverse reactions.
8. Patients who dropped out of the study on their own volition, because of reasons unrelated to the study (e.g., moved, personal reasons).
9. Patients discontinued by the investigator because of safety considerations (e.g., adverse reactions, unacceptable benefit to risk ratio).
10. Patients discontinued by the investigator because of other reasons (e.g., lack of cooperation, poor compliance).

Some of these categories may overlap, may not be relevant for a study, and/or may have to be redefined. Once all relevant patient categories to be analyzed in a study are chosen, it is essential to determine which type(s) of data analysis will be used. For example, will the "last observation carried forward" approach be used, will all data be presented, or will multiple analyses be conducted? After these choices are made the data may be analyzed with the tests and procedures considered most valid. Relevant within-treatment groups, between-treatment groups, subgroup analyses, and other comparisons will be conducted.

Preparing Statistical Reports for an NDA

A few general points are listed that should be considered when preparing statistical reports of clinical studies which will be included in an NDA.

1. Reports should present a detailed account of all protocol modifications and/or violations. Reasons for these digressions should be presented.
2. Patients in a study who do not meet the inclusion criteria should be identified in the statistical report. Explanations should be given in the medical report, although an abbreviated explanation may also be given in the statistical report.
3. All relevant baseline variables or combinations of variables should be used to compare treatment groups, even if the data appear to show no differences.
4. It is important to include an accountability section (e.g., the number of patients at each stage of the study).
5. Data should be analyzed separately from each study site whenever possible.
6. A statistical rationale should be given when data are pooled to use a single statistical analysis.
7. All patients who do not complete the study should have relevant data

listed (e.g., treatment group, time on drug, dosage at time of withdrawal, amount of drug taken, concomitant drugs, adverse reactions if any, reason(s) for dropping out or discontinuation, plus other relevant information).

8. Results of any interim analyses conducted should be discussed, plus the reasons for conducting an interim analysis.
9. It is important for statisticians to avoid presenting a clinical interpretation of the results. This issue is discussed in *Guide to Clinical Interpretation of Data* (Spilker, 1986).

5

Integrating Efficacy Data from Multiple Studies

Data from multiple clinical studies on a single drug may be combined in several ways. The least integrated manner is merely to arrange sets of data obtained from each study alongside each other and to combine the data solely through discussion of the conclusions reached for each set of data. At the opposite extreme, the data from all studies may be combined into a global (i.e., single) data set so that a single unified interpretation may be developed, as well as separate interpretations of each subset.

Various other possibilities for combining data lie between these two extremes of the spectrum. For instance, only similar data of identical parameters may be combined. This is commonly done with laboratory parameters on samples collected at comparable times after drug initiation, administration, or termination. It may also be done for data obtained using standard tests of efficacy.

Dissimilar data may be combined if they were obtained for similar parameters. One means of accomplishing this is to convert or transform some or all of the variables so that all data have a common basis. For example, data collected on the same efficacy test derived with different equipment in different studies could be converted to a qualitative scale to indicate whether the patient improved, remained unchanged, or deteriorated. Alternatively, a five-point (or larger) scale could be created and all data could be converted to fit this scale and then combined. This particular example is not completely satisfactory because much of the potential value obtainable from quantitative data is lost when they are converted to qualitative data.

A more satisfactory approach is to create ranges that may be used to combine dissimilar data. For instance, if patients have been able to tolerate a drug for different lengths of time (e.g., 3 days to 3 months) then broad categories may be utilized to create an appropriate number of categories in which all patients' responses may be entered, with only minimal loss (in most cases) of the quantitative value in the data. In this case, data may be presented from patients who received a study drug for 0 to 2 weeks, 2 to 4 weeks, 4 to 8 weeks and 8 to 12 weeks, rather than using a specific number of days or weeks that could, in theory, place each patient in a separate category.

It is obviously easier to integrate data from studies that utilize identical or similar protocols and methods of obtaining and measuring efficacy data than from studies using different protocols. It is important to design protocols and data collection forms with an eye toward eventual integration of efficacy (and safety) data. If that has only been done to a limited degree (or not at all) and many studies have been conducted, then the integration of data will be more difficult.

One of the first steps to consider in integrating efficacy data is to evaluate the general results and relevant aspects of all studies to be combined. A useful approach is to list all studies by name or number on the left column and to list all of the important elements about each study that are of interest along the top of a spreadsheet format. These elements may include the number of patients treated, the doses of drug tested, the frequency of dosing, the duration of the study, whether a placebo group was included, plus any other pertinent features of the study design. On the same or different table indicate overall results in terms of efficacy. Table headings could include measurements made, equipment used, tests conducted, plus synopsis of the data resulting from the evaluations.

From these tables a number of combinations of studies may suggest themselves, such as combining studies in newly diagnosed patients, in patients receiving no concomitant medications, pediatric (or geriatric) studies, mild or severe disease, inpatient or outpatient, oral or parenteral therapy, and so forth. A further breakdown of these studies by key elements or data may be made, whereby similar data within each study would be combined. Examples of efficacy data that may be combined across studies are given in Table 5.1. Examples of sample tables used to combine data across studies were published by Guy (1979). Selected uses of clinical data are listed in Table 5.2.

Tables may be used to present general overviews of data across many studies or specific subgroup analyses within individual studies. Group means for baseline and overall or final treatment periods may be presented in addition to group means for each dosage level and each time treatment effects were measured. Multicenter studies should usually have results presented for each separate investigator to evaluate whether site-related differences occurred.

The above approach may be defined as a "forward approach," i.e., starting out with a large amount of apparently dissimilar data and seeing the ways one can extract pertinent parts to combine together.

Another approach to combining various types of efficacy data is to use the "backward approach." In this system one determines at the outset where one desires to end up. This may take the form of a specific format of a conclusion, figure, or table of data one wishes to generate, or alternatively an entire series of blank tables and figures may be created. With these specific endpoints in mind it is possible to go through available reports and data

TABLE 5.1. *Examples of efficacy data that may be combined across studies*[a]

1. Specific values or scores obtained in standardized tests or any tests that are used in a standard way. These tests measure physical performance, laboratory measures, or other objective parameters. Data combined across studies may be chosen as either one or more values for each test. If one value per patient per test is used, it may be the first value obtained, last value obtained, mean value, median value, or modal value of all applications of the test. Other choices may be made but should be defined in advance. If multiple values from a single patient's test are combined across studies, consultation with a statistician is strongly advised to insure that appropriate methods and approaches are followed
2. Data from patient diaries (e.g., number of events, maximum or mean intensity of events, maximum or mean duration of events, scores of events using an arbitrary scale, number of entries)
3. Data from efficacy scales obtained and measured by written tests or verbal interviews (patient and/or investigator completed)[b]
4. Clinical global impression scores (patient and/or investigator completed)
5. Scores of disease severity
6. Percentages of patients improved or cured at different time points
7. Drug formulations, dosing regimens, and combinations of drugs used by patients where maximum efficacy was observed
8. Dosages found to elicit a maximum therapeutic effect

[a] Raw data should be combined whenever possible, before converting it to percent response or by another data transformation where the nature of the effects measured become less clear. Normalization of data is one statistical method of transforming data that usually causes little distortion of raw data. Patient populations should be similar for defined characteristics in the studies being combined.

[b] If different scales were used in different studies to measure efficacy, then broad categories (e.g., improved, unchanged, deteriorated) are a possible (though often undesirable) means of transforming data so that dissimilar data may be combined.

on clinical studies to cull out those parts that may be pieced or combined into the final tables or figures.

If all studies provide the necessary pieces to create final tables and figures then the "forward approach" works well. The choice of a system to combine data usually depends on the nature of the individual conducting this effort as well as the specific type of available data. But, if small or large portions of the tables or figures are found to be missing when everything is put together, the options to consider should be discussed with a statistician. Other options are discussed in Chapters 5 and 8 of *Guide to Clinical Interpretation of Data* (Spilker, 1986).

When combining certain parameters across studies it is important to confirm that they are measuring, or refer to, the same thing. For example, investigators may look for different attributes or rate the same attributes differently in assessing their Clinical Global Impressions (CGI). The best means to help standardize this parameter is to create operational definitions and examples for the investigators to use. This will hopefully prevent or at least minimize the problem where multiple investigators in the same (or

TABLE 5.2. *Selected uses of clinical data that are collected*[a]

1. For preparation of regulatory submissions (e.g., IND, NDA)[b]
2. For preparation of reports (e.g., review of the study or project)
3. For preparation of an article for publication
4. For assistance in monitoring future studies
5. For providing clinical guidance and/or decisions for future studies or patient treatment (e.g., what dose should be used)
6. For comparison of results with those from other studies (a) for general interest, (b) to address specific questions, (c) to support a theory or belief, (d) to challenge a theory or belief
7. For providing information for advertising and/or other marketing activities
8. For exploring new indications, formulations, or product line extensions
9. For providing an enlarged data base to assess safety and to have the information available for dissemination
10. For addressing a specific question about efficacy, safety, and/or pharmacokinetics
11. For generating a new hypothesis for additional studies

[a] A set of clinical data may be useful for two or more of these objectives.
[b] IND, Notice of Claimed Investigational Exception for a New Drug; NDA, New Drug Application.

different) study apply different criteria. Review the definition(s) of CGI and other relevant parameters at both individual and group prestudy meetings with investigators. Examples of how demographic data may be combined across studies (or in a single study) are given in Tables 5.3 to 5.5. Suggestions for preparing NDA sections of efficacy data are listed in Table 5.6.

TABLE 5.3. *Demographic characteristics of individual patients in a study or studies*

Patient number	Treatment	Age (years)	Sex (M,F)[b]	Race (W,B,O,*)[c]	Height (cm)	Weight (kg)
Group 1[a]						
101						
102						
103						
104						
etc.						
Group 2						
201						
202						
203						
204						
etc.						

[a] Each group could represent patients from different centers in the same study or from patients enrolled in different clinical studies.
[b] M, male; F, female.
[c] W, white; B, black; O, oriental; and *, other. If other, specify.

TABLE 5.4. *Demographic characteristics—combined patients across multiple centers*

Parameter	Center 1[a]				Center 2				Combined centers			
	Drug A ($n =$)	Drug B ($n =$)	Placebo ($n =$)	Total ($n =$)	Drug A ($n =$)	Drug B ($n =$)	Placebo ($n =$)	Total ($n =$)	Drug A ($n =$)	Drug B ($n =$)	Placebo ($n =$)	Total ($n =$)
Age[b]												
Mean												
S.D.[c]												
Range												
Sex												
Male												
Female												
Race												
White												
Black												
Oriental												
Others[d]												
Height (cm)[e]												
Mean												
S.D.												
Range												
Weight (kg)[e]												
Mean												
S.D.												
Range												

[a] Instead of individual centers, data could be combined by groups of centers, age group of patient (e.g., 2–11 years, 12–18 years, and above 18 years), type of study, or other categories.

[b] Age could be divided into decades or broad groups (e.g., below 18, 18–65, above 65). Age is given based on the date treatment was initiated.

[c] S.D., standard deviation.

[d] Specify the identity of "others" in a footnote.

[e] Height and weight percentiles could be used instead of raw data. Alternatively, the median percentiles could be given in this table.

TABLE 5.5. *Demographic characteristics—combined patients by center*

Study category[a]	Study number	Total no. of patients	Sex		Race				Age		
			Male	Female	White	Black	Oriental	Other[b]	Below 18	18–65	Above 65
Pharmacokinetic											
1.											
2.											
Dose-ranging											
1.											
2.											
Double-blind											
1.											
2.											
Open-label											
1.											
2.											
Long-term treatment											
1.											
2.											

[a] Multiple studies are generally listed within each category.
[b] Specify "other".

TABLE 5.6. *Suggestions for preparing NDA sections of efficacy data*[a]

A. Relating to statistical analysis and presentation
   1. Present group means for baseline and overall treatment periods for drug and placebo groups (e.g., number of patients at each week of study, means at baseline and treatment, difference and categorization of the patient's response as excellent, good, fair, or poor)
   2. Present daily (weekly, monthly) breakdown of the treatment period and possibly stratify patients on basis of their disease severity
   3. Present a list of concomitant drugs taken by all study patients
   4. Present a list of prior drug therapy used by patients in the same format as that used directly above
   5. Analyze efficacy parameters by important variables (e.g., age, sex, race) that may be considered to influence the results
   6. Analyze and present data separately for each investigator who participated in a multicenter study and had a sufficiently large population of patients

B. Relating to document preparation
   1. Present clinical studies in as similar a format as possible
   2. Each final medical report should be preceded by a one-page and a five-or-more-page summary. The one-page summary should include (1) title, (2) investigator(s) name(s) and address(es), (3) a phrase describing the study design, (4) number and type of patients, (5) test drug schedule, (6) safety results, (7) efficacy results, and (8) conclusions. The longer summary would expand on each of these points
   3. Use an objective style that does not promote the drug but judges it fairly and presents it in a reasonable manner
   4. Present data side by side whenever possible for placebo, study drug, and active control groups
   5. Have separate individuals track progress on each part of the NDA, write final medical reports, review final medical reports, and prepare the expanded summary. The purpose is to prevent delays in NDA preparation

C. Relating to formatting and administration
   1. Group clinical studies of the same type together (e.g., clinical pharmacology, controlled studies for indication(s) pursued, uncontrolled, other)
   2. Provide a list of (1) study titles, (2) number of investigators, (3) total number of patients, (4) number of patients on each treatment, (5) duration of treatment, (6) NDA volume, and (7) page number
   3. Include information that is believed to be useful to a reviewer, even though it may already be present in another section of the NDA
   4. Delay submission until a relatively complete package of data may be submitted. Additional data in NDA amendments often markedly delay reviews
   5. References to other documents should contain specific date, volume, and page numbers (e.g., to a drug master file). Attach actual copies of documents referenced if they are particularly important. Do not reference documents that the FDA has previously rejected
   6. Insure that all pages are correctly numbered and that all references to other sections of the NDA and all indexes are correct

D. General comments plus communications with the regulatory agency
   1. A small number of large studies is easier to present and review than a large number of small studies
   2. Indicate whether there were previous discussions with the FDA relating to the study design, conduct, or analysis. If so, provide a synopsis of the situation and agreement (if any). This will help the reviewer understand the background and context of the study
   3. Indicate which studies support the desired claims of efficacy (and/or safety)

[a] Several points could be considered in more than one section.

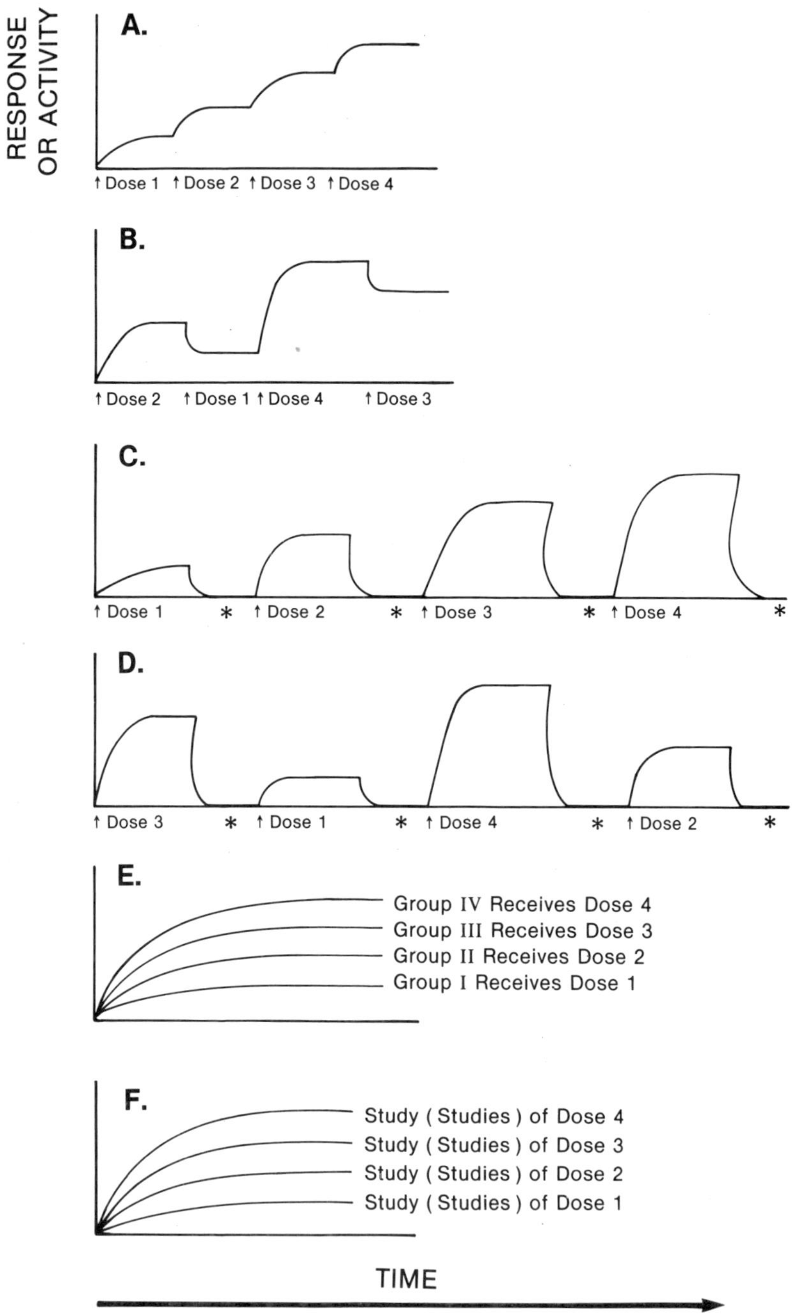

FIG. 5.1. Types of studies that may generate data for creating dose–response relationships. The same dose–response curve may be created from any of these six graphs (graphs not drawn precisely to scale). Asterisks denote periods of washout. **A:** Cumulative doses

TABLE 5.7. *Types and characteristics of dose–response relationships*

Type of dose–response relationship[a]	Number of groups of patients	Number of doses per patient	Washout between doses[b] (*)	Order of presenting doses
A	1	≥2	No	Cumulative
B	1	≥2	No	Random
C	1	≥2	Yes	In order of ascending dose
D	1	≥2	Yes	Random
E	Multiple (one study)	1	No	Single dose or fixed range per group
F	Multiple studies	1	No	Single dose or fixed range per group

[a] The letters refer to dose–response relationships illustrated in Fig. 5.1.
[b] The "*" in Fig. 5.1 indicates that time was allowed for a washout period between doses.

If the preparation of an NDA appears to be too formidable a task for a small (or even large) group to handle, each of the separate components and subcomponents should be identified and assignments should be made to complete each. Dividing a single mammoth task into a series of smaller tasks usually allows an individual(s) to cope better with the challenge. When more individuals are assigned to a task, it is usually easier to complete when they work together as a team. The team concept helps many people maintain their interest and enthusiasm while working on difficult or tedious tasks. It is extremely important for the individual who organizes the effort to either have had previous experience in assembling an NDA or to have contact with experienced individuals.

Dose–Response Relationships

One goal of integrating data from multiple studies may be to construct a dose–response relationship of the study drug. Various types of studies and data that may each be used to generate the same dose–response relationship are illustrated in Fig. 5.1. Characteristics of these figures are described in Table 5.7.

administered to a group of patients in a stepwise manner without washout (in one or multiple studies). **B:** Doses administered in a random order to patients, without washout (in one or multiple studies). **C:** Progressively increasing doses administered in a stepwise manner with washout periods between each dose (in one or multiple studies). **D:** Doses administered in a random order to patients with washout periods between each dose (in one or multiple studies). **E:** Each patient in a group receives a single dose and several groups in one study each receive different doses. **F:** Each patient in a group (or study) receives a single dose and several groups in different studies each receive different doses.

It is possible to conduct dose–response evaluations in a single patient, single study, or multiple studies. The choice of approach to follow depends on the characteristics of the study drug, the disease, or problem being treated and on the availability of patients. It is undesirable statistically (and often clinically) to construct a dose–response relationship where each dose was tested in a different study or studies. Doses studied must be carefully chosen to be within an appropriate range. If they are too low they may be below or at the threshold of the dose–response curve; likewise, if the doses are too high they may be at (or beyond) the peak or plateau phase of the dose–response curve. In addition, they must cover an appropriate range so that a dose–response relationship may be observed.

In dose-escalation studies that are conducted to develop a dose–response relationship, only those patients who do not respond to a given dose are given a higher dose. This is a highly ethical design because all data may be used and each patient contributes to the dose–response evaluation, even if they drop out of the study. This approach is also similar to the way patients are often treated in a clinical practice. In addition, inter- and intra-individual variability are distinguishable and one can obtain a population dose–response curve. On the other hand there are some potential problems with this dose-escalation method for obtaining a dose–response evaluation, primarily because simple pooling of data may produce biased results. A statistician should be consulted for techniques to minimize or eliminate such biases.

If a patient is responding positively to treatment the protocol should specify whether he should be given still higher doses. Forced escalation is not usually done because physicians rarely would increase the dose further in clinical practice unless the patient's response was inadequate; and, one of the major goals of Phase III studies is to approximate usual clinical practice. In addition, it could be considered below ethical standards to raise the dose of a patient already benefiting from therapy to a point at which new adverse reactions or more intense ones could occur.

Two additional cautions about using the dose-escalation techniques are that (1) the natural history of the disease may change over time and (2) effects may be attributed to drug when, in fact, these effects are not drug related. Also, it is possible to increase the dose when no effect is observed, but the patient may not yet be at a steady state pharmacokinetically and/or clinically at that particular dose. Therefore, it is advisable to have a minimum period required before a patient's dose may be raised to the next higher dose or dose range.

If no dose–response relationship is observed with a drug it may be a true effect or it may mean that (1) inappropriate efficacy parameters were used, (2) the efficacy parameters were inappropriately measured, (3) the data demonstrate great variability, (4) the doses chosen to study were all at the plateau part of the dose–response relationship, or (5) the doses were too close together to illustrate the shape of the curve.

In addition to dose–response relationships to illustrate and evaluate a drug's efficacy, dose–response relationships may be used to illustrate safety parameters. A dose–response curve may be constructed for each adverse reaction, using each of the following as a parameter on the ordinate: percent of patients affected, median effect observed, maximum effect observed, or another measure of the intensity of the response. A different approach is to present all significant or frequently observed adverse reactions on a single dose–response curve by indicating the dose at which each of the effects is known to occur. This approach would be useful to illustrate that different adverse reactions usually occur at different doses.

The issue of the shape of the dose–response relationship at low doses of carcinogens or teratogens is actively debated in the fields of toxicology and oncology. The implications are quite significant as to the true shape at very low doses of drugs. If the true shape of the dose–response curve was linear and without a threshold dose (i.e., the curve passed through the origin), it would mean that there is always some risk of that drug causing cancer, even at relatively low doses. A supralinear dose–response curve (i.e., curved above a straight line, but meeting the line at its two endpoints), starting at the origin, would have the same interpretation. A linear dose–response curve with a threshold dose would mean that there is a dose below which there is no risk of the drug causing cancer. A sublinear dose–response curve (i.e., curved below a straight line, but meeting the line at its two endpoints) with a threshold dose would have the same interpretation.

Placebo Effect

Another goal of combining data from multiple studies is to evaluate the nature of the placebo effect. The magnitude and time course of this effect is important to evaluate but may not be apparent in a single study. Various types of time courses of a placebo response are illustrated in Fig. 5.2. If this information is known or estimated prior to a study, it can help determine the optimal duration of a study that is necessary to separate drug and placebo effects. There are obviously several other factors that influence the duration chosen for a study. More extensive discussions of the placebo effect are included in the other two books of this series.

Patients Who Fail Therapy

A potential means of improving efficacy may result from careful analysis of why patients fail therapy. It is therefore important not only to determine

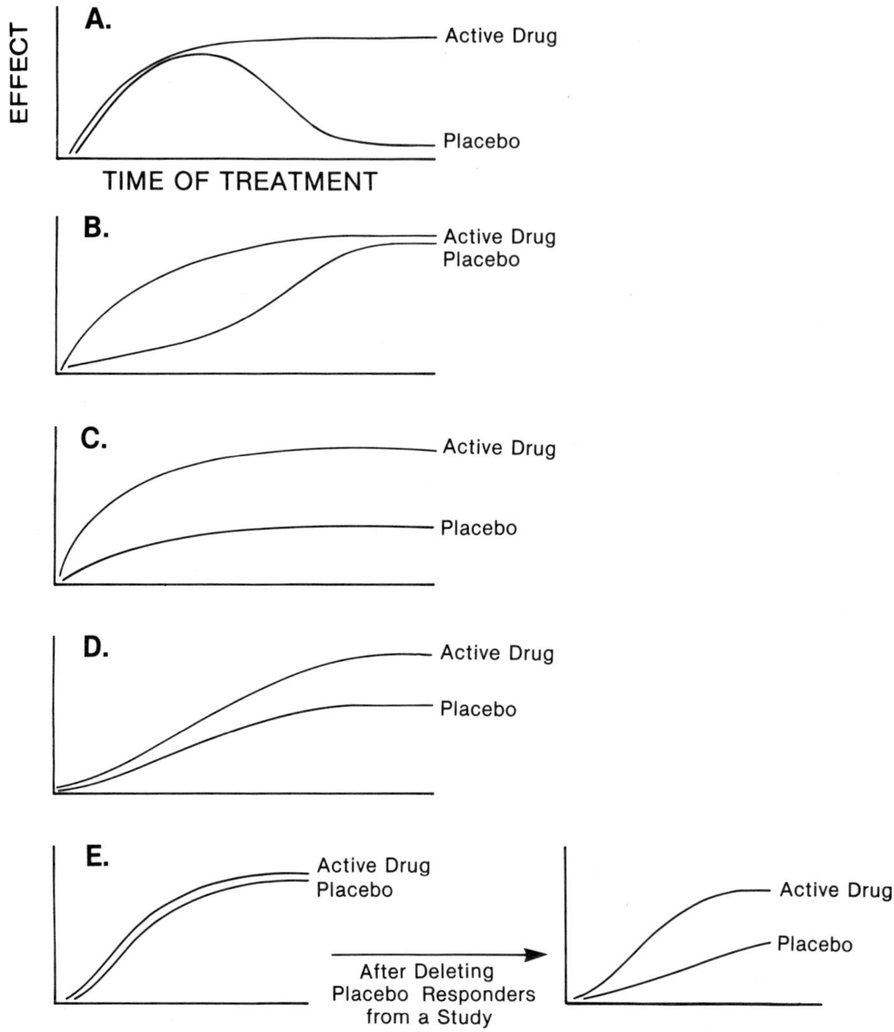

FIG. 5.2. Time course of placebo response. Five patterns illustrate selected means to separate placebo and drug effects. This information, if known historically, may help determine the appropriate design and duration of a clinical study. When the situation on the left of part E is expected, all patients may be placed (single-blind) on placebo and evaluated at a predetermined time. All responders are then discontinued. Remaining patients are then placed double-blind on either study drug or placebo to give the curves on the right.

the number and percent of patients who fail therapy but also to determine why they fail and the amount of time it takes for them to fail after drug is initiated. Reasons given may relate to the rigors of the protocol and not to the drug. Reasons may also relate to factors that may be modified (e.g., taste of the drug, frequency of dosing, adverse reactions from rapid peak concentrations), which will allow the study to be completed successfully. In an extreme case, a suitable means of evaluating a drug may be elucidated. It is important to explore this issue for clues to help both current and future studies to be conducted successfully and to better interpret data from completed patients and studies.

6

Integrating Safety Data from Multiple Studies

Introduction • Laboratory Data • Adverse Reactions

INTRODUCTION

It is important to determine how much safety data are adequate and necessary to collect in clinical studies in terms of both scope (i.e., the number of different parameters and tests to evaluate) and depth (i.e., the amount of data required for each parameter). The answer to this question depends on the (1) characteristics of the drug, (2) previous clinical experience and data available on the drug, (3) disease being treated, (4) regulatory considerations, (5) safety of alternative therapy, and (6) the time in history that is being discussed.

Requirements in the quantity and quality of data necessary to demonstrate safety of a new drug have steadily increased over recent decades, and the requirements of many national regulatory agencies differ. One may address the question of how much data to collect by establishing the scope and magnitude of the safety data that a prudent physician in the relevant country would desire to know prior to prescribing a new drug for a patient. It is also possible to address this question by attempting to second guess the relevant regulatory authorities on the amount of data required for approval.

LABORATORY DATA

Detailed laboratory data from normal volunteers and patients should be relatively extensive. These examinations include evaluation of clinical chemistry and hematology analytes in blood (even for topically applied drugs) and routine urine analytes. Specialized tests suggested by the specific actions of a drug or by its chemical relationship to other known drugs should also be evaluated. Except in unusual circumstances, a minimum of approximately 100 patients should be evaluated with broad screening tests, in addition to the normal volunteers who are evaluated in Phase I studies. There are exceptions to this generalization. For example, some orphan drugs for a rare disease will never be able to enroll 100 patients, and if over-the-counter status is sought for a marketed drug then many more than 100 patients will be required to establish a reasonable level of safety.

In addition to a broad battery of tests, a more limited laboratory examination should be conducted on a much larger group of patients, including those who are part of various special populations (e.g., decreased renal function). This more limited series of tests should include common chemistry, hematology, urine, and other tests suggested by the nature of the drug and prior data obtained.

If the above data suggest that abnormalities may occur as a result of the drug, then those parameters should continue to be closely monitored, until the reason for the abnormality is determined (e.g., a concomitant drug) and evaluated. If the reason is not found, a sufficient characterization of the abnormality and its clinical importance should be achieved. Issues regarding risk-to-benefit considerations are discussed in Chapter 27 of *Guide to Clinical Interpretation of Data* (Spilker, 1986).

It is important during Phase I studies of most new drugs to evaluate normal individuals who do not abuse drugs or alcohol. These groups of abusers generally have a higher rate of abnormal laboratory results and are usually less reliable in complying with a protocol. Nonetheless, it is common for normal individuals to have one or more laboratory parameters fall outside the normal range and for this event to be clinically unimportant. The abnormality is often not reproducible. If abnormalities that were not noted at baseline occur during the study there may be a strong suspicion that they are related to the study drug. In many cases these changes may be anticipated because of the study, patient, or drug characteristics. It may require additional evaluations to establish whether the abnormalities were actually related to the study drug or to another factor(s) (e.g., concomitant drugs, protocol violation).

Categorizing Abnormal Data

In comparing laboratory data from several studies it is possible and usually meaningful to categorize the data by degree of abnormality, in addition to the generally all-or-none question of whether the data are defined as abnormal. One means of categorizing abnormalities is by the percentage deviation both above the top of the normal range and below the bottom of the normal range. Various categories that classify degrees of abnormality may be created. One such example is to choose ranges of 20 to 40% above normal values, 41 to 60% above normal values, and so on. Alternatively the actual laboratory units of measure may be used (e.g., 201–400 mg/deciliter, 401–600 mg/deciliter, and 601 mg/deciliter and above). Similar categories would be created for percents or values below normal values for most laboratory analytes. There are a few biochemical parameters where abnormalities are not considered to exist when a value is below the range of normal (e.g., serum cholesterol).

Apart from establishing broad categories as described above, there are several other ways to classify laboratory results. These include categorizing:

1. Values that extend beyond an expanded normal range, so as to include only those values that are clinically important abnormalities.
2. Differences of before and after drug values that are greater than a fixed percentage of the normal range.
3. Differences of before and after drug values that are greater than a fixed percentage of the baseline value.
4. Values greater or less than a fixed number (e.g., platelets >500,000, platelets <100,000).
5. Patients with a specified group of laboratory abnormalities indicative of a specific organ dysfunction (e.g., renal analytes, hepatic enzymes).
6. Patients whose laboratory abnormalities are characterized by the investigator as probably or definitely drug related.
7. Abnormalities that have been confirmed by repeating duplicate samples or have been reported as abnormal on at least two separate occasions. Any of the above categories may be used with this additional criterion.
8. Duration of abnormality after drug treatment is discontinued. The time for the return of an abnormal value to the normal range (or to baseline) may be used as a parameter.
9. Association of the degree of abnormality with (1) dose of drug given, (2) duration of treatment, (3) total quantity of drug given, or (4) another parameter.

Another approach to the categorization of abnormal data is to concentrate on the patients whose abnormalities are defined as clinically important by the investigator. An important positive aspect of this approach is that this evaluation brings clinical judgment into the assessment and presents a measure of the clinical importance of the abnormality. This allows a better perspective of the laboratory value(s) rather than merely stating the fact that a value is abnormal. This later statement often has no clinical importance. There may be several problems, however, with using this approach. First, using clinical judgment introduces a subjective evaluation that often differs among different physicians. Second, the physician may not have sufficient information on which to arrive at a well-based conclusion as to whether the abnormality has clinical importance. Third, another physician evaluating the patient and abnormality at a subsequent visit may arrive at a different conclusion.

Presenting Data on Laboratory Abnormalities

If both objective and descriptive judgmental approaches are used to present abnormalities it will increase the likelihood that an accurate clinical impression will be created. It is important to categorize laboratory abnormalities by magnitude (i.e., degree of abnormality) and according to other parameters (e.g., duration of abnormality), as well as incorporating an investigator's clinical judgment as to the clinical importance of an abnormality. The degree of association between the drug and the abnormal event is often best assessed by the sponsor, because much more information on the drug is available to them than to a single investigator.

Some of the basic approaches to presenting laboratory data are to illustrate statistically significant (1) within-group changes, (2) changes within prespecified categories, (3) detailed within- and between-group changes, and (4) specific data on individual analytes. Various tables may take the reader or reviewer progressively from tables, figures, and descriptions of (a) general cross-study presentations of data to (b) overall study data, to (c) specific within(and combined)-study analyses, and finally to (d) specific patient data.

Other crucial issues to consider in presenting data relate to (1) whether or not the abnormality is reversible, (2) the time required from discontinuation of the drug until the effect is reversed, and (3) whether rechallenge with the drug leads to reoccurrence of the abnormality. These considerations have a resemblance to Koch's postulates for confirming that a specific disease results from a specific type of bacteria. A description of several commonly used methods to present laboratory data in publications or regulatory submissions are shown in Table 6.1. Specific examples of a few are illustrated in Tables 6.2 to 6.4. Additional tables and figures are illustrated in the appendix of *Guide to Clinical Studies and Developing Protocols* (Spilker, 1984).

Transformations of Laboratory Data

There are various proponents of different methods of data transformation as a technique to more easily combine laboratory data across patients and across studies. Transformations of data are intended to eliminate any influence of different normal ranges or different analytical techniques at different laboratories. Sogliero-Gilbert et al. (1986) and Abt and Krupp (1986) each present their own version of data transformations of laboratory data. Sogliero-Gilbert et al. (1986) propose two concepts for "simplification of lab data monitoring and interpretation." First, they propose normalizing data by dividing each value by the upper limit of the normal range for the particular laboratory in which the data were obtained. This means that all analytes have an upper limit of 1.0 for normals, a lower limit of 0, and all transformed values are positive. Their second concept is a multivariate scoring system that determines a number from normalized values for a functionally related group of analytes (e.g., liver function group). This number is called a "Genie Score" and the authors of this article state "Just as the Genie in Aladdin's lamp made Aladdin's work easier, so the Genie Score

TABLE 6.1. *Methods of presenting abnormal laboratory data in publications or regulatory submissions*[a]

1. Plot or tabulate the overall number of abnormalities for each parameter in each study and cumulatively for all studies
2. Conduct subgroup analyses to determine the influence and associations of age, sex, race, and other relevant patient factors
3. Tabulate (or plot with histograms) the number and severity of abnormalities observed with different drugs or treatments. Compare number and percent of patients on each treatment with different degrees of significant increases above normal (and those with decreases below normal)
4. Define categories of mild, moderately, and severely intense abnormalities and plot or tabulate number of abnormalities in each category
5. Tabulate data based on whether the baseline was normal or abnormally high (or low) with laboratory values obtained during treatment (normal, abnormally high, or abnormally low)
6. If multiple values were obtained, tabulate the number of patients with all values normal, those with no two successive values abnormal, or those with two or more successive abnormalities. Further describe data in the latter group
7. Transform data to standardized scales[b]
8. Describe noteworthy abnormalities in the text, presenting sufficient details

[a] Approaches to developing and presenting summary statistics of overall and abnormal results are provided in the appendix of *Guide to Clinical Studies and Developing Protocols* (Spilker, 1984). The term abnormality must be carefully defined. It is sometimes used to denote all values outside the normal range or only those values that are outside the normal range by a prespecified amount.

[b] If this technique is used it should be followed for all studies on a drug.

TABLE 6.2. *Significant within-group changes for laboratory values in clinical studies*

			Week 2[b]			Week 4			Week 6		
Category	Laboratory test[a]	Study no.	I or D[c]	Change[d]	P	I or D	Change	P	I or D	Change	P
I: Drug (Dose A)[e]											
II: Drug (Dose B)											
III: Drug (Dose C)											
IV: Placebo											

[a] Depending on the number of abnormalities reported, a separate table could be prepared for each laboratory test where significant abnormalities were observed. The normal ranges for each test should be listed.

[b] Each time period of the study may be listed separately.

[c] I, increase; D, decrease.

[d] The units of the parameter may be listed as well as some measure of variability.

[e] A dose range may be specified.

TABLE 6.3. *Summary of patient's laboratory values/changes on drug*[a]

Treatment group	Pretreatment status	Number of patients during treatment at week *X* (or weeks *X* to *Y*) who were: Below normal	Normal	Above normal	Total
Drug (low-dose range)	Below normal				
	Normal				
	Above normal				
	Total				
Drug (high-dose range)	Below normal				
	Normal				
	Above normal				
	Total				
Placebo	Below normal				
	Normal				
	Above normal				
	Total				

[a] Each analyte (e.g., glucose, creatinine, bilirubin) would be listed on a separate sheet. This series of charts could be prepared for each study or for combinations of studies.

introduced here will simplify the management and assessment of the lab parameters''. Abt and Krupp (1986) propose that laboratory data obtained in multicenter studies be combined by transforming data from each center into percent-scaled values from 0% to 100% for the upper range of normal at each site. The author strongly disagrees with the concept of transforming laboratory data for reasons given below.

These methods and other transformation techniques often allow data to be combined more easily, but the process of interpreting the data becomes more complex and difficult. Depending on the specific transformation used the data themselves usually have little or no meaning to clinicians who are experienced in interpreting data presented in actual units. Clinicians develop a ''feel'' for the data based on the specific analyte measured, its degree of variability within (and between) most normals and patients, and their knowledge and experience with accepted interpretations. For example, potassium is tightly regulated by the body, laboratory measurements are highly accurate if the blood is not hemolyzed, and small increases or decreases in mEq/L (milliequivalents per liter) often have a marked clinical importance. Glucose values, on the other hand, vary widely during the course of a day and depending on when a sample was taken and under which circumstances, there would be less clinical importance if values changed to the same degree as for potassium.

It is not reasonable at the present time to expect clinicians to develop a ''feel'' for how to interpret data transformed in each of various ways pro-

TABLE 6.4. *Summary statistics of laboratory analytes*[a]

Study no.	Investigator	Treatment group	No. of patients[b]	Pretreatment			Week X[c]			Change from pretreatment[d]		
				Mean	Median	±S.D.	Mean	Median	± S.D.	Mean	Median	± S.D.
	A	Drug[e]		Q	S							
		Placebo		R	T							
				Difference	Difference							
	B	Drug										
		Placebo										
	C	Drug										
		Placebo										
	etc.											
	Total	Drug										
		Placebo										

[a] Each analyte (e.g., glucose, creatinine, bilirubin) would be listed on a separate sheet and expressed in units measured.
[b] If the number of patients is not the same at each time point then the number of patients at each time point should be listed.
[c] This could be an end of treatment value, average of a few weeks, or defined differently.
[d] Statistically significant differences could be shown for (1) change from pretreatment within a group, (2) differences between treatment groups at a given time period, or (3) differences between investigators.
[e] Different doses or dose ranges could be presented separately for analytes that were affected by drug.

posed. The interpretation of a change of 10% or a doubling of the value in one system would obviously differ from the same change in another system. Clinicians at regulatory agencies would have an extremely difficult job if many companies submitted laboratory data transformed with different techniques. If one transformation does become popular and accepted over time, then that particular method would certainly be a useful approach for standardizing the combination of laboratory data in a study as well as across studies.

ADVERSE REACTIONS

Safety data include much more than just laboratory data. Probably the most well known area of safety relates to physical and psychological adverse reactions to drugs. These effects are often particularly difficult to combine and integrate from multiple studies or even in some cases from within a single study. A few representative approaches to this issue will be described.

Obtaining Adverse Reactions

In the most simple case, several clinical studies may have been conducted on relatively few patients, as in certain orphan drug applications. In this situation a tabular presentation of adverse reactions may be prepared with a relatively complete description of each moderate or severe adverse reaction that occurred.

It is extremely important that adverse reactions, especially serious ones, be diagnosed accurately throughout the world. This is not only so that patients may be promptly and appropriately treated but also to insure that, when data on the cases are combined and incidence figures are created, all cases of a certain adverse reaction really did have the same problem. Another reason why adverse reactions must be diagnosed accurately is that the benefit-to-risk ratio of a drug may change when a serious adverse reaction is reported. This could affect the drug's use or may even cause it to be withdrawn from the market. Criteria to use in identifying some adverse reactions such as seizures are generally well understood. But, under circumstances where no direct observations of a patient have been made, it may be difficult or impossible to know if a seizure has actually occurred. In addition, certain adverse reactions (e.g., various type of rashes) are labeled differently by different physicians, depending on their knowledge of the medical area, the state of knowledge in the particular field of medicine, and other factors. It is thus important to carefully define the criteria for any serious adverse reactions that may be anticipated to occur and to have a specialist consulted on all serious or potentially serious adverse reactions that lie outside the investigator's area of expertise.

In combining data on adverse reactions from different clinical studies it is usually important that the means of obtaining the adverse reactions was similar. If unsolicited comments were collected in one study, a general probe used in a second study, and a specific list of symptoms read to patients in a third study, then simply adding the results to determine incidence figures would probably be highly misleading. In Phase IV postmarketing studies data are often obtained in many different ways and by many different physicians, but in studies conducted during Phases I to III, attempts should be made to standardize methods of collecting data on adverse reactions.

Categorizing Adverse Reactions

In most new drug applications (NDA) submitted to regulatory authorities, 500 to 3,000 patients are evaluated. Within each NDA, different types of clinical studies have usually been conducted and highly diverse adverse reaction data accumulated. These adverse reactions may be categorized in numerous ways, including (1) type (e.g., behavioral, cardiovascular, topical, neurological), (2) severity (e.g., mild, moderate, severe), (3) counteractive treatment provided (e.g., discontinued drug, increased surveillance, prescribed an antidote), (4) duration of effect (e.g., weeks, months, number of occurrences), and (5) degree of association with the drug (e.g., possible, probable, definite, unknown). Adverse reactions present at baseline which did not worsen during the study should be separated from those which emerged or worsened during the study. Steps to follow when patients report adverse reactions are given in Table 6.5.

Presenting Data on Adverse Reactions

Tables A.21 to A.31 in *Guide to Clinical Studies and Developing Protocols* (Spilker, 1984) present an approach that illustrates one means of presenting such data. Those tables were intended to represent compilations of all adverse reactions from a 10-site multicenter study but may also be viewed as representing a compilation of data from 10 separate clinical studies.

There are several types of clinical studies where adverse reaction data are not appropriate to combine together. An obvious example is when some studies were conducted in children and others were conducted in adults. Also, if one (or more) study was conducted in severely ill patients and the other studies were all conducted in mildly ill patients (for whom the drug was intended) then it might be preferable to present the data separately from the severely ill patients. Many adverse reactions observed in severely ill patients may not be directly attributable to the drug, and those that were attributable to the drug might have occurred because of the nature of the patient population studied.

TABLE 6.5. *Steps to follow when patients report adverse reactions*[a]

1. Quantify the rate (incidence), intensity (severity), duration, and total number of episodes
2. Obtain information on related events and determine possible causes[b]
3. Consider countermeasures[c] to deal with adverse reactions
4. Establish a reminder system to contact the patient for a follow-up visit. Suggest that the patient contact the clinic or investigator if the problem persists, recurs, or worsens
5. Consider additional follow-up by telephone, letter, or by scheduling another visit
6. If the adverse reaction is severe or serious, complete an FDA 1639 form[d] or UK "yellow card"[e]
7. Contact the sponsor for severe and/or unexpected adverse reactions if the study is sponsored
8. Contact the Institutional Review Board (IRB) if the adverse reaction is severe[c]

[a] The flow of information for patients reporting serious adverse reactions is shown in Fig. 21.3.
[b] As part of determining the cause of the adverse reaction, it may be relevant to ask the patient for his/her opinion.
[c] See list in Chapter 22 of *Guide to Clinical Studies and Developing Protocols* (Spilker, 1984).
[d] See Fig. 21.4. This form is completed by either individual physicians or drug companies.
[e] See Fig. 21.5. This form is completed by either individual physicians or drug companies.

The approach described in the appendix of *Guide to Clinical Studies and Developing Protocols* for presenting data is extremely laborious to compile and evaluate. It is also not usually followed in the highly detailed manner described for most multicenter studies initiated in academic centers. Rarely does one encounter this level of detail in clinical publications. A detailed style is adhered to, however, for the majority of regulatory submissions on new drugs in the United States.

Creation of a single large data base in a computer is usually essential in order to easily combine data on adverse reactions from multiple studies. A single data base allows future reanalyses of the data should that become necessary, and also allows new adverse reaction data to be easily integrated with existing data.

Another style for presenting adverse reactions is referred to as the "Summary Style". In this scenario, it is assumed that a great deal of data has been collected on adverse reactions. These data could be presented in the exhaustive manner described above, but for various reasons a general overview is desired.

In the "Summary Style" of presenting adverse reactions, tabulations are made of the incidence of all observed adverse reactions. This can be either on paper or with the aid of a computer program (e.g., Lotus 1,2,3). The left-hand vertical column could list all of the observed adverse reactions and the horizontal headings could list each of the studies. The number of patients entered in each study could be entered in parentheses under the study titles. After data are entered in this table, a column could provide both total numerator and denominator figures for each adverse reaction. These totals could also be converted to a percent incidence. Separate tabulations could also be made of all serious adverse reactions attributed to the drug. These two tables would provide a broad view of adverse reaction types, incidence, and severity that could be interpreted in the text of a report. Separate summary tables of adverse reaction durations and also patient outcomes (e.g., died, nonreversed, reversed) could be prepared.

Calculating the Incidence of Adverse Reactions

The incidence of a specific adverse reaction usually relates to the rate of its occurrence. In its most simple form, it is the number of patients with the adverse reaction divided by the number of patients treated with the drug. This ratio may be converted to a percent by multiplying by 100, but most commonly both the numerator and denominator are presented.

There are many other ways of presenting incidence figures of adverse reactions. The most appropriate way depends on the particular therapeutic area and situation (e.g., duration of treatment, severity of the adverse reaction, whether patients have one or multiple episodes). The value of these ratios will often differ for a drug evaluated in Phase II or III versus a drug evaluated in Phase IV. Moreover, the quality of data used to establish the ratio also markedly differs between these two categories of studies (see Chapter 13 for additional discussion of this point).

Some of the possible means of presenting incidence figures are listed below:

1. $$\frac{\text{Number of patients with the specific adverse reaction who received drug for at least } X \text{ days (or weeks)}}{\text{Total number of patients who received drug for at least } X \text{ days (or weeks)}}$$

2. $$\frac{\text{Number of episodes (events) of the specific adverse reaction reported in a study}}{\text{Total number of possible episodes (events) of the specific adverse reaction which could have been reported}}$$

3. $$\frac{\text{Number of patients with severe adverse reactions of a specific type}}{\text{Total number of patients treated with the drug for at least } X \text{ weeks}}$$

TABLE 6.6. *Combining safety data across studies to develop a profile of an adverse reaction using the example of EKG abnormalities*

Study	Proportion of patients with EKG abnormalities	Severity of abnormality	Duration of abnormality	Number of reports in study[a]	Countermeasure	Comments
A	0/17	—	—	0	—	
B	1/34	Mild	1 hr	2	None	On placebo
C	1/40	Moderate	1 week	5	Surveillance	Did not occur on rechallenge
D	1/14	Mild	Persistent	14	None	Occurred at baseline too
E	4/56	Severe	Unknown	14	β-blocker	See Report X
		Mild	Persistent	7	None	None
		Moderate	Unknown	2	Surveillance	None
		Moderate	1 week	5	Surveillance	None
F	2/17	Mild	Unknown	7	None	PVCs possibly associated with drug
		Moderate	Persistent	14	Surveillance	On placebo
Totals:	9/178	Mild = 4 Moderate = 4 Severe = 1	Unknown = 3 Persistent = 3 1 hr = 1 1 week = 2	Range = 2–14 Total of 70 reports in 9 patients	None = 4 Surveillance = 4 β-blocker = 1	One report issued

[a] A maximum of 14 reports for each abnormality were possible per patient in these studies (i.e., each patient's EKG was evaluated on 14 separate occasions).

4. $$\frac{\text{Number of patients with severe adverse reactions of any type}}{\text{Number of patients with mild, moderate, or severe adverse reactions}}$$

5. $$\frac{\text{Number of patients with a specific adverse reaction that is severe}}{\text{Total number of patients in the study treated with the drug}}$$

6. $$\frac{\text{Number of patients treated in the clinical practice who had the adverse reaction to the drug}}{\text{Total number of patients treated in the practice with the drug}}$$

7. $$\frac{\text{Number of patients with the specific adverse reaction}}{\text{Total number of patient years of treatment with the drug}}$$

8. $$\frac{\text{Number of episodes of the adverse reaction lasting over } X \text{ hours}}{\text{Total number of episodes possible}}$$

For ratio number 7 the total number of patients treated is also important to present, so that this ratio may be adequately understood. Without this information the reader could not determine whether one patient year represented 365 patients treated for one day each or one patient treated for the entire year. For ratio number 8 (and 2) the total number of possible episodes equals the total number of patients in a study multiplied by the number of clinic visits or times when adverse reaction reports are collected.

Note that some of these ratios are more appropriate to a clinical study and others to clinical practice. In any report of adverse reactions the most appropriate ratios must be determined. It may be relevant to present several different ratios in a report, in order to convey a more accurate impression of the data. The ratio may also be based on the patient's age, sex, race, type of disease, or dose of drug given. Other approaches to either calculating the incidence rates of adverse reactions or to illustrating their characteristics are possible.

Data from other evaluations of safety (e.g., physical examinations, electrocardiograms, microbiology, immunology) may be combined from multiple studies using methods described above. Some specific examples are presented in Tables A.1 to A.20 of *Guide to Clinical Studies and Developing Protocols* (Spilker, 1984) and in Table 6.6 of the present book. Many related issues on adverse reactions are discussed in Chapter 8 of *Guide to Clinical Interpretation of Data* (Spilker, 1986). Additional methods that could be used to integrate safety data from multiple clinical studies are described in Chapter 5 of the present book.

7

Potential Ethical Issues in Single and Multiple Studies

Universal Standards • Individuals Involved with Ethical Issues • Ethical Considerations Related to Study Design • Ethical Considerations in Protocol Development • Ethical Considerations in Conducting a Study

UNIVERSAL STANDARDS

The *Guide to Clinical Studies and Developing Protocols* (Spilker, 1984) indicated some of the international societies and groups that have been actively involved in attempting to define universal standards for ethical conduct by physicians. Some of these groups have evolved a series of codes for ethical behavior. An early code is the famous Hippocratic oath, which interestingly is not presented in many medical school programs and is only read at graduation at others. The Helsinki doctrine, which was approved by the World Medical Association, is an important example of a recent ethical code (see Appendix). These doctrines place responsibility for ethical conduct in drug investigation directly on the physicians involved.

Three basic points will be made relating to ethical considerations in the design and conduct of clinical drug studies. The first point is that ethical questions involve all individuals and groups connected with a clinical study, not just investigators and sponsors. The second point is that ethical questions are an important consideration in most aspects of a clinical study, from the initial steps of developing the study design through to the analysis, interpretation, and publication of results. Third, ethical questions are not issues that are either merely present or absent, but range from the obvious to those where the presence of ethical considerations is strongly debated. Many ethical issues are not black or white and lie in a gray middle range.

The term "ethics" is used in a broad context that includes and overlaps with legal responsibilities in some instances and with routine obligations of a drug study's sponsor in other cases. Some of the major ethical issues in drug studies concern informed consent and ethical review committees or Institutional Review Boards (IRB) at the institution where the clinical study is to be performed. These issues have been widely discussed in the medical literature and will not be dealt with in detail in this chapter. Additional details relating to clinical studies were presented by the Committee for the Protection of Human Participants in Research (1982) and published by the American Psychological Association.

INDIVIDUALS INVOLVED WITH ETHICAL ISSUES

The first point to discuss relates to the conclusion that virtually all people and institutions involved in any aspect of a clinical study must deal with at least some ethical questions. Examples of the types of ethical issues dealt with by eight different groups will be described. The ethical involvement of each group generally varies somewhat from study to study.

1. The Principal and Assistant or Co-Investigators

As physicians, investigators have a professional responsibility to maintain the highest ethical standards possible. These standards are enforced by State Medical Boards, peer review, and by regulations of the hospitals and medical schools at which they practice medicine. Specific ethical responsibilities of investigators toward their patients are to insure (1) that the protocol adheres to appropriate and acceptable procedures, (2) that the protocol is approved by the relevant IRB, (3) that the patient gives a valid informed consent, and (4) that the protocol is followed according to appropriate and proper medical practice. The investigator has the ethical responsibility of notifying the patient of any relevant information that arises during the conduct of the study which might affect the patient's informed consent.

2. The Institution of the Investigator and Its Ethics Committee

There are specific regulations in the United States governing the makeup of IRBs (see 21 CFR 56). The IRB acts as the major ethical overseer of the study and usually requires the investigator to provide periodic reports describing progress of the study, as well as information on any serious or unforeseen events. In some situations the investigator's clinical department must also approve the protocol. If the investigator uses facilities maintained by the institution to conduct the study, then the group that operates that facility (e.g., a Clinical Research Unit) may also require the right to approve the protocol used.

3. The Investigator's Staff

The major ethical issue involving the investigator's staff is the manner in which they carry out the aspects of the protocol that are assigned to them.

This relates to all matters, including contact with study patients where there would be significant consequences if their performance did not meet an acceptable standard. Protocol violations caused by the investigator's staff may range from minor incidents to issues of serious negligence.

4. The Staff of the Institution(s) Who Will Participate in the Clinical Study

The staff at the institution who participate in the study (e.g., physicians who provide medical consults or evaluate electrocardiograms, staff who perform and interpret X-rays) must follow commonly accepted medical standards in meeting their responsibilities. This also applies to all personnel at sites other than those where the study is taking place (e.g., at laboratories where biological samples are sent for analysis).

5. Staff at the Sponsoring Institution

For those studies that are sponsored by a different institution than the one where the study is conducted, it is important that the sponsoring staff adhere to appropriate standards in each of their roles relating to the study. These roles include those related to study design, study initiation, monitoring, study termination, data analysis, data interpretation, publication, and all interactions between the various people and groups involved in the study.

The sponsor chooses the investigator for a study. It is important to choose investigators who will maintain high standards. If this issue is not a concern of the sponsor, then the entire ethical conduct of the study may be severely compromised. Monitors who follow the conduct of the study must be cognizant of the standards that are followed by investigators, staff, and patients.

6. The Regulatory Agency

Protocols that are sent to a regulatory agency must be ethically sound, and it is the agency's responsibility to insure that appropriate standards are maintained. In this manner, the regulatory agency acts as a safeguard to back-up the formal and informal review processes that have already occurred at several points in the protocol's approval process. In a sense, various regulations promulgated by the agency govern the previous steps in protocol approval (e.g., having an IRB approve each protocol, use of good laboratory practices, use of good clinical practices) and thus the agency influences various ethical issues throughout the design and approval process.

Regulatory agencies in different countries adhere to different ethical standards. This may create a variety of difficult and often complex situations for companies that perform studies in several countries and also submit regulatory dossiers in many countries. Many of the issues discussed in the rest of this chapter become more complex when standards and customs of different countries come into conflict.

7. The Patient (Plus the Patient's Parent(s) or Legal Guardian(s) When Relevant)

From an ethical perspective, the informed consent is one of the most significant issues relating to a clinical study. In signing an informed consent, a patient accepts the responsibility of complying with the terms of the study. Patients who are minors but above the approximate age of seven should be asked for their assent to participate in the study, in addition to obtaining the legally required informed consent from their parent(s) or legal guardian(s).

There may be an ethical question as to whether patients who could otherwise afford to pay for and receive more expensive and perhaps medically "preferable" treatment should be enrolled in a study. Their enrollment would be acceptable if they are fully informed about alternative treatments.

8. The Press and Other Media

Important clinical studies are often reported by the press. The press has the responsibility to present data and conclusions honestly and not to distort or alter conclusions and interpretations of the study. This may occur inadvertently when the medical language of the study is changed to make it more easily understood by the public.

ETHICAL CONSIDERATIONS RELATED TO STUDY DESIGN

The second and third major points concerning ethical issues discussed in this chapter are related and will be discussed together. The second major point is that most aspects of a clinical study involve ethical considerations. The third point is that ethical questions that arise in regard to clinical studies are not merely present or absent. Instead, they range from clear ethical issues to issues whose connection with ethics may be strongly debated. A wide range of issues to illustrate these points will be presented in the discussion that follows.

Almost all of the ethical considerations described are directly or indirectly under the control or influence of the investigator conducting the study and/or the sponsor(s) of the study. If the sponsor believes that the ethical conduct of the investigators and/or patients are substandard then the sponsor has both the right and obligation to terminate the study. Issues raised in analyzing and interpreting results of studies, as well as publishing data, will not be covered in detail. Many of the problems and issues in each category will be described, but possible solutions to most of these issues will not be presented.

Eight areas that relate to ethical issues raised in developing a study design will be described.

1. Is There a Need for the Study?

The actual need for conducting a clinical study should always be established prior to starting the study. There are sometimes simple alternatives to conducting a drug study, such as conducting a literature search or discussing a topic with experts in the field. To conduct a study that is not truly necessary is contrary to commonly accepted standards.

2. Is It Ethical to Include a Placebo Treatment Group?

There are many occasions when the ethical acceptability of including a placebo treatment group in a study is raised. The outcome of discussions and the guidelines used to assist a decision vary in some cases from country to country, even for the same study drug, conditions, and rest of the study design. For example, the West Germans generally believe that a drug must have the potential to offer patients benefit before it is acceptable to enroll them in a study, and also do not believe in using a placebo if an alternative treatment is available. This view is not as strictly held in the United States. Many aspects and considerations of this general issue are complex and will not be presented or discussed.

3. Choice of an Active Control

When a pharmaceutical corporation compares the activity of an investigational drug with a marketed drug the choice of the marketed drug may raise important issues. For example, there may be a dilemma for the company if the drug chosen for comparison with the study drug is also made by the same company. If unanticipated adverse reactions appear with the marketed drug it could have a negative impact on the sales of that drug. To avoid a potentially compromising situation some companies as a matter of practice do not compare an investigational drug with one of their marketed or other investigational drugs.

4. Has the Study Eliminated Obvious Types of Bias and Deceit?

Biases may be introduced into a clinical study at any stage. It is the responsibility of both the sponsor and investigator to minimize bias. As major and minor biases manage to enter a study, the less value the study generally has. At a certain point, biases of sufficient magnitude will have compromised a study's value to the extent that it is unacceptable to continue.

In the past patients were sometimes given placebo medication without their knowledge. This deceit is generally unacceptable today and informed consents should indicate the probability that a patient will receive placebo. There are, however, circumstances where certain types of deception may be condoned, but such studies should be approved by IRBs.

A few examples of deception are described below. No judgment is made by the author as to whether these should have been condoned. One treatment group in a study to evaluate stress reduction by oxprenolol received a placebo but were led to believe they received an active drug (Landauer and Pocock, 1984). In another study 80 patients were given a placebo liquid that was described to 40 patients as an "energizer" and to the other 40 as a "tranquilizer" (Dinnerstein and Halm, 1970). A third type of deception occurs where patients are given an active drug, but they or others are told that a placebo has been given. An example occurred in a study with mentally retarded patients who were given active drug, but the institution staff were told that the medication was a placebo (Breuning et al., 1980).

5. Has Sufficient Attention Been Given to Sample Size?

In well-designed clinical studies that involve significant resources and numbers of patients, it is scientifically unacceptable to guess at the number of patients to enroll, even if this is done by experienced individuals. The data used to generate the number of patients required in a study is often based, however, on assumptions that involve less than certain information (i.e., on educated guesses). A well-controlled study with too few patients will have minimal scientific value, and an important treatment difference may fail to be detected. Thus, it is not ethically acceptable to enroll patients in such a study. Another problem that may occur if too few patients complete a clinical study is that a false-positive or false-negative result may occur. Although a false-positive (or false-negative) result may occur in all studies, the chances of its happening are higher in studies with too few patients.

When establishing the basis for determining sample size it is important to consult a statistician and to carefully consider: (1) Which variables are to be measured? (2) What size difference is important to detect? (3) What is the previous experience with the drug?

6. Is the Statistical Power of a Study Adequate To Show an Effect If It Is Present?

Power is defined as the probability of detecting the difference that is looked for, if it is present. It is the goal of any study to have a high power, i.e., a high probability of detecting a difference between treatments if one actually exists. A power of at least 80% (0.8) to detect clinically relevant differences is usually considered an adequate value for most controlled studies. If a study with a low power is designed, there may be little chance of actually finding the difference sought, and it may be below commonly accepted standards to enroll and treat patients in such a study.

7. Are the Patient's Chances of Receiving an Active Drug Acceptable?

Some statisticians advocate that all patients should have at least an equal (i.e., 50%) chance of receiving an active drug rather than a placebo. Patients are usually more willing to enroll in a drug study where their chance of receiving an active drug is great. The relative importance of the patient's feelings in determining the ratio of group size in a study relates to a large degree on the particular disease studied and the severity of its symptomatology. A patient with severe chronic pain will be less willing to enter a study where the chances of receiving placebo medication are 50% than where the chances are about 10%. When the chances of the patient receiving the active drug are relatively low, it may be ethically unacceptable to enroll and treat the patients in a study.

8. What Types of Patients Are To Be Entered into the Study?

Normal Volunteers Versus Patients

In Phase I clinical studies where the initial safety of a drug is to be tested, it is often possible to perform the study with either normal volunteers or patients with the target disease. Phase I studies usually involve little risk to volunteers or patients despite the fact that these people are the first humans ever to receive the new drug. Johnsson et al. (1984) stated that 157 studies were conducted using 1,325 normal volunteers between 1980 and 1982 at Hässle and there were no serious adverse reactions to drugs. Only one case of drug-related sequela was reported in 29,162 normal prison volunteers tested over a 12-year period in 805 protocol studies conducted in the United States (Zarafonetes et al., 1978). Cardon et al. (1976) surveyed 331 investigators who had conducted research on 133,000 human volunteers and patients over the preceding three years. Injuries were reported in 3.7% of the subjects. Of these injuries 80% were reported as trivial, 19% as temporarily disabling, and about 1% as fatal or permanently disabling. The total of 57 cases that were fatal or permanently disabling (out of 133,000 subjects) primarily occurred after cancer chemotherapy. This rate is less than risks of accidents in everyday life.

The death of a volunteer in a Phase I study was so noteworthy that it was written up in the *Lancet* (Darragh et al., 1985) and discussed in an editorial and several subsequent letters to the editors on February 9, 1985 (pages 343 and 344). An important point is that the volunteer had a psychiatric history and had received a depot neuroleptic the day prior to the study. If this were known, he would have been considered unsuitable for the study. This points out the need for careful evaluation of all prospective participants in Phase I studies.

Currently most Phase I studies are performed with normal volunteers. There is, however, a growing belief that it may be appropriate to use patients in Phase I studies to test new drugs for safety. This may be especially true in epileptic patients who metabolize drugs differently than do normal volunteers. Another example where patients may be used for Phase I studies relates to the use of drugs with expected toxicity, such as evaluating the safety of new anticancer drugs that are potentially toxic. In this situation it is usually not acceptable to enroll normal volunteers in a Phase I study.

Inpatients Versus Outpatients

There are various studies where either inpatients or outpatients may be enrolled. In reaching a decision on which group to enroll it is important to know if (1) the drug has been well tested, (2) the pharmacological profile is well understood, and (3) it is safe enough to give to outpatients. Also, is it ethically acceptable to allow patients with the disease being studied to function as outpatients during the study?

Types or Groups of Patients Who Require Special Consideration

Special ethical considerations are raised in studies performed on infants, children, pregnant women, lactating mothers, prisoners, the mentally retarded, psychotic individuals, or other persons who are unable to fully protect their own rights. A major ethical problem encountered with these groups relates to the difficulty of obtaining a freely given informed consent.

ETHICAL CONSIDERATIONS IN PROTOCOL DEVELOPMENT

Fifteen separate categories relating to protocol development are discussed.

1. Inclusion/Exclusion Criteria

A major area of any protocol involves inclusion/exclusion criteria. These criteria influence and control the types of patients enrolled. A number of specific types of inclusion/exclusion criteria are described that may raise ethical considerations on how these criteria are applied to patients who may enter a clinical study.

Sex of the Patient

It is required in studying most investigational (and many older) drugs to exclude all women of childbearing potential until appropriate reproductive and teratology studies have been performed in animals. In pediatric studies it is usually unacceptable to continue a female patient in the study after her first menses.

Age of the Patient

In both pediatric and adult studies there are usually important ethical issues raised about which age to set as the lower limit for patient enrollment. There is also increasing concern about conducting clinical studies in the older population. There are various constraints about the health status of older patients that should be considered. Publications of ethical committees about their deliberations and decisions regarding inclusion of children and older patients in studies would be valuable. Their conclusions would assist individuals developing protocols as well as other ethics committees who must discuss and approve such protocols.

Pregnancy and Lactation

There is a general prohibition against evaluating drugs in pregnant or lactating women in studies that are not specifically designed for this population. A pregnancy waiver is sometimes required from women of childbearing potential prior to enrollment in the study. This waiver usually states that the patient is not currently pregnant and will either refrain from sexual relations or will utilize contraceptive methods approved by the investigator for the duration of the study [e.g., See Fig. 22.12 in *Guide to Clinical Studies and Developing Protocols* (Spilker, 1984)]. If an investigational drug is being evaluated and a female participant in a clinical study becomes pregnant the woman must be immediately discontinued from the study. In addition, it is imperative to closely follow the course of her pregnancy and to evaluate the newborn infant.

Sensitivity to a Study Drug

It is not ethically acceptable in most situations to enroll patients in a clinical study if they have a high risk of experiencing a hypersensitivity reaction to one of the drugs or tests used in the study.

Concomitant Drugs

Although it is usually desired to study most drugs as monotherapy, it is not always ethically acceptable to do so. The basic reasons for studying a drug as an "add-on" medication are that (1) the efficacy and/or safety of a drug have not been adequately tested or (2) other drugs are available that are demonstrated to be efficacious and the patient should not be denied use of one or more of those drugs. As more information becomes known on a new drug, it often becomes more acceptable to evaluate it as monotherapy.

Previous Drug and Nondrug Treatment

There may be ethical reasons to exclude from a study patients who were previously treated with certain drugs or treatments. For example, if a mild analgesic is being evaluated, it would not be acceptable in most situations to include patients if they were previously given strong analgesics and failed to improve.

Washout Period of Nonstudy Drugs

Whenever patients are being taken off one treatment and a different treatment is to be initiated, a period of time must elapse to eliminate or minimize the influence of the original drug or treatment on the subsequent treatment. This interval is referred to as the washout or drug-free period. Previous treatment effects often persist beyond the time of the drug's known biological activity. The nature, intensity, and duration of possible carryover or residual effects of a drug must be considered in determining the length of time that is necessary for an adequate washout period.

Many patients with numerous diseases cannot tolerate the drug-free period required for an adequate washout of a drug. An ethical dilemma may be created when patients need constant drug treatment and investigators cannot take patients off certain drugs for an adequate washout period. If the patient is not drug free for an adequate period there may be a residual drug effect that may alter the data obtained with the new drug tested. One solution is to eliminate consideration of the first several weeks on the new drug because of the possible carryover effect. This assumes of course that the previous treatment was discontinued when the new drug was initiated.

History of Other Diseases

It is not generally ethically acceptable to include patients with certain diseases in a study, when those diseases would place them at a significantly higher risk than a patient who does not have those diseases. An exception is made when the anticipated benefits are believed to outweigh the risks. Individuals with many specific diseases are generally excluded from early studies of a new drug until adequate data are obtained on how various types of patients are affected, and an initial profile of the drug's safety is available.

Present Clinical Status

It is generally considered below currently acceptable standards to enroll patients with clinically *unstable* acute or chronic disease(s) unrelated to the study disease in a study. Even patients with *stable* chronic disease(s) unrelated to the study disease are often excluded from a study, especially Phase II studies. Both the minimal and maximal severity of illness required to enter the study are important to define, in order to enroll patients with an appropriate range of disease and disability.

Patients with clinically significant emotional problems or retardation are often excluded from clinical studies, unless the study is designed specifically to include them.

Participation in Another Drug Study

Some patients engage in the unethical practice of enrolling in multiple drug studies at the same time. Examples have been noted where patients were enrolled simultaneously at two sites of a multicenter protocol, as well as cases where patients were enrolled simultaneously in two separate studies.

Some volunteers or patients enroll in studies one right after the other. They usually do this for financial gain, to obtain temporary housing, or for other reasons. This is especially common in Phase I clinical studies. Carryover or residual effects from the preceding study may occur that would confound the data obtained in the present study. Strict entry criteria about participation in other studies within *X* weeks are intended to minimize or prevent this problem.

Institutional or Environmental Status

Certain studies are conducted with patients who reside in institutions or nursing homes, or who constitute a specific population (e.g., patients visited by a public health nurse). They may sometimes be coerced into entering or continuing with a study, raising obvious issues regarding the validity of their informed consent.

Occupation

It may not be acceptable to include patients in an outpatient study if they are engaged in occupations involving the use of dangerous machinery. This may include patients who must drive a car. This is especially relevant when it is expected that there is a high probability of sedation, disorientation, or other effects on the central nervous system resulting from use of the study drug.

Litigation

Some diseases or problems such as cervical pain or back pain due to trauma are associated with a high incidence of litigation. In cases where there may be secondary gain to the patient if he/she does *not* improve with treatment, the beneficial effects of a drug may be compromised or completely unobserved if a patient with pending litigation is entered into a study. It is not a satisfactory ethical situation when patients have conflicting motives vis-à-vis improvement at the time of entering a study.

Another aspect of litigation relates to patient compensation for drug-induced injuries. This issue was addressed in the United Kingdom by the Association of the British Pharmaceutical Industry and a series of guidelines was issued (Association of the British Pharmaceutical Industry, 1983).

2. Choice of Efficacy Parameters

There are usually limits on the amount of resources available to conduct any study. In certain situations it might be medically desirable but financially impossible to utilize specific equipment. If, as a result, some or all important parameters cannot be measured in a study, then it may not be ethically justifiable to conduct the study.

3. Individuals Conducting the Tests

It is sometimes relevant to enumerate the individuals (by function) in the protocol who are permitted to perform certain tests. In addition, it may be relevant to specify the qualifications or credentials required of these individuals in terms of degrees, certification, and/or training. It is ethically unacceptable to have incompetent or poorly trained personnel (or investigators) conducting clinical drug studies. This holds for all individuals in roles that may affect either the patient's care or the collection, analysis, and interpretation of data obtained.

4. Choice of Safety Parameters

Some of the ethical considerations and issues that relate to safety include the following: (1) proper tests must be chosen to insure the patient's safety, (2) tests must be properly performed at appropriate time intervals, and (3) if problems occur the patient must be promptly and appropriately treated. If any toxicity is either anticipated or considered possible, then a specific attempt should be made to evaluate patients for their risk of having problems occur. Patients at high risk should be excluded unless there are strong reasons not to do so.

5. Modifying Dosing Schedules

When it becomes apparent during a clinical study that a patient is experiencing difficulties with a study drug it may be necessary to modify either the dose of a drug or the frequency of dosing. The most common safety reason requiring a dose modification is the occurrence of an adverse reaction. It is ethically desirable to determine the procedures, prior to initiating the study, that describe how this situation will be handled. If systematic plans for modifying doses have not been written into the protocol, then different patients who require dose adjustments may be treated differently. This situation might compromise the integrity and value of the data collected and of the study itself. In studies using fixed doses of a drug, dosage adjustments are usually unacceptable and patients who experience adverse reactions may have to be discontinued from the study.

6. Compliance

Patients who fail to comply with the requirements of a study are not meeting the responsibility that they accepted when they agreed to participate. This occurs to varying degrees in most studies and a great variety of tests have been developed to monitor patients for their extent of compliance. Many of these tests are straightforward (e.g., counting the number of pills remaining in medicine bottles that patients bring to clinic), but some other techniques raise ethical concerns about invasion of patient's privacy. These techniques must be discussed with a patient prior to the study and preferably are included in their informed consent. One example is where a member of the clinical team, such as the nurse, visits the patient's home at an unannounced time to collect a blood, urine, saliva, or other biological sample in which the amount of study drug will be measured.

Some of the reasons for poor patient compliance may be due to problems with the study that raise ethical considerations for those responsible for the study design or implementation. For instance, the requirements of the study may be too painful, stressful, or demanding on the patient.

7. Patients Lost to Follow-up

If adequate information is not obtained on how to locate patients enrolled in a study they may become lost to follow-up. This could pose ethical problems if patients had to be contacted during or after the study about an issue that could affect their health. Methods of locating missing or lost patients are given in Tables 22.43 and 22.44 of *Guide to Clinical Studies and Developing Protocols* (Spilker, 1984).

8. Patients Discontinued from a Study

After a patient is discontinued from a study because of a medical problem it is the responsibility of the physician in charge of the study not to discharge the patient from his/her care until the patient's condition has returned to its prior state or the patient is transferred to the care of another physician. Frequent causes of patient discontinuation include adverse reactions to the drug and abnormal laboratory or test results.

Patients who are discontinued from a study because of adverse reactions may be rechallenged with the drug at a later time under certain conditions. These conditions include: (1) the benefit outweighs the risk, (2) the abnormality was relatively mild, or (3) the information to be gained is considered substantial and the risk to the patient is relatively minor. If a patient is to be rechallenged, an additional informed consent should be obtained.

9. Early Study Discontinuation

A study may be discontinued early for either positive or negative reasons. Negative reasons for discontinuing a study include: (1) observation of serious adverse reactions, abnormalities in laboratory examinations or in vital signs that create an unacceptable risk for at least some of the patients to continue in the study, (2) failure to enroll an adequate number of patients, (3) failure of the investigator and/or staff to maintain adequate clinical standards, (4) failure of the investigator and/or staff or patients to comply with the protocol, (5) termination of the study drug's development by the sponsor, (6) unacceptable changes in personnel or facilities at the investigator's site, and (7) determination that no statistically significant result can be obtained.

There are also a number of positive reasons for discontinuing a study early. The major reason is that beneficial effect of treatment is observed which raises ethical concerns for patients who are not receiving this treatment. If early termination for ethical reasons is considered possible at the outset of a clinical study, then criteria should be established to define conditions under which the study would be terminated early.

It is the investigator's responsibility to prepare patients for the study's discontinuation once that course has been chosen. The investigator must inform patients in some manner about the results, arrange for continuation of their medical care, and collect the final data to be incorporated into the data collection forms.

10. Medical Emergencies

Patients may be given a wallet card indicating that they are in a clinical study. The card should contain the name and telephone number of the investigator, coordinator, and/or other individuals who could be reached at any time. Another issue is the situation where a patient is in a double-blind study and a medical emergency arises. It is imperative that a rapid means of breaking the study blind be devised for all studies. Information on treating drug overdose should be provided to all investigators by a sponsor prior to a study. Information known to the sponsor for treating any serious adverse reactions should also be provided to all investigators, if that information might eventually be included in the drug's labeling.

11. Amount of Data To Collect

Collecting either too little or too much data in a clinical study may raise ethical issues. Too little data may lead to the situation where data generated are inadequate for appropriate statistical analyses and clinical interpretation. In this situation the study objectives are inadequately addressed. The opposite extreme occurs when the vast amount of data generated interferes with the conduct of the study. In such cases the quantity of data collected may actually prevent the study from being completed.

12. Instructions for Patients, Investigators, and Study Personnel

During the initiation and conduct of any clinical study, many different types of instructions must be provided to patients, investigators, and study personnel. Although these do not need to be provided in a written form, it is essential that at least some communication is made. It would be unacceptable, for example, if patients went home, developed study-related problems, and could not readily contact appropriate members of the study team.

13. Continuation Protocols

An important ethical consideration in studies of investigational drugs that have a specified duration is, will patients who have benefited from treatment be allowed to continue receiving drug after the study is completed? If so, a continuation protocol is generally provided. Many questions relating to the necessary qualifications for patients to enter a continuation protocol have ethical implications. One dilemma relating to the design of a continuation protocol for patients completing a double-blind study is whether patients who are receiving a placebo should be entered and remain on placebo in the continuation protocol. If these patients are either switched to active drug in an open-label continuation study or are not entered in the continuation study because they had been on placebo, then the blind of the ongoing double-blind study will be jeopardized and may be broken. If the continuation protocol is also double-blind there will be numerous ethical issues to consider (e.g., how long may a patient be treated with placebo).

If a continuation protocol emanates from a sponsor, then periodic review of data generated in the continuation protocol should be conducted by the sponsor. The sponsor should reserve the prerogative to cancel any continuation protocol if the drug's development is discontinued, or for other reasons. Otherwise, the sponsor may be caught in the obligation of having to "indefinitely" supply a drug to a small number of patients, even though the drug is no longer being developed and will never be marketed. There is also a potential issue if the sponsor removes the only drug that has benefited certain patients, and no suitable alternative therapy is available. Most sponsors would continue to provide the drug under these circumstances.

14. Large Multicenter Studies

There are a few ethical issues involved in large-scale multicenter studies that are not present in smaller studies. The larger scale of the study requires more monitors and usually more monitoring groups concentrating on specific aspects of the study. There may be a special group appointed with the responsibility of insuring high standards at each site. This group will react to any ethical problems observed.

15. Confidentiality of the Data

There are several types of confidentiality associated with clinical studies. Confidentiality relates to information supplied by the sponsor to the investigator and to the IRB, in addition to information in the patient's medical record generated in the study. This subject raises numerous ethical concerns in terms of deciding which, and from whom, information is confidential, as well as how the confidentiality will be maintained and under which conditions it may be breeched. Discussions of confidentiality in protocols and informed consents must be consistent with FDA regulations and with the policies of IRBs and sponsors.

Physicians involved in either a sponsored or unsponsored double-blind controlled study should not be made aware of results of interim analyses. If they are cognizant of one treatment being markedly better than another, it may be ethically difficult or impossible for them to continue treating seriously ill patients with a less effective drug or placebo.

ETHICAL CONSIDERATIONS IN CONDUCTING A STUDY

Four aspects of conducting a study which have ethical implications will be briefly mentioned.

1. Recruiting and Screening Patients for a Study

There may be a temptation for investigators or sponsors in some Phase II and III studies to stimulate patient enrollment by offering overly generous inducements. It is unacceptable to offer a relatively large sum of money or other nonmedical inducements to patients so that their primary motivation to enroll in a study is for financial gain. This view must be modified for Phase I clinical studies, plus selected other studies (e.g., pharmacokinetic studies) where financial benefit is accepted as the primary motivating factor for many volunteers.

During the screening phase of a study it is important for all data to be available on patients prior to enrolling and treating them. Otherwise, unanticipated abnormalities may be reported after the patient has been treated with a study drug that would have excluded the patient from the study. The patient may be at high risk of a problem or may have developed adverse reactions that could have been avoided.

2. Providing Information to Referring Physicians

It is a responsibility of investigators to provide relevant study data and other information to colleagues who have referred patients for the study. This usually takes the form of a letter or possibly a telephone call. This practice should be followed both as a matter of professional courtesy and as part of the responsibility of temporarily caring for another physician's patient. If the study has a significant effect on the patient's disease, then an account of all clinically relevant events and data should be communicated to the original physician.

3. Protocol Violations

Both investigators and sponsors must be sensitive to the issue of protocol violations. Although many minor deviations do not raise ethical issues, it is obvious that some deviations will raise significant dilemmas. These problems must be dealt with on a case-by-case basis in a prompt, sensitive, and effective manner.

4. Conducting a Study

During a study many questions usually arise which were not anticipated during the development of the study design and protocol. Many of these questions may raise ethical concerns.

In conclusion, the numerous examples have demonstrated that a wide range of ethical issues may arise in any part of a clinical drug study. Once an issue is accepted as an ethical concern, there are many complex questions about that issue which are subject to many interpretations and solutions. These matters affect all individuals and institutions involved in a clinical study.

Section II

Considerations for Planning Special Types of Clinical Studies

8

Planning Surgical Studies

Introduction • Differences Between Surgical and Drug Studies • Types of Surgical Studies • Designing Surgical Studies • Placebo Effects and Sham Operations • Management of Surgical Studies • Methodologies Used in Surgical Studies • Evaluation of Drugs During Surgery

INTRODUCTION

There has been a heated debate for many years as to the proper role of randomized and well-controlled studies in surgery. This chapter will not rehash each of the pros and cons of that debate, but will assume that it is both ethical and desirable to perform such surgical studies whenever possible. One argument supporting this view relates to the benefits for society. If a study involving 100 patients (50 in each of two treatment groups) can evaluate whether a questionable surgical procedure is of value, it is considered unethical to avoid this study and subject large numbers of future patients to an operation that might be ineffective or even harmful. This assumes that all patients who enter the study are fully informed and agree to participate. The other side to this debate claims that a number of patients may be unnecessarily subjected to sham surgery or a less than state-of-the-art surgery just to evaluate a point on which most surgeons may agree.

The history of surgery contains many examples of procedures which attained acceptance and were later shown to be without medical value. Many of those operations, which have been discarded in recent decades, were rejected on the basis of controlled studies. Some of the stories about these events have been well documented and illustrate the great value that randomized studies may have in differentiating between useful and nonuseful surgeries. A classic example involved reputed benefits of the internal mammary artery ligation for improving the clinical status of patients with angina pectoris. This procedure became a national fad for a period during the 1950s. The true value of this particular surgery was not adequately assessed until two randomized controlled studies were performed, which included patients who underwent sham operations (Cobb et al., 1959; Dimond et al., 1960). This story is recounted well by Beecher (1961). One of the most salient points from the study of Dimond et al. (1960) is that objective evidence of clinical improvement (improved T-wave changes in the electrocardiogram) was apparent in a patient who had received a sham operation. In addition, there were numerous reports of subjective improvement in the sham operated groups. Some other examples of accepted surgeries which were eventually rejected include: (1) prefrontal lobotomies for treating aggressive and/or schizophrenic patients, (2) laparotomy for tuberculous peritonitis or pelvic inflammatory disease, and (3) colectomies to cure epilepsy (Beecher, 1961).

These few examples make one wonder if some surgical procedures being used today are essentially no better than placebo, or may actually be detrimental to patients. By posing this question the author does not presuppose that any specific procedures are suspect. Nonetheless, surgeons with open critical minds should retain a healthy skepticism in their evaluation of currently used methods. The origins of some well-established surgical procedures may have been based originally on authoritative statements rather than on scientific evidence, even though many surgical procedures have been subsequently validated.

Most surgeons previously believed that a retrospective analysis of a large series of patients who underwent a particular surgery would provide sufficient information to assess the value of that operation. Many surgical publications were of this type of retrospective review of a particular surgeon's (or group of surgeons') experience. The evidence has been overwhelming that even large series of surgical experiences often do not provide the correct interpretation of a particular operation's efficacy (Moses, 1984). There is a growing tendency away from this approach in surgery as a means of validating a particular operation.

DIFFERENCES BETWEEN SURGICAL AND DRUG STUDIES

Surgery itself has various objectives, which may be summarized in five categories:

1. To treat and cure an acute illness.
2. To treat and cure a chronic illness.
3. To treat a disease that is otherwise fatal and thus prolong life.
4. To palliate a slowly progressing disease.
5. To palliate a rapidly progressing disease.

In any particular comparison between a single surgical study and a single drug study, the differences in protocol design and in patient outcome may be either minimal or substantial. There is no simple list of characteristics that may be used to evaluate or address all comparison studies. Nonetheless, many surgical studies may be differentiated from most drug studies by one or more characteristics. For instance, surgery usually consists of a one-time operation or procedure that is irreversible, although multiple surgeries are sometimes required as part of a single treatment or study. Drugs on the other hand, are usually taken multiple times to treat a problem.

Although some surgical studies measure parameters postsurgery prior to the patient's discharge and do not require follow-up visits, most surgical studies include a follow-up period of evaluation after the patient has been discharged from the clinic or hospital. Obtaining adequate data during this period is often difficult and, depending on the length of follow-up, may be compromised by patient's (1) lack of cooperation, (2) moving to a new location, (3) death, or (4) loss to follow-up for other reasons. Although the length of the follow-up period may be determined prior to the surgery, it is often unstated in the protocol (if a follow-up exists). The number of patient visits during this period is also usually left unstated in the protocol, as well as the specific parameters and tests to measure at each visit.

The majority of drug studies have clearly defined endpoints that are measured, and most studies are completed at a certain point in time. After a study is completed and drug treatment is discontinued, patients are not continued in the same study during a long-term follow-up period. In some surgical studies, however, patients are continued for an indefinite period (i.e., follow-up period) after the surgery has been completed. When patients are enrolled for a one-year or even longer drug study, the number and schedule for all clinic visits (as well as the specific tests to be performed at each visit) are usually described in the protocol.

The term "endpoint" is often used differently in medical and surgical studies. In medical studies, an endpoint is usually a parameter that is measured to gauge the effect of the treatment or intervention. Endpoints are developed within certain categories of parameters (e.g., pharmacological, clinical, quality of life, physiological, biochemical) and a study may include any number of endpoints. In surgical studies, an endpoint usually refers to either a certain time after the surgery and/or a certain clinical event that occurs (e.g., rehospitalization for the same problem, reoccurrence of the same problem, a new episode).

Many surgeries have a greater risk associated with them than is associated with taking most drugs. Immediate risk is generally more apparent in surgical studies than for drug studies. Risks include the potential for damage to nerves, muscles, and blood vessels during most surgeries (e.g., perforation, massive bleeding) as well as after the surgery is completed (e.g., bleeding, wound dehiscence). In addition, there are risks inherent in the use of both general and local anesthesia and risks of infection. Occurrence of new diseases or problems may develop post-surgery which are related or unrelated to the original problem that necessitated the surgery.

Surgery also requires a greater degree of technical skill than is associated with providing most drugs to patients. Finally, surgical expertise for any specific operation requires special training, whereas special training is usually not necessary before a drug study is initiated. Surgical expertise varies greatly among surgeons and may be expected to influence the outcome of many surgical studies. Even for a single surgeon, his skills will be greater when performing certain operations. The technical skills of investigators in drug studies are generally less critical to the outcome than are the technical skills of a surgeon. These distinctions are broad generalizations and numerous exceptions exist.

TYPES OF SURGICAL STUDIES

Although it is logical to consider a surgical study as a comparison of two surgical treatments, this chapter views surgical studies more broadly by identifying a number of comparisons that may be made under the general heading of surgical studies. It is certainly possible to limit consideration of surgical studies to one (or more) of the types of possible studies. These studies are listed in Table 8.1.

It is apparent from this list that the surgery conducted is paramount in some studies and not in others. Most of the considerations described in the following sections on surgical study designs are concerned with those studies where one type of surgery is being compared with another, or where surgery is of major importance in the study.

Types of surgical studies may also be described according to the study designs used. The major controversy in this respect relates to the use of randomized controlled surgical studies. This topic has strong advocates and critics and the interested reader is referred to the literature, including the following articles by proponents of these studies: Spodick (1973), Gilbert et al. (1977), Haines (1983), and Baum (1983); and by the opponents of this

TABLE 8.1. *Types of studies involving surgical procedures*

1. Evaluation of drugs or anesthetic agents used during surgical procedures (e.g., neuromuscular blocking agents)
2. Evaluation of a disease treated either by surgery or drugs (e.g., angina, peptic ulcers)
3. Evaluation of a disease (e.g., cancer) treated either by surgery or nondrug modalities (e.g., hyperthermia, radiation)
4. Comparison of two (or more) surgical procedures (e.g., new versus old method, modified versus original method)
5. Evaluation of one surgical procedure (usually a novel technique) compared with historical controls
6. Comparison of a surgical procedure performed with and without medical (or other) adjunct therapy
7. Evaluation of equipment used in surgery (e.g., cauterizing machine, stereotaxic device) or medical devices (e.g., prosthetic heart valves), either used or implanted during surgical procedures
8. Evaluation of surgical materials (e.g., adhesives, suture materials, drapes, pins, staples) used during surgery

approach: Bonchek (1979), van der Linden (1980*a*,*b*), and Byer (1983). The article by Bonchek elicited a flurry of letters defending randomized surgical studies (Loh, 1979; Chalmers and Sacks, 1979; Fowler, 1979; Folland et al., 1979). Bonchek later expanded discussion of his position (Bonchek, 1982).

Gilbert et al. (1977) reviewed the surgical literature and reported that about one-half of the surgical innovations evaluated with randomized studies demonstrated improvements, and that less well-controlled studies tend to yield more positive results than do well-controlled studies. Van der Linden (1980*a*,*b*) suggested that patients should be randomized to different surgeons who would perform the surgery they do best, rather than having the surgeon perform two different operations, one of which might be performed with less interest and possibly with less skill.

DESIGNING SURGICAL STUDIES

This topic primarily concentrates on those design aspects of surgical studies where differences from medical studies are likely to exist. Since considerations of single surgical studies were not described in detail in *Guide to Clinical Studies and Developing Protocols* (Spilker, 1984), some considerations of individual studies are included in this chapter. Various aspects of study design particularly pertinent to surgical considerations are divided into a number of separate topics. These topics are listed below, and one is described in more detail (number 2):

1. Basic considerations (Table 8.2).
2. Identifying endpoints and parameters to measure (Table 8.3).
3. Preoperative considerations (Table 8.4).
4. Operative considerations (Table 8.5).
5. Postoperative considerations (Table 8.6).
6. Short-term outcomes (Table 8.7).
7. Long-term outcomes (Table 8.8).
8. Training and technique of personnel (Table 8.9).

There is a great range in the definition of "standard surgical procedure" (DeCosse et al., 1980). Many of the details that make up the presurgical, surgical, and postsurgical procedures must be identified in a protocol to help insure uniformity between surgical procedures and also to insure uniformity of care given to different patients. An example of a presurgical issue that should be clarified in a protocol is bowel preparation. This may be done by mechanical means, elemental diet, antimicrobial agents, or any combination of these techniques. Another example relates to the number of lymph nodes biopsied during surgery. This number (or range) should be identified in the protocol and associated with the level or stage of the patient's disease. A typical postsurgery issue would involve identifying the technique of stim-

TABLE 8.2. *Basic considerations in surgical studies*

1. Consider including a placebo or sham operation in the study design
2. Determine the nature of the control group (e.g., historical control, placebo, standard surgery)
3. If a crossover design is contemplated (e.g., for a surgical procedure that is repeated, devices used in a repeated procedure, medical versus surgical study in the same patient) evaluate whether patients will generally be willing to accept a second leg of treatment
4. Determine the magnitude of the difference between treatment groups needed to convince most surgeons to alter their clinical practice
5. Consider how tightly the protocol should be designed and how much flexibility is acceptable
6. Consider patient referral patterns and the treatment that referring physicians expect their patients to receive
7. Determine which parameters are to be used to establish the diagnosis and magnitude of the disease, condition, or problem
8. Consider whether multiple subsets of patients are to be included (e.g., cancer patients with different stages of one type of cancer)
9. Consider whether it is possible to have the patient evaluated independently, especially if the surgeon and patients will not be blinded to the study treatment
10. Consider whether the patient's medical status may be monitored and controlled by a single internist at each study site, who should remain blind to the patient's treatment
11. Monitor the surgeon's technique by a head surgeon or a quality control monitoring group
12. Incorporate a period of training into the study as a "pilot study"
13. If the objective of the study is to evaluate a new method or type of surgery, determine whether the goal is to establish a high standard of performance which others may try to emulate, or to establish a standard that most surgeons can readily achieve and perform on a routine basis
14. Determine whether patients can be randomized to different surgeons who each perform the type of surgery they are most familiar with
15. Determine whether an algorithm may be useful in designing the study[a]

[a] A comparison of surgical emergencies treated with and without an algorithm was published by Hopkins et al. (1980).

ulating respiration (to prevent atelectesis) which is to be used, plus the frequency and other details of its use. Another issue involves whether prophylactic treatment to prevent deep vein venous thrombosis will be included as part of the study, along with the details of this treatment.

Identifying Endpoints and Parameters to Measure

All surgical patients may be followed for a specified time (e.g., 10 weeks or 10 years) after surgery. In the situation where this duration is relatively long (e.g., 10 years), most published data include all patients who have been followed for at least a minimum period of time, although the durations for the individual patients will vary. If the follow-up period is relatively short

TABLE 8.3. *Suitable parameters used to evaluate surgical procedures*

A. During surgery
   1. Technical ease or difficulty of surgery
   2. Amount of practice required to "perfect" the surgical technique
   3. Duration of surgery
   4. Rate and nature of severe complications plus treatments given
   5. Rate and nature of moderate and mild complications plus treatments given
   6. Number and expertise of staff required to assist during surgery

B. After surgery
   1. Morbidity and/or mortality rates
   2. Improvement in physiological, pharmacological, biochemical, pathological, clinical, and/or other endpoints
   3. Length of hospital stay
   4. Total cost of hospitalization and total cost of the disease over an *X*-year (*X*-month) period
   5. Quality of life at predetermined time points
   6. Cosmetic appearance before and after surgery
   7. Need for additional surgery or treatment
   8. Amount of patient anxiety and stress prior to and after the surgery
   9. Type and amount of drugs required to treat the patient's problem before and at specified times after surgery
   10. Rate and nature of complications plus treatments required for these complications
   11. Performance of patient on standardized tests (e.g., treadmill) before and after surgery
   12. Clinical global impression rated by investigator
   13. Clinical global impression rated by patient

TABLE 8.4. *Preoperative considerations in designing surgical studies*

1. Describe acceptable preoperative care (e.g., specific preoperative drugs, doses, time of administration relative to surgery)
2. Determine whether the procedures for obtaining informed consent should be standardized
3. Determine if a blind (single or double) is possible or necessary. If so, determine how it will be implemented and maintained
4. Determine whether contact between surgeons and patients should be limited or avoided in single-blind studies
5. Determine whether the surgeon's level of enthusiasm should be controlled or measured
6. Determine whether to measure each patient's anxiety and how this may be done
7. Determine whether to alter dosages of drugs patients may be taking
8. Determine type of bowel preparation (if relevant)
9. Specify patient's diet

TABLE 8.5. *Operative considerations in designing surgical studies*

1. Specify which anesthetic(s), neuromuscular blocking agent(s), and other drugs patients may receive during the operation
2. Specify types of dosing of neuromuscular blocking agents (e.g., by bolus or by constant infusion). Specific doses or dose ranges may be identified
3. Specify instrumentation and equipment required to be present in the operating room. Specific models and numbers required may be identified
4. Specify the calibration and use of the instrumentation and equipment
5. Specify relevant synthetic and biological materials to be used in the operation (e.g., suture materials)
6. Specify the pathological and/or X-ray or other examinations to be conducted during the operation

TABLE 8.6. *Postoperative considerations in designing protocols for surgical studies*

1. Describe both required and acceptable postoperative care and monitoring procedures in the recovery room
2. Describe both required and acceptable postoperative procedures and care after the patient leaves the recovery room (e.g., respiratory care, diet, activity)
3. For outpatient surgical procedures, indicate the time that patients must remain in the clinic or office prior to discharge
4. Provide instructions of how the patient should behave at home and how they should handle and care for potential problems that may be anticipated. Provide a telephone number for patients to use
5. Determine whether some or all patients will be placed in a special program postoperatively (e.g., occupational therapy)
6. Indicate how long a follow-up period is essential to include in the study and how long a period is desirable

TABLE 8.7. *Potential factors to measure in assessing short-term outcomes after surgery*[a]

1. Amount of blood loss during surgery
2. Duration of surgery from the opening incision to closing the wound
3. Number of patient failures
4. Degree of improvement observed and measured
5. Rate of complications during and after surgery
6. Severity of complications during and after surgery
7. Rate of mortality and reasons for death
8. Number and severity of episodes of the medical problem requiring surgery
9. Improvement in laboratory parameters
10. Improvement in rehabilitation therapy (e.g., physical therapy, occupational therapy, other forms of therapy)

[a] Short-term is defined as the period from initiation of surgery to the time of patient discharge from the hospital. Outcomes in high- and low-risk patients as well as in other groups of patients may be compared.

TABLE 8.8. *Potential factors to measure in assessing long-term outcomes after surgery*[a]

1. Length of follow-up
2. Number of patients lost to follow-up
3. Number of readmissions to hospital[b] and length of stay during subsequent admissions
4. Risk of mortality
5. Estimate of survival time
6. Covariates associated with long-term survival
7. Number and severity of episodes of the medical problem requiring surgery
8. Interval of time between episodes
9. Degree of improvement
10. Percent of patients improved by preset quantities or amounts
11. Improvement in laboratory parameters
12. Degree of functional disability
13. Improvement in rehabilitation therapy (e.g., physical therapy, occupational therapy, other forms of therapy)
14. Factors that place patients in either a high- or low-risk group
15. Total costs of health care for each treatment group

[a] Long-term is defined as beginning at the time of patient discharge. The termination of this period will depend on the specific surgery. Each of the specific times at which measurements are to be made should be determined prior to the study (e.g., annual examinations).
[b] Only for reasons relating to the disease treated by the previous surgery.

TABLE 8.9. *Considerations of training and technique of personnel in designing surgical studies*

1. Specific qualifications may be indicated for surgeons who actually perform the surgery in a study (e.g., residents, board-certified specialists)
2. Specify the required skills for the rest of the surgical team (e.g., anesthesiologists, pathologists, scrub team)
3. Specify the required training in the techniques to be evaluated (e.g., each surgeon to have conducted a minimum of *X* operations with an operative mortality of less than *Y*%, training for *Z* months, skills approved by the head surgical monitor)
4. Specify whether a single surgeon must perform all operations or whether a group of surgeons may operate and have their results combined
5. Determine whether a single anesthesiologist or group of anesthesiologists will assist during the operation
6. Determine whether to measure the skills of the surgeon for each type of surgery included in the study
7. Determine whether the surgeon uses conventional dissection or "no-touch" dissection techniques
8. Determine whether a surgeon's preference for one of the test surgeries is a basis for assigning that type of surgery to the surgeon or for replacing him with another surgeon

(e.g., 10 weeks), then publications usually include patients who have all been evaluated for approximately the same period.

Another type of endpoint that is sometimes established in surgical studies relates to (1) the occurrence or reoccurrence of certain adverse reactions, (2) rehospitalization, (3) exacerbation of problems related to the patient's disease, (4) death, or (5) other clinical occurrences. Any of these endpoints may be used to mark the termination of a patient's participation in a study. If the surgery is primarily (or even secondarily) concerned with cosmetic appearance of the patient, then photographic depiction of the before and after appearance may be used to derive cosmetic endpoints. Photographs of control patients who were selected before their surgery was performed should be included for comparison purposes. Cosmetic endpoints such as 1+ to 4+ may be defined and independent surgeons kept blind to the patients' treatment may be used to rate all photographs.

In addition to these endpoints it is important to identify the parameters (e.g., mortality, postoperative sepsis) that are to be included in a study to evaluate and compare treatments. A number of parameters that are more suitable for surgical, as opposed to medical, evaluation are included in Table 8.3.

Control Populations

The concept is alien to some surgeons who are used to evaluating new therapies without recourse to including a control population. It is clear, however, that more and more surgeons understand and accept the necessity of including control populations in surgical studies. There are also more surgeons who recognize the benefits that control populations offer in the field of surgery. This change in attitude is possibly related to recent changes in the training of surgeons. Training of surgeons is considered in Table 8.9.

Control populations may include a (1) no-treatment group (for open studies), (2) sham-operated group (see section below on placebos and sham operations), (3) standard accepted surgery, or (4) unmodified form of surgery. Murray (1986) has advocated the use of large banks of observational data serving as a control population for comparing results of new surgical techniques. He describes a large international data bank that exists for severe head injury. This recommendation has value for some areas of surgery, but would not be suitable for all areas and can never provide data as strong as those from randomized controlled studies. Other forms of control are to identify two groups of patients in the study whose results will be compared, although this type of comparison is usually weak in the degree of control it offers. This approach is similar to a subgroup analysis addressing questions such as: (1) Do men and women react similarly to the operation? (2) Is the operation equally effective in children as in adults? (3) Do patients with severe cardiovascular compromise tolerate the operation as well as patients with a normal cardiovascular system?

PLACEBO EFFECTS AND SHAM OPERATIONS

There *is* a beneficial result from surgery that may be attributed to a placebo effect and to sham operations. The evidence supporting this statement is strong, and some of it will be summarized below.

In the case of sham operations, Dimond et al. (1960) and Cobb et al. (1959) used sham operations in double-blind studies and demonstrated that the sham procedures had positive subjective and objective effects on anginal symptoms. Ruffin et al. (1969) used a sham freeze in the double-blind evaluation of gastric freezing for treatment of duodenal ulcers. No difference in patient response to the sham and real freeze was observed.

A placebo effect has been widely attributed to surgical intervention and is partly responsible for both objective and subjective improvement observed after surgical treatment. Beecher (1961) estimated that the magnitude of the placebo response in surgery was the same (about 35%) as that observed in medical studies. The placebo effect was also enhanced by the enthusiasm of the surgeon. One way in which this occurs is when the surgeon alleviates or decreases the amount of anxiety a patient feels and encourages the patient to be optimistic about the outcome. This form of bias may easily enter the study and should be controlled and possibly evaluated (if a question of the bias arises) through patient interviews and/or questionnaires.

MANAGEMENT OF SURGICAL STUDIES

The management of well-designed surgical studies is similar to the management of well-designed medical studies. A few points of particular importance to surgical studies involve monitoring procedures. Monitoring may be performed by a designated surgeon who supervises, evaluates, or otherwise oversees surgical activities at one (or multiple) study site(s), or by a team of surgeons and/or nonsurgeons who review and oversee the quality and consistency of the surgical study.

It is extremely important for surgery to be conducted by surgeons who are patient oriented rather than surgically oriented. Surgeons chosen for studies should be well-trained physicians who are both experienced and interested in pre- and postoperative care. If the surgeon(s) chosen, however, are less interested in pre- and postoperative care than performing the surgery it may be relevant to appoint a specialist in internal medicine to manage (or monitor) patient care. The potential advantages of this approach are several. First, it insures a greater degree of consistency if a single nonsurgeon (or small number of nonsurgeons) take care of all patients in a study. Second, routine postoperative clinical care is usually allied with internal medicine. Third, this approach will tend to minimize or eliminate any influence of investigator enthusiasm on results, especially if the internal medicine physicians are blind to patient treatment. On the other hand, the internist usually lacks a great deal of detailed physiological understanding of the surgical procedure and the insight that accrues with having done the surgery.

Costs of a Study

A special aspect of surgical studies that is indirectly associated with management are costs of a study. This is often an important factor in determining whether a particular surgical procedure becomes widely used, especially when alternative medical treatments are possible. Costs of a treatment include more than determining the total hospital bill for patients in two or more treatment groups. Costs do not merely refer to the cost of performing the surgery, but to a determination and comparison of the overall costs of the comparison treatments. This often becomes an important factor that relates to how well new surgical techniques are accepted.

There are many types of costs associated with treatment and several are highly complex and subjective. Costs relate to direct medical costs, indirect costs, and nontangible costs. These are discussed more fully in Chapter 23. Costs of treatment include the time in lost productivity resulting from the disease or condition and how this time is affected by each of the treatments evaluated. It is clear that a more expensive surgical treatment may be cost effective if patients are able to return to productive work sooner than patients who undergo a less expensive operation.

It is often important for costs of several types to be monitored in a study, especially if the study is evaluating a novel surgical technique. If costs are compared between two surgeries it should generally be on the basis of "per successful operation." This term must be carefully defined in terms of survival plus a specific quality of life for a specific period of time. Therefore, all patients who are operated on and die or who have an unsuccessful outcome in terms of established criteria are counted in with the costs of that surgery. This prevents an apparently inexpensive surgery with a poorer outcome from seeming to be much more cost effective.

METHODOLOGIES USED IN SURGICAL STUDIES

Some of the considerations for reporting surgical results are listed in Table 8.10. Except in some unusual situations, most surgical studies do not involve placebo control groups. An active control may be readily incorporated into most evaluations of new surgical techniques or procedures, but even this practice is not as widespread as it could be. The active control included in

TABLE 8.10. *Reporting results of surgical studies*[a]

1. Report number of surgeries performed by each surgeon
2. If possible, describe the results obtained by each surgeon
3. Report the nature, number, and time of all specimens obtained during surgery and the pathologist's report
4. Describe monitoring systems used and the results of the monitoring

[a] Relevant factors listed in Tables 8.4–8.9 should be reported in a publication or report and will not be repeated in this table.

a study is usually the standard surgical procedure, performed under conditions as identical as possible to the investigational surgical technique. Use of an active control has several advantages in an investigational study, especially when patients are randomly assigned to receive either the new or standard technique.

Many new surgical procedures do not develop *de novo*, but rather evolve slowly through a series of small steps from established procedures. It is often neither practical nor necessary for a surgeon to approach an Institutional Review Board (IRB) for permission to perform a slight modification of a standard technique. In most situations the surgeon modifies an existing technique on his/her own initiative. Some surgical procedures are performed in many different ways. When a further modification is later considered and evaluated, the surgeon again might not approach the IRB. Eventually, a totally new procedure may have evolved and the surgeon will publish the results, using historical data from his/her prior experience as a control, or through reference to published literature for control data.

It is not firmly established which modifications of surgical procedures require IRB approval. A possible guideline is that any modification that places patients at an increased risk during or after surgery should be submitted to an IRB. At a certain point in developing minor modifications of a known method the surgeon should formally initiate a controlled study that will not depend upon historical data to evaluate the surgery. It is understood that this suggestion is not always realistic or possible.

One alternative to a completely randomized approach is to assign different surgeries to the surgeons who perform them best and to randomize patients to different groups and therefore different surgeons. Another alternative is to alternate patient assignment or to assign every third or fourth patient to the standard surgical procedure group. Surgery would be performed by surgeon(s) A. An independent surgeon (surgeon B) who is blind to patient randomization could be used to evaluate patients. If the two surgeries could not be blinded for an independent surgeon, then the independent surgeon (or surgeon A) could evaluate patients and code or describe surgery results on preprinted forms. These forms could then be evaluated by yet a different surgeon (surgeon C) who was blind to patient treatment.

There are some surgical procedures where it is generally acceptable to compare new results with historical controls. For example, where there is a significant and consistent improvement in survival compared to well-documented historical controls or a significant and consistent decrease in surgical or disease complications, then one may use historical controls. Nonetheless, one must be wary of this approach because the rates of mortality and morbidity resulting from surgery, or even the natural history of a disease, often change over the years and apparently valid historical data will turn out to be invalid.

EVALUATION OF DRUGS DURING SURGERY

A common type of drug study performed during surgery relates to prophylaxis against infection. Patients are treated with either a study drug, active control, or placebo at a defined time during the surgical procedure, and the occurrence of infection (defined by precise criteria) is measured and evaluated during a subsequent period. Patients may be randomly allocated to treatment groups, there may be double-blinding of the study with a "double placebo" technique, and the study may be conducted at a standard as high as any double-blind medical evaluation.

Other drugs evaluated during surgery (e.g., anesthetic agents, neuromuscular blocking drugs, vasopressors) should also be evaluated in a rigorous and well-controlled manner. Methods for their study are described elsewhere in this series.

9

Planning Studies to Evaluate Medical Devices

Types of Devices • Designing Protocols • Differences Between Developing Devices and Drugs

With the passage of the Medical Device Amendments in 1976, the field of medical devices entered a new era. These amendments were incorporated in the Federal Food, Drug, and Cosmetic Act and require materials used in medical devices, as well as the devices themselves, to undergo comprehensive testing. The regulations were intended to raise the standards for introducing new medical devices on the market and to better insure the safety of the American public. The statutes pertaining to medical devices are found mainly in Sections 501 to 521 of the Act.

TYPES OF DEVICES

Definitions and Examples of Class I, II, and III Medical Devices

Medical devices have been divided into three classes, which are defined in section 860.3 of the Code of Federal Regulations.

Class I devices are the least hazardous and are subject to the "general controls" that had been used to regulate devices prior to the Medical Device Amendments. These controls include rules concerning good manufacturing practices, labeling, purity, banned devices, recalls, records kept, and reports. Devices are in Class I if they are not intended to support or sustain human life or prevent impairment to human health and do not present a potentially unreasonable risk of illness or injury. Class I devices make up about 29% of all types of devices and include elastic bandages, surgeon's gloves, manual surgical instruments, nasopharyngeal catheters, enriched culture media, and tongue depressors.

Class II devices are subject to specific performance standards, which the FDA has developed or will develop. Most of these have not yet been written. General controls alone are deemed insufficient to provide reasonable assurance of their safety and effectiveness. Class II devices (63% of the total) have some risk associated with them. Examples include flexible laryngoscopes, surgical drills, stomach pH electrodes, arthroscopes, chin prostheses, and electrocardiogram machines.

Class III devices are subject to premarket approval. A device is in Class III if its safety and effectiveness cannot be assured by performance standards. All devices that (1) are life supporting (or sustaining), (2) are for a use which is of substantial importance in preventing impairment of health, or (3) have a potential for causing risk of injury or illness are in Class III. New devices are automatically placed in Class III until the manufacturer or importer successfully petitions the FDA to reclassify it. Class III devices (8% of the total) require premarket approval from the Food and Drug Administration (FDA) before they may be marketed. These devices include many orthopedic implants, artificial organs, intrauterine devices, tracheal prostheses, and herpes simplex serological reagents.

Classifications Based on Use

Although medical devices have been divided into three classes based on the degree of risk, there are also other means of classifying devices. A general classification may be used which relates to their use. In this classification there are four types or categories of devices.

Type I—Internal devices. These devices are introduced into, or penetrate, the body for a month or less (e.g., cannulas, needles, i.v. catheters, drainage tubes); or for greater than a month (e.g., heart valves, orthopedic prostheses, surgical clips).

Type II—Topical devices. These devices may be subdivided, depending on whether they come in direct contact with skin (e.g., surgical dressings, tapes, cast materials) or mucous membranes (e.g., catheters placed in the urethra, tubes placed into the trachea).

Type III—Indirect devices. These devices come in contact with drugs, fluids, or other substances that enter the body (e.g., oxygenators, hemodialysis machines, syringes, transfusion apparatus).

Type IV—Noncontact devices. These devices do not come in contact with the body or with substances that enter the body, but do come in contact with devices that contact the body (e.g., instrument trays, operating-room table covers).

Another classification of many medical devices could be made, depending on whether the device is intended for one-time use or limited number of uses, or is indefinitely reusable. Another aspect of this classification would be whether the device were intended for only a single patient's use, or for use in multiple patients.

Combination Products: Devices and Drugs

Although most medical devices are clearly devices and not drugs, there are some that have both characteristics and may be considered as a combination product. For example, a wound dressing or bandage that is placed on the skin is a medical device. But, if it is impregnated with an antibacterial agent, growth factor, or other bioactive chemical it could be considered as a combination product. This type of product is not necessarily difficult to study and evaluate, but identifying the regulations that apply to its approval could pose numerous complex issues that may not be easily resolved with a regulatory authority.

DESIGNING PROTOCOLS

Types of Investigators and Studies

When designing protocols for studying a medical device it is usually relevant to consider who the intended user will be. If the device will be used by nurses and non-MD therapists, it is important to include them in evaluations, as well as including relevant medical specialists. The investigator(s) must be provided with preclinical data as well as clear written instructions (and oftentimes training) in the device's use, in addition to warnings, hazards, and other information. Although studies may be scientifically or marketing oriented, as with drug studies, there is probably a higher percentage of medical device studies than drug studies that are marketing oriented. This probably results from the fact that regulatory requirements are generally much less stringent for medical devices.

The two major stages of testing involve (1) an initial pilot stage where the device's design and materials are being developed and tested and (2) a multicenter stage where safety and efficacy of the final product is evaluated. The former stage is analogous to early Phase II studies in evaluations of new drugs, and the latter stage is analogous to Phase III studies. Adequate testing must be conducted with the final medical device, regardless of the amount of testing with the pilot product. Most controlled studies use a parallel study design. Crossover designs may be considered for a small number of medical devices (e.g., comparison of filters used in a dialysis machine).

Choosing Parameters

Although there is temptation to evaluate every parameter of interest and to obtain all or most of the answers to development questions in a single study, this is not usually possible. When designing clinical studies it is important not to attempt to make any study all-encompassing. An attempt to do so may actually slow progress with development of the device (or drug) and could even create problems, resulting from a complex study that attempted to achieve too many answers. This situation may lead to further studies that would explore problems raised in the overly ambitious study.

The need of many patients for a Class III medical device is often certain (e.g., heart valve replacement, hip replacement). In such cases it is generally unethical to consider including a placebo treatment group in a clinical study. Therefore, clinical studies depend heavily on the patient's baseline values to evaluate the effects of the device. When open-labeled studies are conducted and no blinding is used, greater reliance should be placed on objective measures of change (e.g., ejection fraction) or semiobjective measures (e.g., distance the patient can walk without pain in a given period). Subjective parameters (e.g., quality of life measures) are usually more susceptible to influence by a placebo effect than are objective measures. Use of subjective measures should therefore be deemphasized whenever possible, unless they are validated parameters or there is no other choice. When one product is compared with another the parameters evaluated must be comparable.

Control Groups

The literature on the clinical evaluation of medical devices is much smaller than that for most drugs. The quality of reported studies varies enormously, and most studies suffer from lack of a control patient group that received a comparison medical device. Studies commonly describe a group of patients who received a device and present before and after values for certain tests and parameters. There is usually no adequate control. One reason for this failure may be that the sponsor of most of these studies (i.e., device manufacturers) often do not wish to directly compare their device against a competitor's. In addition, it is rarely ethical to include a placebo or sham-operated group as a control. Placebo controls are often not necessary or possible in testing certain medical devices. Many situations in which Class II and III devices are used are not amenable to observing a placebo effect (e.g., the patient may be unconscious, the interaction between patient and device may be minimal or nonexistent). There are several types of comparisons which may be used to evaluate medical devices (Table 9.1), and special considerations for designing protocols (Table 9.2) which illustrate differences between medical devices and drugs.

Double-Blind Studies

There a number of techniques whereby two or more medical devices may be effectively tested and compared in a double-blind manner. One process is to have two (or more) surgeons each implant or insert different devices

TABLE 9.1. *Types of comparisons that may be made in studies of medical devices*

1. Device A versus device B—usually performed single-blind
2. Device A versus drug B—usually performed single-blind
3. Device A versus surgery B
4. Device A versus no treatment
5. Device A versus placebo device—preferably performed double-blind
6. Device A versus other treatment modality (e.g., radiation)

and to have an independent surgeon (who is kept blind) review all patients. Each surgeon may implant only one type of device, or may be permitted to implant all of the devices being compared. In the latter situation, devices should be implanted in a random order. Since many surgeons will have preferences as to the devices they use and also will be more experienced in implanting certain devices, they will generally prefer being assigned to implant only one type of device. Since differences in surgical skill rather than the device implanted may influence patient outcome, it is preferable to have several (or many) different surgeons each implant one specific device and a different group of surgeons each implant the other device studied. Alternatively, all surgeons may be trained in the device's use so that they each achieve a minimum standard of technical competence. A third possibility is to measure and grade the skills of each surgeon and to consider this in the evaluation of the results.

If multiple hospitals are involved in a study of a medical device, it is often necessary to control for differences in hospital care. This may be done by having at least one surgeon at each hospital assigned to insert device number 1 and a different surgeon or group of surgeons at each hospital chosen to insert device number 2. It is also important to insure that all patients meet

TABLE 9.2. *Special considerations in designing protocols for medical devices*[a]

1. In a double-blind study it may be necessary to blind the identity of the device used. This may be done by disguising its outside appearance or by having the device inserted by one physician and having the patient evaluated by another physician
2. Describe all increased risks that patients may experience in the study. Indicate how these risks will be minimized
3. Label all devices appropriately, including the phrase "CAUTION: INVESTIGATIONAL DEVICE LIMITED BY FEDERAL LAW TO INVESTIGATIONAL USE"
4. Indicate appropriate methods of disposition of both used and unused devices
5. Describe all functional tests of range of motion, correction of deformity, relief of symptoms, and other criteria of improvement
6. Provide written instructions for use of the device, plus warnings, hazards, and contraindications[b]

[a] These points are in addition to relevant considerations for designing protocols for drug studies.

[b] Evaluate the clarity of the instructions and their comprehension by potential users.

standard criteria to enter the study, to eliminate the possibility that surgeons at one hospital select patients differently than surgeons at another hospital.

Other Tests

In addition to the clinical testing of the device in humans, it is necessary to conduct many other types of tests. These include studies of shelf life (i.e., stability) and biocompatability. This latter term relates to the studies that demonstrate no untoward effects when the device remains in contact with skin, blood, mucous membranes, or other parts of the body for a prolonged period. Sterility tests must often be performed for medical devices.

Adverse Reactions

When commonly expected types of complications from a medical device are known, the data collection form may list these for the investigator to check off. Although this practice is not as common in clinical studies evaluating drugs, there are a number of advantages and justifications for its use in tallying "adverse reactions" due to medical devices. For example, the number of likely adverse reactions resulting from medical devices are usually fewer than for drugs and may be more precisely described.

Federal regulations in the United States require manufacturers and importers of medical devices to report device-related serious injuries and deaths to the FDA. Physicians and other health professionals are encouraged to report their experiences to the manufacturer, directly to the FDA Product Monitoring Branch, or indirectly to the FDA via the Problem Reporting Program administered by the United States Pharmacopeia. A newsletter of world medical device news (*Clinica*) is published by George Street Publications in Surrey, United Kingdom.

DIFFERENCES BETWEEN DEVELOPING DEVICES AND DRUGS

Medical devices are a much more heterogeneous group of products than drugs in terms of their design, use, and purpose. Many devices never come in direct contact with patients, some have only brief direct contact, others attach to the skin or are inserted in the body for varying periods and then removed, and some become a permanent part of the patient. Each type of medical device has to be preclinically tested prior to its use. Implants, prostheses, and other devices must pass preclinical tests to confirm that they function electronically and mechanically in a reliable manner before they can be used in patients. Many of these devices must be sterilized after such tests are complete.

Device Companies and Drug Companies

The companies that develop and market most medical devices include a greater proportion of small companies than those that develop new drugs. Device companies generally have extremely small regulatory affairs departments and have relatively large marketing and research and development groups.

A major difference between medical device companies and drug companies is that the goals of the device companies are more closely associated with specific needs of their customers. Device companies determine the specific needs of the users and often work closely with clients to develop prototypes of new products. Drug companies are more dependent on inherent attributes of the drugs they discover or license to determine which specific indications to pursue.

EDUCATION OF INVESTIGATORS

Most investigators in studies testing new medical devices have to be educated about the correct use of the device. This is often a major issue and there is a period of learning necessary before the device is able to be used properly and efficiently. Therefore, it is necessary to either provide education and/or training prior to initiating the protocol or else to conduct the protocol in two stages. Data from the first part (pilot or training part of the protocol) would not be used to evaluate the device. Data from the second part of the study would be of major importance. Objective criteria should be established to determine when the investigator is allowed to proceed from the first to the second part.

These considerations do not usually occur in drug studies, especially when drugs are given orally. Investigators or their staff may have to be taught how to operate certain equipment used to measure parameters of safety or efficacy, to assay for drug levels in biological fluids, or to perform other aspects of a study unrelated to drug administration. In unusual situations, technique may also be important in drug delivery (e.g., placing radiocontrast dyes to perform myelograms, inserting depots of drugs, placing tubing from infusion pumps into intrathecal spaces, performing epidural or other types of anesthesia).

Modifying Devices and Developing a Final Product

Many device manufacturers do not create a final version of a medical device *do novo*, but proceed through a series of modifications. Many devices are continually being modified during their development and each clinical study may actually test a somewhat different device. After a device is finalized it must be evaluated in a new and separate study. It is not acceptable to state, in an application for marketing approval of a device, that each part was tested separately in different studies so that the entire device does not have to be studied in a new study. It is possible that the whole may differ from the sum of its parts. This principle holds for Class I and II medical devices, as well as for Class III devices.

When problems occur with devices, the company may involve many different groups to help resolve the issue, just as with drug development (e.g., consultants, investigators). But device companies also involve design and other engineers to resolve many issues, whereas these people are rarely involved in a comparable role in developing a new drug. Engineers are involved, however, in the manufacturing aspects of both drugs and devices.

Although drugs are provided without charge in almost all drug studies, companies sometimes sell new devices to physician/investigators who will then use them (e.g., implanting them in their patients) in a study. This is a major reason why investigators often want to make changes in the design and/or use of a device. This may or may not be desirable from the company's perspective, but many investigators are chosen because of their reputation as a thought leader or opinion setter in a specific field. The investigator may have his or her own way of testing the device and in such situations exerts greater control on the design and conduct of the study than does the sponsor of the study. This approach used to be more prevalent in the past in the drug industry than it is at present. See Chapter 20 for a discussion on old-fashioned and modern approaches to monitoring, which describes an analogous situation.

10

Developing Orphan Drugs for Rare Diseases

Introduction • Classifications of Orphan Drugs • Incentives and Disincentives for Corporations to Develop Orphan Drugs • Stimulating Development of New Orphan Drugs • Orphan Drugs Under Development in the Pharmaceutical Industry

INTRODUCTION

From the perspective of the drug industry, orphan drugs represent a heterogeneous group of drugs that differ from each other in various ways: (1) patent status, (2) whether they are investigational drugs or are already marketed, (3) whether they are used only to treat rare diseases or both rare and common diseases, (4) degree of clinical usefulness, (5) availability to physicians, (6) cost to develop, and (7) commercial potential. It is therefore difficult to generalize about orphan drugs because each has its own set of characteristics and problems. Most orphan drugs also differ from nonorphan drugs in several ways (Table 10.1).

The decision to develop an orphan drug is usually based on a combination of complex factors. Information about many or most of these factors is incomplete at the time that the decision must be made to develop (or not to develop) an orphan drug. More than 25 drug companies in the United States are presently developing new orphan drugs. There are many incentives and disincentives for their development, and these are described later in this chapter.

CLASSIFICATIONS OF ORPHAN DRUGS

There are estimated to be 4,000 rare diseases (or conditions), many of which are not presently treatable with effective drugs. Although the term "orphan drug" is generally used to describe all drugs used to treat rare diseases, a close look at orphan drugs reveals a wide variety of drugs that are or may eventually be used to treat rare diseases. To illustrate this point, two classifications of orphan drugs are mentioned. The first classification,

TABLE 10.1. *Comparison between characteristics of orphan and nonorphan drugs*

Orphan drug	Nonorphan drug
1. Used in a limited patient population	1. Used in a large patient population
2. Often used only by a few specialists	2. Generally used by a wide variety and/or number of physicians
3. Often loses money for the manufacturer	3. Are more likely to make money for the manufacturer
4. May require fewer patient exposures to obtain approval for marketing	4. Usually require a "standard"[a] quantity of data prior to approval

[a] The definition of the term "standard" depends on the identity and nature of the disease targeted, the nature of the drug, the specific regulatory agency involved, and numerous other factors.

consisting of four categories, is an easier and more practical approach to use when describing orphan drugs.

1. Marketed drugs on or off patent used *only* to treat a rare disease.
2. Marketed drugs on or off patent used to treat *both* rare and common diseases.
3. Investigational drugs being actively evaluated in humans for treating a rare disease.
4. Investigational drugs that are available from a company for treatment of a rare disease, but which are not being actively developed for a New Drug Application (NDA).

A second, more detailed, classification of orphan drugs consists of 18 separate categories (Spilker, 1985). This detailed classification illustrates the heterogeneity of orphan drugs.

Both of the above-mentioned classifications are complicated by many factors, a few of which are listed below.

1. There are various nonofficial definitions of an orphan drug as well as definitions in federal laws and regulations; furthermore, the interpretations of these definitions may also change with time.
2. Most drugs and compounds that may be placed in a particular category will not always remain in the same category. Research ideas are often translated into investigational compounds, and eventually some investigational drugs are marketed while on patent and finally go off patent. Another example is when a drug that was originally marketed for a rare disease is later found to be useful in the treatment of a more prevalent disease, or vice versa.
3. An investigational formulation of a drug (e.g., intravenous) may be found to be useful for a rare disease, whereas the marketed formulation

(e.g., topical or oral) may not be as useful or as effective for the rare disease.

4. The classification of orphan drugs described refers to prescription drugs. There may be a number of over-the-counter (i.e., nonprescription) drugs that are useful for some or all of the symptoms associated with certain rare diseases. There are a different set of considerations for these drugs, which are not discussed in this chapter.

INCENTIVES AND DISINCENTIVES FOR CORPORATIONS TO DEVELOP ORPHAN DRUGS

There were incentives for pharmaceutical corporations to develop orphan drugs long before the Orphan Drug Act was signed into law in the United States in 1983. This Act significantly improved some of those incentives and provided new ones as well. In addition to the incentives that will be described below, there are a number of disincentives, most of which were not addressed by the Orphan Drug Act. The major incentives and disincentives are described from the perspective of a pharmaceutical corporation in the United States.

Incentives for Development of Orphan Drugs

1. In the United States, the term "rare disease or condition" includes, but is not limited to, diseases or conditions affecting up to 200,000 patients (i.e., prevalence). This is an eminently fair and reasonable definition. Moreover, the definition allows one to consider drug development for a subgroup of a more common disease, if a drug is found to be only active in a subgroup of a total disease population.
2. Marketed drugs can qualify for orphan drug status for new indications that are specific to rare diseases.
3. In the United States, drugs that may qualify for orphan drug designation are those which are intended for populations larger than 200,000 patients, but the sponsor cannot recover sufficient revenues to cover costs of research, development, and distribution.
4. Companies may recover additional clinical research costs for drugs originally developed for major indications but where efficacy was limited to treatment of a rare disease. Tax credits are given for clinical studies on orphan drugs conducted between the time of designation of orphan drug status and approval of the drug's NDA.
5. Marketing exclusivity for 7 years post-NDA approval may be obtained on an unpatentable orphan drug for a specific rare disease indication. This provides some financial benefit to the sponsor and helps recoup costs.

6. Orphan drug status potentially provides an opportunity to obtain more clear information from regulatory agencies on requirements for an NDA on the specific drug than is achieved with most nonorphan drugs.
7. Given the increased attention recently focused on this area, it is possible that an NDA application for an orphan drug will obtain a more rapid regulatory review than if it did not have that designation.
8. If a company wishes to move into a new therapeutic area and has the potential to develop an orphan drug at the outset, then it may be viewed as a means of enabling sales representatives to achieve easier access to offices of specialists in a new therapeutic field.
9. Publicity of new orphan drugs will enhance the image and prestige of the company in both the lay and professional community.
10. It is never possible to preclude the possibility that an orphan drug may eventually be used to treat a common disease. There is always some hope that an orphan drug may become highly profitable.
11. Development of certain orphan drugs may expand a current product portfolio in a specific therapeutic area. This would allow a company to advertise and promote a more complete range of therapeutic, diagnostic, and/or prophylactic products within that area.
12. If the company has few drugs of major commercial potential under development, then orphan drugs may provide scientific stimulation on a meaningful drug and also utilize efforts of the staff while a drug for a more common disease is being sought.

Disincentives for Development of Orphan Drugs

1. The tax credits for developing an orphan drug will usually have little impact on the total cost of a drug's development. Major financial costs of developing a drug often occur in areas where no reimbursement via tax credits are given under provisions of the Orphan Drug Act (e.g., toxicological studies, patent requirements, formulation studies, development of a practical route for chemical synthesis). Clinical studies may be less extensive in developing an orphan drug and thus cost less than for most other drugs. Other development costs, however, may not be less for an orphan drug than for a nonorphan drug. It is thus ironic that the tax credits are given in the one area (clinical studies) where lower development costs are generally expected for an orphan drug.
2. A company may encounter difficulties in obtaining marketing exclusivity on an orphan drug if a pending patent is rejected or awarded to another company. An approved orphan drug may not be easily marketable if another company owns the patent. If the patent situation is not clear at the time of regulatory approval, then a company takes a

great risk if it sells the drug. If the patent is later awarded to another company, the first company may have to pay punitive damages that are greater than the amount of their sales.

3. A company that allocates its resources to developing an orphan drug is not allocating them to developing drugs needed by larger patient populations. Since drugs for large populations are potentially more profitable than orphan drugs, there is a lost opportunity cost in developing orphan drugs.
4. When a marketed drug (off patent) is being sold by generic companies and is found to be useful for a rare disease, it will probably be unprofitable for the primary manufacturer to conduct studies to demonstrate the drug's activity. This is because marketing exclusivity will be unenforceable if a generic manufacturer is already selling the same drug for a more common indication. It may also be unnecessary for the company to study the drug because physicians may legally use the drug for the rare disease without a formal NDA being approved. In addition, it may be impossible to obtain an NDA approval if the drug is not sufficiently active in a high enough percentage of patients with the rare disease.
5. The time required to develop new drugs for some orphan indications (e.g., epilepsy) is long, the problems encountered are usually tremendous, and the costs to develop these drugs are among the highest of all classes of drugs. Given the enormous potential for difficulties, it is uncertain when initiating development of drugs for orphan indications that success will be achieved.
6. The anticipated current and future competition and anticipated market share for a proposed orphan drug must be evaluated. If there are drugs presently used to treat a rare disease, a new drug must be compared with them in terms of both safety and efficacy. The need for the orphan drug should be assessed since there is a great difference between a drug that will be the only treatment for a rare disease and a drug that will offer limited benefits in treating a rare disease where alternative therapy is available.
7. If the sponsor of the orphan drug is not the original developer and current manufacturer, there may be great difficulties in obtaining necessary development and toxicology data from the original developer that must be submitted to the government to obtain approval to market the drug. This is because the original NDA may only be referenced with the consent of the NDA holder.
8. It is not certain that the Internal Revenue Service will actually grant all relevant tax credits and, if they do, which definition and clinical costs of an orphan drug they will use.
9. Postmarketing studies may be required by the Food and Drug Administration (FDA) as part of the NDA approval of an orphan drug. Since

the tax credits for clinical studies on orphan drugs stop at the time that the NDA is approved, there is no reimbursement for any postmarketing studies. These studies are usually extremely expensive, and the relatively small patient population treated with orphan drugs may make studies to monitor these patients even more costly than usual.

10. The possibility of liability exists for any new drug. The magnitude of this risk will vary for each drug. But, there are no reasons to believe that liability of a manufacturer for an orphan drug will be any less than for a more widely used drug. Certainly there are no regulations stating that orphan drugs may be less safe than nonorphan drugs.

After reviewing the incentives and disincentives of developing orphan drugs listed above, a number of substantial questions remain. One of these concerns the activities of the Orphan Products Development group at the FDA. It is yet unknown how efficiently and effectively this group is in (1) granting drugs orphan status, (2) providing information to companies on requirements for approving an NDA, and (3) helping other groups within the FDA to expedite the NDA review process. Initial experiences suggest that they are able to rapidly approve orphan status of new drugs, but are relatively ineffective in regard to points 2 and 3 for most orphan drugs.

Costs and Activities Associated with Orphan Drug Development Which Are Not Covered by the Orphan Drug Act

1. Preclinical studies conducted prior to initiation of clinical studies.
2. Nonclinical biological studies conducted after initiation of clinical studies.
3. Technical development costs.
4. All clinical studies conducted prior to the approval of the orphan drug application.
5. Administrative costs.
6. Patent costs.
7. Marketing costs.
8. Manufacturing costs.
9. Other support costs.

STIMULATING DEVELOPMENT OF NEW ORPHAN DRUGS

It is generally inefficient and not cost effective for a drug company to establish many highly specific animal models of rare diseases in their own laboratories to evaluate marketed drugs and promising chemical leads or to screen potentially interesting compounds. Yet, there are occasions when testing chemical leads or marketed drugs for potential activity in treating rare diseases is of interest to a pharmaceutical company. There is no single document available that provides information on most animal models suitable for evaluation of potential drugs for rare diseases. Likewise, the names and addresses of leading experts involved in most rare diseases are not readily available.

To optimize the development of new orphan drugs within the pharmaceutical industry, it would be valuable to have a list of selected rare diseases and information about those diseases. This document would provide additional opportunity and stimulus for collaboration between researchers in the pharmaceutical industry and academia. Information collected on individual rare diseases should include data on (1) animal models, (2) names and addresses of the most qualified researchers and leading experts, (3) names and addresses of relevant volunteer organizations, (4) drugs or chemicals presently used to treat the disease, and (5) any known chemical leads for treatment that are not patentable (either specific chemicals or classes of chemicals could be listed). Additional categories of information should be considered for inclusion.

This list would have to be updated regularly. The information obtained would *not* list priorities among diseases or drugs, nor would it include information of specific interest to patients or treating physicians. Although much of this information already exists, it is currently fragmented and not readily available. This type of activity is not currently part of the mandate of the National Information Center for Orphan Drugs and Rare Diseases (NICODARD). This information would be sent to interested academicians, government agencies, volunteer organizations, individual pharmaceutical companies, and associations.

Potential uses for this information include:

1. Pharmaceutical companies with an interest in a specific disease or types of disease could privately pursue contacts with academicians or others. The companies could inquire about screening compounds for activity or about collaborating on a research project.
2. Academicians would readily see which orphan diseases did not have appropriate animal models or experts to serve as champions of that disease. The list might stimulate development of valuable new methodological techniques or encourage new champions. Little or no coordination of these activities would be required by the government.

It is proposed that a government agency such as the National Institutes of Health, the Department of Health and Human Services, or NICODARD prepare and disseminate this list, since the drug industry is not generally considered to be in an appropriate neutral position to undertake that role and most academicians would not have sufficient time nor resources to devote to this effort. The National Organization for Rare Disorders (a volunteer group) could also play an important role in this activity.

It would also be desirable if academicians could contact pharmaceutical companies to explore possible collaborations on projects of mutual interest. It is unlikely that most pharmaceutical companies have specifically explored their own research interests in all rare diseases or would be willing to have this information made public. On an individual basis, however, a frank discussion between an academician and company could occur after a statement of confidentiality was signed. In this situation the individual academician would have to explore company interests one company at a time and might find it difficult to identify the most suitable company to collaborate with. Possible solutions to this dilemma should be sought since there are many academic scientists who seek to identify an industrial partner for collaborative research or drug development.

ORPHAN DRUGS UNDER DEVELOPMENT IN THE PHARMACEUTICAL INDUSTRY

How Are New Orphan Drugs Discovered and Developed?

There are usually no substantial differences between the specific processes used for developing drugs for rare diseases or common diseases. Orphan drugs (as all drugs) are discovered and developed through a variety of mechanisms. A company does not generally set up a program to discover drugs for a rare disease such as hairy cell leukemia. Instead, it sets up research programs to study biological activities in specific areas such as muscle metabolism, receptors, enzymes, or branches of medicine (e.g., immunology). The company may also establish therapeutic targets such as specific diseases or groups of diseases.

The company usually develops and creates animal models to screen compounds for interesting biological activity. If a compound with an interesting biochemical and/or pharmacological profile emerges, then a series of possible diseases will be considered against which the specific compound might be active. This list usually includes both common and rare diseases. During the clinical testing program, it is not uncommon for companies to sponsor a pilot study in a rare disease to evaluate a compound's activity, or to make their drug available to an investigator who has reason to believe that the new drug might have activity in a rare disease.

One can never know with certainty which diseases a drug will eventually be used to treat. Many newly marketed drugs are given to patients with diseases or conditions other than the one for which they are approved, to evaluate the total spectrum of the drug's activity. This often leads to serendipitous results, such as the discovery that the antiviral drug amantadine, originally approved to prevent and to treat influenza, also had activity in patients with Parkinson's Disease. This effect was unknown prior to marketing.

A different perspective or orphan drugs emerges by retrospectively examining drugs that have been marketed, rather than looking prospectively at drugs under development. Many drugs have been approved and marketed for multiple indications, and some of these indications would qualify as rare diseases. Yet, most drugs used to treat both rare and common diseases are virtually never thought of as orphan drugs. A few examples include the use of propranolol for idiopathic hypertrophic subaortic stenosis (IHSS) and cimetidine for the Zollinger–Ellison syndrome. Many of these indications were detected after the drugs were marketed for more common diseases. There are also examples of drugs that were marketed for a rare disease which were later found to have a more widespread market for another indication (e.g., carbamazepine, which was originally sold for tic douloureux was later found to be active in treating patients with partial and other types of epileptic seizures).

Establishing Efficacy and Safety Data

One of the greatest difficulties in developing an orphan drug involves the conclusive demonstration of the drug's efficacy. Patients with a rare disease are generally geographically dispersed, and unless they are brought to large referral centers, it is not possible to enroll a sufficient number of patients to conduct a well-controlled clinical study. Evaluating a drug in a few widely scattered patients may be possible if a clear and objectively measurable endpoint exists. If the prevalence of the disease is much less than 200,000, it will be necessary to conduct multicenter studies in Phase II. Phase I studies may be conducted in normal volunteers if the drug is relatively nontoxic.

If clinical improvement is difficult to measure, then obtaining convincing efficacy data will pose major problems because of the low incidence and prevalence of the disease. It is especially difficult to evaluate dose levels, frequency of dosing, and other important clinical factors when few patients are available to enroll in a study. A shortage of available patients also means that parallel double-blind placebo-controlled studies are usually impractical. Crossover studies require fewer patients than do parallel designed studies, but the former design is often not suitable. Thus, innovative designs that seek to optimally utilize all available patients must be sought. Special considerations in designing protocols for studies of drugs for orphan diseases are indicated in Table 10.2.

In multicenter studies each center may call a central location when a patient is available to enter the study. Depending on the number of centers and required speed necessary to start patients on therapy, drug may either be kept available at each center or flown to the site from a central location. Patients may be assigned to treatment in a double-blind study by a central coordinator at the sponsor or at one of the study sites. Each patient may

TABLE 10.2. *Special considerations in designing protocols for studies of drugs for orphan diseases*

1. The number of available patients may be limited and their geographical location may require special procedures to insure adequate enrollment
2. Inclusion criteria often must be more lenient than in other studies in order to include a greater proportion of available patients
3. Providing funds for transportation and meals or actual transportation may help minimize patient drop-outs
4. Patients may be given reminders by cards at one clinic visit to inform them of their next appointment. Telephone calls and/or mailed reminders may also be useful to minimize the number of missed appointments
5. Depending on the availability of useful alternative therapy, a financial inducement for patients may be required to obtain sufficient enrollment. The magnitude of this inducement must be determined for the study after careful consideration of its projected effects on the patients and their family, but all patients must receive the same amount
6. The most knowledgable and experienced investigators in the field should be chosen to conduct the study
7. A volunteer patient organization may provide valuable information that will help in designing the study, identifying potential patients for the study, and identifying potential investigators
8. Cooperation may be provided by a government agency (e.g., NINCDS[a] for certain epilepsy studies, National Cancer Institute for certain anticancer studies)

[a] NINCDS, National Institute of Neurological and Communicable Diseases.

be treated in a dose–response manner or, alternatively, patients may be initially placed in a cohort that receives the lowest dose of the test drug or placebo. When the total number of patients enrolled reaches a predetermined number, a new cohort is begun, to receive the next highest dose or placebo. With both of these study designs relatively few patients are needed to generate data that provide a dose–response relationship.

Significant problems may also exist in the evaluation of the safety of an orphan drug. Patients with rare diseases desire drugs for treatment which are as safe as most other drugs. This raises an important issue when there are an inadequate number of patients with a rare disease to enroll in the clinical studies that are necessary to establish safety within a reasonable period of time.

The smaller number of patients used to establish the safety of orphan drugs is not necessarily a significant drawback, because the initial safety data on any drug are usually the most important. Also, patients with the disease could be followed for a period after the drug is marketed, to develop further the safety profile of the orphan drug.

The benefit-to-risk ratio must be considered in any discussion on the safety of new drugs. It is possible that an orphan drug would be approved by the FDA on the basis of data from fewer patients than the number required for most nonorphan drugs. Thus, the probability of observing rare but serious adverse reactions at the time of marketing is usually less for orphan than nonorphan drugs.

Current Status of Drug Industry Activities and Perspectives on Orphan Drug Development

To obtain an impression on current industry-wide development of orphan drugs, a questionnaire (Fig. 10.1) was mailed to the Head of Research and Development at each of 102 companies, chosen from the 121 members of the Pharmaceutical Manufacturer's Association (PMA). Nineteen of the subsidiary companies that belong to PMA were not contacted. Sixty-one responses were received. Of these, one company refused to participate, and 10 replies indicated that their companies do not develop new drugs (e.g., medical device company). Fifty responders answered the questions and their responses are shown in Fig. 10.1.

This questionnaire was not validated, and it may contain questions that were either unclear or misleading. It had a different purpose than the questionnaire used by Representative Waxman at the hearings on the Orphan

RESULTS OF QUESTIONNAIRE

1. Is your company developing any orphan drugs for Rx use that are currently either investigational or marketed for other indications? — 28 Yes 22 No

2. If you answered "No", would you agree with those companies who do not feel that it is part of their mission to develop orphan drugs?

Agree that it is not part of our mission	8
The "No" reflects a different reason	14

3. What is the total number of orphan drugs that are:

	Total NCEs	No. of Cos.	Total Non-NCEs	No. of Cos.
A. Under development in preclinical stages?	2	2	0	—
B. Under development in clinical stages?	39	18	4	3
C. In the clinic that are already on the market for other indications?	9	7	4	3
D. In the clinic that are only being developed for orphan indications?	24	11	1	1

4. Regarding NCEs, was the Orphan Drug Act a minor or major influence in your decision to develop a drug for orphan indications? — 20 Minor 8 Major

FIG. 10.1 Results of a questionnaire on development of orphan drugs in the pharmaceutical industry (NCEs, new chemical entities; Cos., companies).

5. What types of incentives would encourage your company to develop more orphan drugs? How important are these factors?

On a scale from 0 (No Importance) to 10 (Marked Importance)

	Mean ± S.D.	Range	N
A. Reimbursement for preclinical studies	4.5 ± 3.0	0 — 10	22
B. Reimbursement for toxicological studies	6.1 ± 2.9	0 — 10	22
C. Reimbursement for technical development	5.4 ± 2.8	0 — 10	22
D. Reimbursement for retrospective expenditures	4.5 ± 2.9	0 — 10	22
E. Inclusion of tropical or other diseases that are common diseases in the "Third World" but not in the U.S.	2.5 ± 2.4	0 — 8	22
F. Reimbursement for clinical expenditures made outside the U.S.	5.7 ± 3.0	0 — 10	22

G. Others (written in): Expedited approval (9) (9) (8),

All clinical costs (8), Full reimbursement of clinical costs (10), Goodwill (6) and Tax credit (3).

( ) = Rating given by reviewer

6. Please check the range of your company's most recent annual sales of pharmaceuticals?

Under $50MM <u>9</u> $50 to 100MM <u>8</u>

$100 to 500MM <u>18</u> Above $500MM <u>15</u>

FIG. 10.1 *(Continued)*

Drug Act (Asbury, 1985). Although an in-depth analysis was not possible with the current questionnaire, a number of observations are pertinent.

1. The response rate (60%) was considered excellent. Some of the non-responders are believed to be companies that do not develop new drugs.
2. Several of the negative replies to Question 1 (Is your company developing orphan drugs?) were from companies that do not develop new pharmaceuticals (the exact number is unknown). This means that the percentage of companies that are developing orphan drugs, compared to the total possible number of companies, is somewhat greater than the current numbers indicate.
3. Of the 50 responding companies, 28 stated that they are developing at least one orphan drug for prescription use.

4. Of these 28 companies, 8 (29%) stated that the Orphan Drug Act was a major influence in their decision to develop a drug for orphan indications.
5. Potential incentives for stimulating additional efforts in developing orphan drugs were important to some companies and not important to others. There is a trend, however, suggesting that reimbursement for toxicological studies, technical development, and clinical expenses obtained from outside the United States are the most important three incentives to the companies actually developing orphan drugs.
6. The 15 companies with the greatest yearly sales of pharmaceuticals (i.e., above $500 million) gave responses similar to those of the smaller companies. This indicates that orphan drug development is not solely an activity of the larger pharmaceutical companies, although they clearly contribute to the overall effort.

Orphan drugs are a heterogeneous group of drugs and offer valuable opportunities for pharmaceutical companies in carefully selected situations. Whereas legislators usually approach issues of orphan drugs as if they represent a single entity, pharmaceutical companies approach issues on the basis of the specific characteristics of each drug. It is hoped that additional incentives for orphan drug development will be enacted by Congress.

11

Conducting Studies in Special Patient Populations

Introduction • Conducting Studies in Elderly Patients

INTRODUCTION

There are many operational definitions of "special patient populations" which are appropriate for different situations. The definitions depend to a large degree on the perspective and needs of the person (or group) who is defining the term. In this book, the term is loosely defined and includes those groups of patients for whom drugs are not usually tested or for whom testing is usually not done until later in a drug's development. Even this loose definition has several exceptions, since some special populations may be involved in a drug's testing from the outset. Special populations that are often referred to include: infants, pregnant women, lactating women, blacks, elderly patients, and patients with decreased renal or liver function. A more complete listing of special patient populations is given in Table 14.1 of *Guide to Clinical Interpretation of Data* (Spilker, 1986). Elderly patients are discussed in this chapter as a prototype of the various types of special patient populations. Considerations for pregnant women and infants are also mentioned.

CONDUCTING STUDIES IN ELDERLY PATIENTS

Designing drug studies for elderly patients or most other special patient populations requires an understanding of the manner in which that population differs from other populations and also requires an appreciation of the factors that should be controlled or evaluated. Knowledge of social, physical, psychological, physiological, and other characteristics of the group is essential. Many of these factors are described in Chapter 11 of *Guide to Clinical Interpretation of Data* (Spilker, 1986).

The first point to make about elderly patients is that age per se is not a good predictor of drug response. On the other hand, a greater percentage of elderly patients than younger adults have (1) pathological changes such as decreased renal and liver function, (2) decreased numbers of certain receptors, (3) altered homeostatic responses (e.g., altered blood pressure reflexes in response to stimuli, as a result of increased deposition of calcium and other substances in arterial walls), and (4) other physiological changes. Thus, it is important to collect data on how a given drug affects the elderly, although it is usually not necessary to study older patients in independent formal studies prior to filing a New Drug Application (NDA) on a new drug. Other relevant factors in considering the elderly as a group are that a higher percentage are disabled, live in substandard housing conditions, live alone, have substandard diets, and exist in an altered physiological and psychological state. This group is at a higher risk of having more clinically important repercussions from adverse reactions to drugs because of their altered state. Data from existing and planned studies should be categorized by age so that any unusual or noteworthy effects in elderly patients may be perceived and subsequently explored to whatever degree necessary.

Designing drug studies for elderly patients is similar to designing studies conducted in an adult population. Nonetheless, there are some practical issues that require special consideration in the elderly, including (1) patient recruitment, (2) physiological status, (3) physical status, (4) parameters to measure, and (5) social status.

Patients may be recruited from nursing homes, where a high incidence of debilitation often exists relative to the elderly patients who live in the general population. Recruitment in a poorer economic area will probably yield a patient group with substandard nutritional habits. Patients who live alone will probably have a higher incidence of loneliness and psychological problems than patients who have a strong support system or are in frequent contact with at least another person in close proximity to their living environment.

The status of an individual's physiological status changes with age [see Chapter 15 in *Guide to Clinical Interpretation of Data* (Spilker, 1986)], and

TABLE 11.1. *Special considerations in designing protocols and conducting studies in elderly patients*[a]

1. Use reminder cards, mailings, and telephone calls prior to appointments
2. Arrange for transportation to and from study site
3. Conduct periodic reviews to insure patient understanding of protocol requirements
4. Conduct periodic checks on compliance
5. Include a sufficient number and frequency of tests of vital status and other safety parameters to insure patient well-being
6. Avoid rigorous demands which might unduly strain some patients
7. Involve family members, nursing home staff, or other individuals to provide assistance and observe the patient for relevant signs and symptoms
8. Consider previous data with the test therapy to determine whether elderly patients are at higher risk of adverse reactions than a younger adult population

[a] These factors are not endorsed for all studies, but should be considered. These factors are often more important issues in elderly patients than in younger adults.

TABLE 11.2. *Special considerations in designing protocols and conducting studies in pregnant women*[a]

1. Involve the patient's obstetrician in the study via direct participation (if possible and convenient) or through frequent feedback of information
2. Insure that demands on the patients are commensurate with their physical and emotional abilities
3. Determine patient's expected date of delivery as accurately as possible
4. Determine the duration of pregnancy (in weeks) permissible at patient entry
5. Determine whether sonograms, amniocentesis, fetal monitoring, and/or other procedures are acceptable or mandatory
6. Determine if any special restrictions on diet or activity during pregnancy, labor, and delivery are relevant
7. Conduct appropriate follow-up of the mother and of the newborn to evaluate any possible effect the study may have had
8. Involve the spouse and other family members to assist in the study (e.g., to observe the patient for any relevant signs and symptoms)
9. Provide arrangements for transportation to and from the study site and, if the patient is near term, to and from the hospital where delivery will take place

[a] Additional toxicology studies may also be performed (e.g., transplacental carcinogenicity studies) prior to the studies beyond those usually done to insure drug safety in this group of women.

TABLE 11.3. *Special considerations for designing protocols and data collection forms for clinical studies on newborn babies and infants*

A. For the mother near and during the time of birth
    1. Previous reproductive history of mother
    2. Type of birth (e.g., Caesarian, forceps)
    3. Type of anesthesia
    4. Medications used by the mother
    5. Details of labor (e.g., duration of each stage, complications)
    6. Details of delivery [e.g., presentation (breech, cephalic), complications (nuchal cord, shoulder dystocia)]
    7. Smoking and illicit drug use
B. For the newborn just before and after birth
    1. Fetal heart rate tracings
    2. Apgar scores at 1 and 5 min
    3. Resuscitation efforts
    4. Examination of newborn
    5. Length and weight
C. For the infant during the first year of life
    1. Events at birth (e.g., prematurity, Apgar scores, type of birth)
    2. Breast or bottle feeding
    3. Percentile of length and weight
    4. Changes in growth performance over time
    5. Time of initiation of solid food
    6. Type of solid food eaten
    7. Family situation (e.g., mother's employment status, number and age of siblings)
    8. Amount and type of stimulation given to the infant

these factors must be considered when designing drug (or other) studies in the elderly. If the population of patients studied excludes some who are debilitated, the physical requirements of the study must be carefully considered. This includes evaluation of the time and effort needed to complete various tests and examinations.

A number of considerations for designing protocols and conducting studies in elderly patients are presented in Table 11.1. A few considerations for designing protocols and conducting studies in other specific patient populations (pregnant women and newborn babies or infants) are listed in Tables 11.2 and 11.3.

12

Planning Pharmacokinetic Studies

Types of Human Pharmacokinetic Studies Used to Profile a Drug • Conducting Pharmacokinetic Studies • Metabolites • Therapeutic Drug Monitoring

TYPES OF HUMAN PHARMACOKINETIC STUDIES USED TO PROFILE A DRUG

This chapter describes the types of studies that are often conducted in humans to profile the pharmacokinetic characteristics of a drug. There is often a close relationship between results of pharmacokinetic and metabolic studies conducted in humans and those conducted in at least one animal species. When numerous animal species have been evaluated in preclinical studies, it is usually uncertain as to which specific species yielded data that will most closely resemble data to be obtained in humans. There is often little relationship between the position of the species on the evolutionary tree and the answer to this question, especially if only nonprimate species have been studied. When pharmacokinetic data obtained in animals are similar to those obtained in humans, there is a greater likelihood that toxicological data in animals will be predictive of the drug's safety in humans.

Pharmacokinetic evaluations of a new drug often begin during the initial clinical evaluation in humans and continue through all three phases of premarketing investigation. The major objectives and types of pharmacokinetic studies are listed in Table 12.1, and studies constituting a pharmacokinetic profile are listed in Table 12.2. It is usually unnecessary to conduct all of these studies on every drug. The exact studies required depend on the (1) biological, physical, and clinical characteristics of the drug, (2) intended use of the drug (e.g., acute or chronic treatment), (3) severity of the disease for which the drug is intended, and (4) issues that arise during evaluation of the drug. These latter issues include questions relating to clinical studies or parameters, toxicology, and technical development. The types of information obtained from pharmacokinetic studies are presented in Table 12.3, and the types of concepts evaluated are listed in Table 12.4.

TABLE 12.1. *Examples of pharmacokinetic study objectives*

To evaluate the:

1. Time course of blood and/or urine levels following a single dose (e.g., oral, i.v.) in a normal population and in patients
2. Time course of blood and/or urine levels during multiple doses, illustrating the ascension and achievement of steady state in a normal population and in patients
3. Routes and rate of elimination
4. Binding of drug to plasma proteins to provide information on distribution and on potential drug interactions
5. Distribution of the drug to various tissues
6. Changes in drug levels when enzymes have been induced with other drugs
7. Effects of a chronically administered drug on the rate of its own metabolism (e.g., induction or inhibition of metabolism)
8. Effects of a drug in patients with compromised renal, hepatic, cardiac gastrointestinal, or other physiological function
9. Screening tests to establish a profile and identify potential problems in the elderly, children, and other special populations
10. Effects of food in general and of specific types (e.g., fats, proteins, carbohydrates) on the pharmacokinetics of a drug
11. Interactions of the study drug with other drugs and nondrugs (e.g., walls or seal of the container, infusion sets)
12. Bioequivalence studies comparing two different dosage forms (e.g., solution and suspension, capsule and tablet), two different salts, or two (or more) different forms of the same drug
13. Comparison of different patients to evaluate interpatient differences
14. Comparison of multiple samples from the same patient to evaluate intrapatient variations
15. Cumulative effects of the drug under steady-state conditions
16. Mass balance study

TABLE 12.2. *Types of human studies involved in establishing a pharmacokinetic profile of an investigational drug*[a]

1. Bioavailability—Comparison of the extent of drug availability in the systemic circulation after oral administration of a solid dosage form with that of an oral solution or an intravenous injection
2. Bioequivalence studies—Evaluate the comparability of two or more dosage forms, salts, or formulations of a drug on the basis of rate and amount of absorption (area under the time–concentration curve)
3. Distribution studies—Obtain biological samples (e.g., biopsies) to detect presence and amount of drug at various times in different tissues and compartments
4. Metabolism studies—Measure presence, quantity, and time course of formation and elimination of metabolites[b]
5. Elimination studies—Measure fecal and urine levels of parent drug, metabolites, and conjugated products

[a] Any of the studies may theoretically be performed using radioactive labeled drug. These studies are especially relevant if assays are not available to measure nonlabeled drug or are not adequately sensitive to detect expected drug levels.

[b] Clinical and biological activities of metabolites are measured in other studies. Numbers 4 and 5 are often combined in the same study.

TABLE 12.3. *Selected types of information obtained in pharmacokinetic studies*

1. Identification and characterization of special populations who are at risk of adverse reactions because of genetic or other factors (e.g., disease states)
2. Identification and characterization of special populations who may not demonstrate a benefit from a drug because of genetic or other factors
3. Association of increased or decreased drug absorption with special patient populations or special patient factors (e.g., age, sex)
4. Association of altered patterns or rates of drug distribution or protein binding with specific factors
5. Identification of drug metabolites
6. Identification of factors affecting drug absorption, distribution, metabolism, or excretion
7. Identification of techniques to treat drug overdosage

CONDUCTING PHARMACOKINETIC STUDIES

There are numerous reasons for conducting bioequivalence studies (Table 12.5). When data are obtained they are usually plotted as (1) concentration versus time and (2) concentration versus effect (i.e., pharmacological activity). Time, effect, and concentration are really three axes of the same relationship and may be plotted on a three-dimensional graph if desired. Criteria to relate concentration of a drug to its effect are listed in Table 12.6, and reasons why a concentration–effect relationship may not be reproducible are given in Table 12.7.

Some individuals advocate a "shotgun approach" to pharmacokinetics where a new drug is evaluated in as many types of patients as possible and in as many ways as possible. This serves to screen the drug for unexpected differences in its profile. Factors evaluated would generally include diet, cigarette smoking, gender, race, gastrointestinal disease, hepatic disease, renal disease, age, pregnancy, and others. Sheiner and Benet (1985) have advocated the use of premarketing pharmacokinetic screens of new drugs in populations of patients, not just in a few selected volunteers or patients.

TABLE 12.4. *Selected concepts evaluated in pharmacokinetic studies*

1. Interpatient variability
2. Intrapatient variability
3. Steady-state kinetics of the drug. This should detect the presence of drug accumulation or altered metabolism
4. Relationship of therapeutic effect with drug concentration in plasma or other fluids
5. Type of elimination mechanisms used to remove the drug and the rate of removal
6. Relationship of drug dose and blood level at various time points after drug is given

TABLE 12.5. *Selected reasons for conducting bioequivalence studies*

1. New formulation of a drug is chosen to replace an older formulation (e.g., new excipients or new salt of the drug are used)
2. New dosage form of a drug replaces an older one (e.g., tablets replace capsules) or extends the product line
3. New physical characteristics of a drug product exist (e.g., increased density of a tablet due to higher compression used in its manufacture)
4. An older supply of the drug is to be compared with a newer one in order to determine the effect of age and "natural" changes in the overall composition
5. Two lots of an active drug are compared where differences are shown to exist[a]
6. A new manufacturing method is used to prepare the drug, or a new manufacturing site is preparing the drug and a question of bioavailability is raised
7. A new manufacturer[b] of a drug desires to compare the new product with a standard

[a] *In vitro* and/or *in vivo* tests may be sufficient to evaluate the possibility of differences [e.g., dissolution tests and other tests that demonstrate that the drug meets United States Pharmacopeia (USP) specifications].
[b] May be a generic manufacturer or a new supplier of a brand name product.

Collecting Biological Samples

The choice of an appropriate number of biological samples to collect and the optimal time points to collect them depends on three types of issues: (1) statistical considerations, (2) pharmacokinetic modeling requirements, and (3) practical considerations.

Statistical considerations are important in deciding how to best cover the time period of interest so that adequate samples are collected to achieve the goals set. For example, it is usually more relevant to collect several samples within the first hour of drug administration and to then slowly start to space out additional collection of samples. Statistical as well as nonstatistical considerations may be used to determine the total number of samples that should be collected on each patient.

TABLE 12.6. *Criteria to relate concentration of a drug to its effect*

1. Plasma samples are obtained at times, which are based on pharmacokinetic properties of the drug
2. The analytical methods used to measure drug concentration are sensitive, selective, quality controlled, and validated
3. There is no tolerance of the receptor sites
4. The drug's action is reversible
5. If clinical effects are clear-cut and the endpoints may be objectively measured the relationship is easier to establish
6. Factors that modify the time course of drug levels in plasma are considered (e.g., metabolites)
7. Total drug concentration in plasma reflects the unbound concentration at receptor sites (i.e., binding must be relatively constant throughout the therapeutic range)
8. Acceptable variability between the magnitude of individual clinical effects

TABLE 12.7. *Reasons for lack of a reproducible concentration–effect relationship*

1. The drug is ineffective
2. Measurement methods of insufficient sensitivity are used
3. Effects of drugs are small or obscured because of difficulties in measuring effects
4. Drug has an irreversible or long-lasting effect
5. Receptor tolerance occurs
6. Variable absorption, distribution, metabolism, and/or excretion
7. Genetic differences in the population
8. Age, sex, or other differences are present in patients studied and influence pharmacokinetics

Developing pharmacokinetic models that fit the data is analogous to choosing clothes to fit a person. It is important to collect enough datum points at appropriate times to cover the drug's profile. The more datum points one has at suitable times, the better the model will fit the drug.

If a drug is being tested in humans for the first time, then it is not possible to make simulations of pharmacokinetic models using data from animal studies, because it is not known which species has a pharmacokinetic profile similar to humans. The first study in humans is basically looking at the pharmacokinetics without knowing what will be found. Later in the life of a drug, data from human studies will be available on which to base simulations and models.

Samples may be collected at the same fixed time points for all patients in a study (e.g., 1, 2, and 5 hr after dosing), or a sequential strategy may be developed. In the latter approach, data from the first patient are used to derive optimal time points to collect samples from the second patient. Data from the first two patients are then used to choose the optimal time points for the third patient. This process may continue throughout the study, or a fixed pattern may be established after a certain number of patients have been evaluated.

Practical considerations include many different types of issues. These include (1) total volume of blood that may be drawn on each patient in the study, (2) degree of inconvenience and bother to the patient (e.g., separate blood draws every 15 min may lead to emotional upset, especially if an indwelling catheter is not used), and (3) inconvenience and bother to staff (e.g., blood draws at 3 A.M. and 5 A.M. or on holidays will often lead to ire). There may be a limit to the number of separate blood draws permitted on each patient because of the quantity of blood necessary to perform duplicate assays. Up to 1 pint of blood may be taken every 8 weeks. It is sometimes necessary to balance the advantage of having duplicate assays performed on a patient versus the benefits of having samples taken at a greater number of time points.

Obtaining all of the appropriate blood samples in outpatient studies is usually more difficult than in inpatient studies because the patient (1) may be unavailable, (2) may not have taken the correct amount of drug, or (3) may have taken the drug too short or too long a period before the time when the sample is to be drawn. When patients collect their own samples (e.g., 24-hr urine) the number of additional factors that may complicate sample collection becomes even greater (e.g., patients may not collect the sample in the correct manner, or at the right time, or the patient may stop collecting samples too soon).

Some Problems Encountered in Pharmacokinetic Studies

Some of the characteristic types of problems often encountered in pharmacokinetic studies are listed below. These problems may affect the conduct of the study or the interpretation of the results. Interested readers are referred to pharmacokinetic texts for additional information.

1. Ability of the assay methods to accurately and reproducibly measure drug levels in biological fluids.
2. Knowledge of the degree to which a drug is bound by protein in plasma in various situations. In some cases the free fraction of drug is markedly affected by certain pathological conditions or other drugs.
3. Differences in activity of optical isomers.
4. Differences in activity of metabolites, whose concentration may be affected by many factors (see section on metabolites below).
5. Type and degree of binding to receptor may affect the clinical time course independent of the drug's general concentration in plasma.
6. Nature of the drug attachment and interaction with receptors may be variable or unknown.
7. Variations in other aspects of drug behavior (e.g., active transport, type of kinetics, tolerance, tachyphylaxis).

METABOLITES

Determining the Importance of Drug Metabolites

The presence of metabolites may be suspected in numerous situations, including when a drug (1) has a highly different duration of effect in different species, (2) is an agonist in one species and a partial agonist or even antagonist in another, or (3) has a bioavailability profile that is markedly different in different species. Each of these reasons also may result from causes other than the presence of metabolites.

When a drug metabolite is identified chemically it is essential to determine whether it has biological activity or clinical importance for the overall

TABLE 12.8. *Selected aspects of establishing a profile of drug metabolites*[a]

1. Chemical identity
2. Quantity produced based on amount found in blood and/or urine (e.g., percent of parent drug converted to the metabolite)
3. Rate of production
4. Biological activities in animals
5. Clinical activity
6. Half-life
7. Presence of cumulation
8. Toxicity (e.g., pathology, clinical chemistry, hematology)[b]

[a] Each of these characteristics may be compared with the parent drug and most are initially determined in animals.
[b] If a metabolite discovered in humans is not detected in the animal species used to evaluate the toxicology profile of the parent drug, it may be necessary to (1) repeat the toxicology studies in a species that produces the metabolite and (2) evaluate the direct pharmacological effects of the metabolite in various animal test models.

project. A preliminary biological profile of each metabolite should be established, but it may not be necessary to complete each profile before deciding that the metabolite has little or no clinical importance. Alternatively, it may be possible to determine that the metabolite's importance is so great (in a negative sense) that further drug development of the parent drug must be terminated. A profile of a metabolite may vary from a superficial characterization of its pharmacokinetic parameters, toxicology, and preclinical properties to a more detailed examination than that given the parent drug. Representative types of biological and pharmacokinetic information that are often desired to profile a drug's metabolite are listed in Table 12.8.

If the metabolite has a profile that is clinically preferable to the parent drug in one or more important characteristics (e.g., less toxicity, longer duration of action), then serious consideration should be given to developing the metabolite as a drug. If the parent drug is already on the market (or close to the market) and the metabolite has significant advantages, then the metabolite may be developed independently and marketed as an improved version of the parent drug. If the parent drug has just started Phase I studies, then switching the development program to the metabolite may be relatively straightforward and highly desirable.

A metabolite that is to be tested in humans is viewed as a separate drug from a regulatory viewpoint. In the United States it is necessary to obtain a Notice of Claimed Investigational Exemption for a New Drug (IND) based on a new set of data for the metabolite before it may be tested in humans. The disadvantage of pursuing development of a metabolite for the market is that it will probably cost almost as much as that spent on developing the parent drug. Separate clinical studies, toxicological studies, and various types of technical development (including formulation development) must be conducted on any metabolite developed, even though it may be chemically (and biologically) similar to the parent drug. Many examples exist where structurally similar chemicals have totally different biological, chemical, and/or toxicological activities.

THERAPEUTIC DRUG MONITORING

Therapeutic drug monitoring refers to the measurement of a drug's plasma level and associating that level with either an acceptable clinical response, an underdose, or toxicity. The possibility of adopting therapeutic monitoring has been evaluated for many, if not most, drugs, but has only been found to be applicable for a small number. The reasons for this failure are numerous and generally relate to the criteria by which an ideal drug and a therapeutic response are associated when performing drug monitoring. The necessary criteria for being able to use therapeutic drug monitoring are:

1. Therapeutic effects of the drug in patients must be able to be measured with accuracy.
2. Free drug concentration in plasma (i.e., drug which is not bound to proteins) should equal free drug concentrations at receptor sites.
3. The drug should not be metabolized to active metabolites.
4. Tolerance should not develop.
5. Drug effects should be reversible.
6. Plasma concentrations above a certain level should represent a drug overdose or toxicity in almost all patients.
7. Drug levels must be measured with accuracy.

One drug that meets these criteria is phenytoin, but many other drugs measured routinely in laboratories fail one or more of these criteria. This is generally why data on their drug levels are less useful clinically than the results of phenytoin measurements. Levels of digoxin, for example, do not accurately indicate whether a patient is under- or overdosed. The same is true for several anticonvulsants and many other drugs. In most cases it is not possible to establish a therapeutic plasma range in which a drug's positive clinical responses occur. The drugs for which data of plasma concentrations are most useful include theophylline, lithium, aminoglycoside antibiotics, phenytoin, and possibly digoxin.

In developing new chronically administered drugs it is almost always worthwhile to evaluate whether a plasma concentration range of a drug may be established which represents the therapeutic range for most patients. If so, and the other criteria listed above are met, then it will provide physicians with a valuable tool to titrate and control patient dosing of potentially toxic drugs. Drugs with a large therapeutic index have little need of this approach, since there is a lesser chance of a therapeutic under- or overdosing and there is also a lesser likelihood of causing toxicity.

Therapeutic Window

This term is applied to the difference between the minimum and maximum doses that may be given patients to obtain an adequate clinical response and avoid intolerable toxic effects. The ratio of these values equals the therapeutic ratio or therapeutic index. The greater the therapeutic index, the greater a drug's margin of safety, and the wider the window.

13

Developing Drugs Worldwide

Organization of a Multinational Company • Worldwide Project Teams • Designing Core Studies • The Case Against Multinational Project Teams and a Core Clinical Package • Multinational Drug Studies • Selected Issues in International Drug Development

ORGANIZATION OF A MULTINATIONAL COMPANY

A simplified view of large multinational companies is described. These models view companies as primarily utilizing a centralized, decentralized, or balanced approach to conducting their business.

In the centralized model, the real power and decisions within the company are made at the company's headquarters. Most important decisions are made by a single leader, a committee, or a combination of the two. The subsidiary sites that conduct research, production, marketing, and other functions are primarily directed from the central site. Modifications of the centralized directives to the subsidiaries requested by local representatives must be approved at the central location.

In the decentralized model, the relative independence and decision making of subsidiary sites is substantial in some or all operating areas. One extreme is where each of the peripheral sites or regions retain autonomy over most of their actions and decide which of the parent company's drugs they wish to develop and/or market. The central site may or may not have a core package of data available to obtain regulatory approval, which is supplemented by studies conducted in the local countries or regions. Financially, the subsidiary may be relatively dependent or independent of the central site. Local laws govern many aspects of company behavior which affect the degree of autonomy possible. Some of the advantages and disadvantages of the centralized and decentralized models are listed in Table 13.1.

The third model contains an approximate balance of centralized and decentralized elements. The areas in which each of the peripheral groups (i.e., subsidiary sites) retains autonomy and in which the central authority pre-

TABLE 13.1. *Pros and cons of centralized versus decentralized forms of corporate management*

A. Centralized management advantages
   1. More clear understanding by all employees in terms of who is setting the corporate course, making decisions, and giving directions
   2. Allows integration of overall strategies
   3. Enables the entire corporation to change direction most easily

B. Centralized management disadvantages
   1. Local territories may lose their identity, image, and control of studies, regulatory submissions, marketing strategies, and other business decisions
   2. Centralized management may not be sufficiently sensitive to ideas coming from subsidiary companies or satellites

C. Decentralized management advantages
   1. Sensitive to local needs in each territory
   2. Allows many units to have some autonomy and to be differentially treated
   3. Permits more rapid decision making and action in response to local issues

D. Decentralized management disadvantages
   1. More duplication of effort occurs, at least some of which is unnecessary and unproductive
   2. More difficulties are present in communications between territories and headquarters and between one territory and another

dominates should be clearly specified. Meetings of regional directors with the overall board of directors or chairman of the board may be a forum where this balance may be established and maintained. The central board of directors may establish policies within which regional and local directors may operate according to clearly established guidelines. Needs of local directors also flow up through the organization in this system.

Another model of multinational pharmaceutical organizations is of a conglomerate consisting of several independent companies. Each of these companies is autonomous and may have its own approach to drug development. Each company within the conglomerate may emphasize a centralized, decentralized, or balanced approach to management.

WORLDWIDE PROJECT TEAMS

The worldwide project team is a group of individuals who plan and execute the activities needed to achieve the goals of worldwide development. Membership on the team will probably include at some point during the life of the project (or perhaps for its duration) representatives of research and development (e.g., preclinical sciences, clinical, toxicology, regulatory, chemical development, technical development, metabolism, statistics), marketing, production, and coordination departments.

Although some companies develop a new drug by utilizing a single international project team, many others operate with separate teams at each independent research and development site in addition to or instead of a worldwide team. Each site may have a project team leader and their own team. The teams may coordinate their activities through various mechanisms (e.g., memoranda, telephone calls, visits) and/or they may each report to a central management group or individual who coordinates their efforts. This individual would generally be part of a matrix system or senior management. An international group composed of some of the members from each site could also function in the role of coordinating the overall activities of the various independent project teams, which are developing all of the company's investigational drugs.

DESIGNING CORE STUDIES

Many multinational pharmaceutical companies are trying to better integrate their international activities and function more as a single worldwide company. One of the issues they are grappling with is the question of whether a core package of studies will increase the efficiency of their drug development on an international scale. A "core package" refers to a group of clinical and nonclinical studies that require only minor revisions to be suitable for submission to multiple regulatory agencies in different countries. The core package contains data from preclinical and clinical studies necessary to answer most or all safety and efficacy questions of major interest (Table 13.2) to a regulatory authority. Locally conducted studies of interest to each specific regulatory agency are generally submitted with the core package.

This issue may be discussed in several contexts, but one of the most important of these relates to the magnitude or size of the core package. The greater the number of studies included in the core package and the more completely they are described, the less likely it is that only minor revisions will be required in order to submit the core package to many regulatory authorities. The smaller the number of studies in the core package, the easier it will be to modify the core package to make it suitable for meeting requirements of multiple regulatory authorities. A smaller core package has greater flexibility than does a larger core package. But, the smaller core package will require a greater number of additional studies, conducted either locally or in another country, to complete each dossier.

Theoretically, it initially appears that a small core package would save less time than would be saved with a larger core package. If the core package is too large it will be impractical and inefficient to use, and if the core package is too small it will not yield the benefits desired. Thus, there is a need for balance in determining an appropriate size of the core package which will

TABLE 13.2. *Example of a core dossier of clinical studies and data*

A. Phase I studies
   1. Single- and multiple-dose tolerance studies
   2. Pharmacokinetics[a] (e.g., effects of single dose, multiple doses, dose–response, drug interactions, bioequivalence; effects in children, elderly, renal compromised patients; effects of food)
   3. Special pharmacology and/or physiology studies (e.g., mechanism of action studies)

B. Phase II studies
   1. Efficacy studies: dose-ranging studies, active drug control with placebo (if possible), and placebo-controlled[b]
   2. Special patient populations (e.g., those with decreased cardiac function, elderly)
   3. Efficacy studies: dose–response studies if ethics prevent use of a placebo[c]

C. Phase III studies
   1. Long-term Phase III studies of up to 1 year (or longer—if appropriate)
   2. Short-term Phase III efficacy studies

D. Studies conducted in all phases
   1. Special safety studies
   2. All adverse drug reactions obtained, with particular reference to incidence data

[a] See Tables 12.1 and 12.2.
[b] Two pivotal studies per indication, including data on the dose–response relationship.
[c] Use of placebo treatment is restricted in certain countries.

decrease time required for multiple submissions and reduce the total work and costs. Finding the ideal magnitude of a core package is complicated by the fact that all drug development programs at a single corporation differ from each other, and the optimal core package size for two drugs will vary widely. The nature and number of the studies in the core package also will vary depending on the particular regulatory agencies to which the dossiers will eventually be sent.

Regulatory Input

Both direct and indirect regulatory input affect the design of a core package of studies. Indirect input results from current regulations in the countries for which the core package of studies is being prepared. Regulations have enormous influence in shaping almost every study on investigational drugs. Regulations are probably the most important single factor responsible for the improved standards in design, conduct, and analysis of clinical studies over the last several decades. Regulatory input will affect both the type and number of studies to be done.

Direct regulatory input refers to statements, suggestions, and directives from regulatory agencies. These may occur at any or all stages of a drug's life. Initial planning and development meetings may be held with regulatory agencies to help plan studies that would be a part of the core package. During the conduct of the studies there will often be regulatory input, especially when an agency has specific questions or concerns to be addressed. While the registration dossier is being prepared, regulatory considerations directly affect the format and manner of data presentation. The type and nature of the direct interactions between regulatory agencies and pharmaceutical corporations during the planning, conduct, review, and approval stages is discussed in Chapter 21. The nature of these interactions varies greatly between different countries. For example, there are traditionally more interactions between a sponsor and the Food and Drug Administration (FDA) in the United States than there are between a sponsor and the Department of Health and Social Security (DHSS) in the United Kingdom.

Making a Core Package System Work

There are innumerable difficulties associated with creating a practical system for developing and using core packages of data. There are also innumerable difficulties for a multinational drug company if a core package system is not used. Once the decision has been reached to utilize a core package system there are a number of principles that will facilitate its implementation and successful outcome.

If a company is initiating or experimenting with a core package system, it may be desirable to choose one or two projects that have a high likelihood of success and are at an early stage of development as test cases. The sponsor will gain invaluable experience using such drugs as models. Initial questions for the project group to consider are listed in Table 13.3.

1. Whenever possible, have a multinational group develop the plan for a drug's development prior to initiating clinical studies. If clinical studies are already in Phase II it may be exceedingly difficult to develop and implement a successful core package system. This is because (1) some appropriate studies may not have been conducted, (2) some appropriate studies may not have been properly designed, (3) some inappropriate studies may have been conducted which have raised new issues to be addressed, and (4) the individuals involved may not have the experience, skills and authority needed to develop and implement a core package for a complex project.
2. It is more efficient in developing a core approach for most drugs to wait until a drug has demonstrated initial efficacy in Phase II studies before implementing many activities requiring detailed coordination between two or more company sites that are each directing the drug's

TABLE 13.3. *Selected questions for an international project group to initially consider*

1. Which dosage form(s) of the compound are to be developed?
2. Which countries will develop the drug and in which order?[a]
3. How will the project team be constituted and who will be in charge?
4. How will the project team operate?
5. How will the overall strategy be developed, reviewed, and revised (when necessary)?
6. How will the plans be developed both nationally and internationally for:
   preclinical studies?
   clinical studies?
   data management?
   coordination of efforts?
7. How will standards be maintained at an acceptable level in each country? Will standardized international monitoring practices be developed?
8. How will this matrix approach be coordinated with ongoing work conducted using line management systems and control?

[a] See Table 13.13.

development. This approach will preserve the company's resources and efforts for those drugs that are most likely to reach the market, since most new drugs that are tested in humans are terminated during Phases I and II.

3. The project team should develop criteria and implement procedures to identify which countries will receive the core package and to determine all of the relevant regulatory considerations from those countries that may influence the design of toxicological, preclinical, clinical, technical development, and marketing studies. The criteria and procedures used for this purpose with other drugs will generally require little or no modification. The team must also be able to incorporate modifications into the core package so that it will meet any special requirements of the regulatory agencies for which it is intended. Table 13.4 describes roles of the regulatory representatives on the project team in planning worldwide regulatory strategies.
4. The medical representatives on the international project team may jointly plan the clinical studies to be included in the core package. This includes planning of the following information for specific studies: (1) indication(s), (2) dosage form(s), (3) study designs, (4) resources and equipment required, (5) locales to conduct studies, (6) specific or general types of investigators to use, (7) number of patients needed per study and per phase, (8) monitoring strategy, and (9) various other factors. Specific considerations for a core clinical protocol have been presented (de Maar, 1986).
5. The relevant representatives from various company sites who are members of the international project team may plan the technical development and toxicological development for the core package. One as-

TABLE 13.4. *Roles of the regulatory representatives on the project team in planning worldwide regulatory strategies*

1. Identify each country's requirements for registration and pricing studies
2. Develop an international dossier to assist local groups in registering the drug
3. Discuss pertinent issues with regulatory authorities
4. Discuss pertinent issues with national opinion makers and local experts
5. Reply to questions on regulatory dossiers from subsidiaries
6. Confirm that dossiers are submitted to local regulatory authorities
7. Reply to questions on dossiers from local regulatory authorities
8. Confirm that each subsidiary understands the role of the project team in providing the dossier, in communicating with the regulatory agency, and in communicating with the local company
9. Determine comparative agents to use in Phase III studies (e.g., in some countries the price a company may charge for a drug is heavily dependent on the drug(s) used as an active control in Phase III studies)
10. Identify appropriate countries in which to conduct Phase II studies
11. Develop or utilize a method of keeping up with changing requirements and situations in relevant regulatory agencies
12. Determine responsibilities of each group that will contribute to the international regulatory submission and to each local dossier

pect of the plan is to determine which parts of the company will have responsibility for which parts of the core package.

6. The amount of documentation relating to a clinical study is a major issue in determining whether the core package system will work. Since the FDA requires more documentation than almost all other countries, the core package system is generally agreed to work best for drug companies that are most familiar with conducting studies that meet FDA regulations. Most of these companies are either based in the United States or have major subsidiaries here.
7. Company representatives in each country to receive the core package must discuss and agree on various issues with the parent organization. These include dosage forms to be developed, indications to be pursued, and technical specifications of the formulation (e.g., dyes, duration of stability, size of capsule or tablet). If disagreements or problems arise and modifications of the development program are requested or required, then these modifications must be factored into decisions regarding the type of product to be made and tested, the target indications, and which countries will be able to benefit from the results obtained (Table 13.5).
8. Most companies believe in tailoring the core package to meet the requirements of the most demanding major regulatory authority. This is generally agreed to be the FDA in the United States, although there are certainly exceptions. In certain situations, standards of the European Common Market should be used as a guideline for organizing the nature of studies to be conducted. If this is done, then separate well-

TABLE 13.5. *Roles of the marketing representative(s) on the project team in planning worldwide marketing strategies*[a]

1. Determine marketing interest in each territory where the drug could be sold
2. Participate in choosing dosage forms, formulations, and capsule colors for all forms of the drug to be marketed
3. Propose and/or discuss which clinical studies would meet common marketing needs in all or most territories
4. Participate in focus groups[b] and roundtable discussions on marketing issues
5. Design a flexible approach that may be used for worldwide promotion of a new drug
6. Consider capabilities of the marketing organization in each territory when designing the strategy and setting goals
7. Assist marketing representatives in each territory to plan the best launch possible

[a] Other roles of marketing representatives on the project team are listed in Table 22.7.

[b] Focus groups conduct interviews with a specific group of potential users (generally physicians) to determine their views and reactions to statements or questions about a product. The questions may relate to a real or hypothetical product.

controlled major Phase II efficacy (i.e., pivotal) studies may be planned for the United States if a New Drug Application (NDA) is to be submitted to the FDA.

9. It is likely that any core package of clinical studies will be inadequate to meet regulatory requirements in all targeted countries. Depending on regulatory requirements, ethics, culture, and other factors of the targeted countries, it may be necessary to exclude one or more countries from receiving the entire core package. It is nonetheless likely that different parts of the core package will be included in the regulatory dossier submitted in each country. Some of the questions for the clinical

TABLE 13.6. *Selected questions for clinical representatives on an international project group to consider*

1. Which studies should be conducted to demonstrate drug safety, efficacy, and pharmacokinetics?
2. How will dose-ranging studies be conducted to evaluate the maximally tolerated dose and also the optimal dose(s) to demonstrate efficacy?
3. Which studies should (hopefully) be the pivotol studies and where should they be performed?
4. Who will prepare the clinical protocols and data collection forms?
5. How will these be reviewed to maximize their usefulness?
6. How will differences in ideas and viewpoints be arbitrated and decided?
7. What standards will be used for the clinical protocols?
8. How can data from studies be rapidly shared among all relevant individuals?
9. How can each relevant group have appropriate input into decision making on expected issues and unexpected problems?
10. Which group will have responsibility for preparing statistical analyses of the results? How will differences of opinion be resolved?

TABLE 13.7. *Levels of detail in reports of a clinical study*[a]

1. Synopsis of one paragraph to one page
2. Manuscript that may be published as an article in the medical literature
3. Comprehensive medical and statistical reports—prepared separately or combined
4. Supportive information (e.g., protocol, listings of adverse reactions, abnormal laboratory data, patient discontinuations, reasons for exclusion of patients from a study, pharmacy records, statistical analyses)
5. Raw data and data collection forms

[a] These are listed in order from the most general to the most detailed and specific. Not all of these data are required by a regulatory agency for all studies. The appropriate amount of data submitted must be determined for each application submitted. See Fig. 13.1 for additional details.

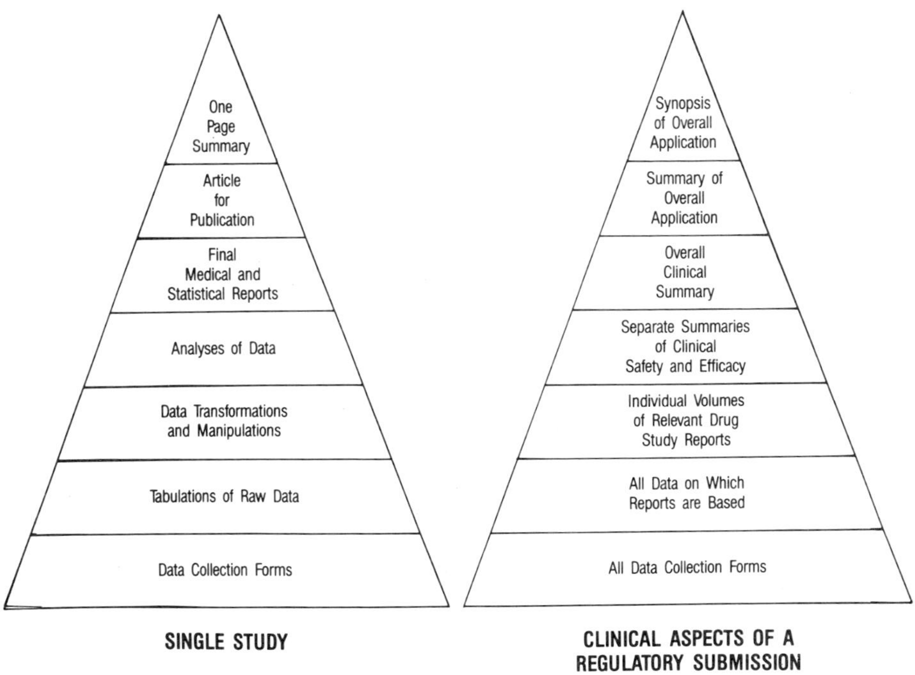

FIG. 13.1. Progressive summaries of clinical data in a single study and in a regulatory submission. The synopsis of the overall application is approximately one to five pages, whereas the one-volume summary is generally 50 to 500 pages. Not all components are necessarily required for a regulatory submission.

TABLE 13.8. *Administrative roles of the project team*

1. Recommend to proceed to full-scale development
2. Inform subsidiaries about new projects
3. Prioritize regulatory submissions based on available information (e.g., market forecasts, regulatory requirements, anticipated availability of data)
4. Develop a plan that addresses medical, regulatory, and marketing considerations
5. Determine the target countries in which the drug will be investigated
6. Recommend to discontinue development in one or more countries
7. Recommend to terminate the project
8. Agree on a plan, methods to monitor progress, and methods to facilitate disputes

representatives on the international project group to consider are listed in Table 13.6. The basic levels of detail in clinical reports which may be submitted to regulatory agencies are listed in Table 13.7. Additional levels are illustrated in Fig. 13.1. This figure shows multiple levels of clinical data and summaries in a single clinical study and in a single regulatory submission. The term pyramid has been used to describe this concept of multiple levels of detail in a single study (Snoddy et al., 1985).

10. Various administrative roles of a project team must be considered, discussed, and determined (Table 13.8) to develop a drug effectively.

Major Types of Foreign Studies from a United States Perspective

Many clinical studies are not entirely United States or foreign studies, but have participation by groups from different countries. Five of the many possible variations are presented (Table 13.9). The activities performed, plus the management and coordination functions differ for each of these major types of studies that are established by the United States company. In the following examples it is assumed that the company in the United States is a subsidiary of a foreign company. If not, then more of the management decisions will probably be made in the United States, unless the foreign subsidiary is given autonomy to make decisions on these issues. A core submission may include several types of these studies (see Table 13.2).

Type 1

The entire management and coordination of these studies are operated in the same manner as studies that are initiated and conducted domestically. One of the few differences is to keep informed the relevant medical regulatory, marketing, and other representatives who are in the country in which

TABLE 13.9. *Major types of foreign (i.e., non-United States) studies conducted by a single company*[a]

Protocol prepared by	Study initiated by	Study monitored from	Final statistical and medical reports[b] prepared by	Data intended for regulatory submission primarily in
1. United States	United States	United States	United States then foreign country	United States
2. United States	United States and foreign country	United States and foreign country	United States and possibly foreign country	United States
3. United States and foreign country	United States and foreign country	United States and foreign country	United States and foreign country	United States and foreign country
4. United States and foreign country	Foreign country	Foreign country	Foreign country then United States	United States and foreign country
5. Foreign country	Foreign country	Foreign country	Foreign country then United States	Foreign country

[a] Numerous variations occur on these types. For foreign-based companies, an additional country (i.e., that of the parent company) may be involved. Other variations would include joint development by two companies, use of a contract organization, and collaboration with a government organization.

[b] Reports and data prepared by one site will be reviewed and may be reanalyzed and/or reinterpreted by the other site (or other sponsor).

the study is being conducted. It is assumed that all regulatory and company permissions have been obtained to do the study in the specific country.

Type 2

The major difference in this type of study compared with Type 1 is that the initiation and monitoring is jointly organized and run. This requires coordination among the monitors and project leaders. The management is the same as for Type 1 studies.

Type 3

In this model all activities are jointly established and conducted. The balance of activities will vary on a given study for each aspect. The study is viewed as a joint venture, although one site usually has more of a leadership role. If the United States has the leadership role, then the major management decisions are usually made here. If the foreign (i.e., parent) country has the leadership role, then management decisions are made there. The coordination functions would be operated semi-independently at each site, but with frequent communication to keep individuals informed and plans up-to-date.

Type 4

In this type of study the balance of activities has clearly shifted to the foreign country, which is now the group playing the greatest role. The original impetus for the study may have come from either the United States or foreign country. Both groups will be involved with management issues, but most decisions will be made by the specific group that "owns" the study, usually after consultation with the other group.

Type 5

In the "all foreign" study, the comparable United States project leader (if the project exists in the United States) or project correspondent (if there is no project in the United States) passively monitors activities on the clinical studies. No coordination or management activities are routinely conducted, except for review of reports generated by the project leader or correspondent to keep management informed.

Overall Coordination and Management Review

Regardless of the type of study, reports prepared for management committees at one site are sent to and reviewed by senior managers at the other site. Thus, important issues relating to clinical studies are usually discussed at both sites, although there is often a time lag before the other site hears about the issue. The magnitude of the time lag depends on the importance of the study and on the importance of the issue.

Coordination occurs at multiple levels between people at both sites, including project leaders, project planners, heads of research, heads of the matrix function, heads of development, plus department heads of all functions involved (e.g., regulatory, medical, statistics, chemical development, pharmaceutics, toxicology).

How Are Core Packages Perceived?

By FDA

It is possible for a pharmaceutical company outside the United States to assemble a core package of data for a drug and to license that drug to a company in the United States. Although the company in the United States has the option, in theory, of submitting the package as is, without conducting any studies in the United States, this approach is not generally viewed favorably by the FDA. Although the FDA has become more willing in recent years to accept foreign data, they apparently prefer that some studies are conducted within the United States. One reason for this viewpoint is that the FDA is less able to conduct an audit of study sites to assure themselves that the studies have been conducted in an adequate and acceptable manner. Other reasons are discussed by Lasagna (1986).

When the FDA views foreign data they prefer to examine a published article by a recognized authority (when available) rather than solely having data reentered in computers and reanalyzed by a sponsor in the United States. The former technique allows them to understand and assess the interpretation of the study from the investigator's perspective, whereas this is not usually possible when the latter technique is used.

By Multinational Companies

The way that pharmaceutical companies view the core package system depends in part on the size of the company and whether the company's headquarters is based in the United States. Large multinational companies either based in the United States or with a large subsidiary here are more likely to favor the core package system than are large multinational companies based outside the United States if they do not have a large subsidiary here. This occurs because it is generally easier to use data from studies conducted in the United States for regulatory submissions in other countries than to use data from studies conducted in other countries for regulatory submissions in the United States. Moreover, companies with a large group in the United States generally have a better understanding than do other companies of how to conduct studies that meet FDA standards.

Each country that is a major market for pharmaceuticals has different regulations. It is uncertain whether the time necessary to complete and submit regulatory submissions, plus the time for regulatory approval, will be significantly diminished by utilizing a core package of data. Differences in dossier format and often content require significant amounts of time to appropriately modify for each new country. Clinical studies conducted in one country may not be acceptable as major or pivotal studies in another.

THE CASE AGAINST MULTINATIONAL PROJECT TEAMS AND A CORE CLINICAL PACKAGE

A worldwide project team is an important mechanism that will help turn a multinational company that is operating inefficiently into a more efficient single international company. But there are also some reasons against using

TABLE 13.10. *Synopsis of arguments against using worldwide project teams*[a]

1. There is a shortage of suitable leaders for these teams in many companies
2. Errors made in strategy by the team may be major ones
3. Committees in general tend to be conservative
4. There is a potential loss of input from advisors from local countries who can often provide valuable information on submitting a dossier and on expediting its approval
5. Trying to develop and complete a worldwide plan may take more time than if a number of subsidiaries developed their own plans that are loosely coordinated with other subsidiaries and the parent organization
6. Many projects are of local interest or are concentrated in only a few territories and do not require a worldwide project team
7. Many projects are too small in commercial potential to justify the effort and expense of a worldwide project team

[a] There are numerous conterarguments to these reasons. The soundness of the counterarguments must be judged by senior research managers.

worldwide project teams (Table 13.10). These considerations should be evaluated each time a new project is adopted, even though there may be worldwide project teams in the same company for other projects.

Despite the obvious appeal and apparent value of a core package of clinical data, there are several reasons that suggest it is not a panacea and has significant drawbacks. Most of the following points may be overcome with a carefully developed core package, but consideration of these issues is often necessary.

1. Regulations differ widely in most countries and the core package may require so much adjustment from country to country that its value may be severely compromised. Some countries require specific study designs to be used for clinical studies conducted in their country and possibly may not accept some of the studies that are included in the core package.
2. Most drugs are developed using different dosage strengths, dosages, formulations, colors, and other specifications for different countries. There are often sound reasons for many of these differences and despite vigorous attempts to standardize most aspects of a drug's development, there are usually certain limitations. For example, the choice of colors for a capsule or tablet may create problems in certain countries because few dyes used to create colors are universally acceptable. There may be sound reasons related to local customs or culture as to why certain colors are undesirable or even unacceptable in some countries. Many excipients are not universally acceptable. Preferred dosage forms often differ between countries (e.g., capsules, tablets, suppositories, liquids). For some products there may be strong desires in some countries to market certain specialized forms (e.g., aerosols, powders, shampoos, lotions, ointments, talcs) and not others.

3. A statistical group in one country may desire to reanalyze and reinterpret data from a study originally performed and analyzed by another subsidiary or the parent company located in a different country. In that situation, the final medical report may differ substantially from the original document. If the study was performed outside the United States, the detailed documentation required by the FDA may not be available, especially if the sponsor is a foreign drug company that is not extremely familiar with FDA requirements or if it has not adhered to those requirements in the study. This may create problems in terms of a core package, especially if different interpretations are reached. Currently, this is less of a problem since the studies may be easily downgraded from pivotal to supportive studies, or in some cases not even described in detail. In some companies, statistical and medical reports are only written once. This is done by the group that ran the study, although input is accepted on the methods to use and results to include from other national groups of the same company.
4. The quantity of data which must be submitted with a regulatory dossier varies between countries. In general, the core package will have to contain both the maximum quantity and quality of data obtained in all studies included. In addition, some countries require more pharmacokinetic data than do others. Some countries require more pharmacy or geriatric data. If each of these supplementary pieces are added to all core packages it may raise problems in the future because of (1) "too much" data in the application increasing the standards expected of all applications, (2) additional preparation time, and (3) longer time for regulatory review.
5. Dose-ranging studies to evaluate safety in humans must be performed in a manner that allows appropriate doses to be chosen which are to be studied for efficacy. These data also permit an understanding of the therapeutic window which is eventually determined. But, dose-ranging studies performed in some countries are based on a different philosophy or goal than in others. For example, dose-ranging studies in normal volunteers in the United Kingdom usually stop at the dose expected to yield efficacy in patients, whereas dose escalation studies in the United States usually continue in volunteers to the point where toxicity is observed. This may lead to differences in doses studied in Phase II studies and eventually may lead to (1) different recommended dosing regimens between different countries and (2) use of different studies to support the recommendations.
6. It is sometimes necessary to use different active controls in different countries. The price that may be charged for a new drug depends, in some countries, on the active drug chosen to compare with the test drug in Phase III studies. Some drug studies may therefore be conducted in one country when they are not suitable for use as part of a

core package for other countries. Moreover, some standard drugs included for comparison purposes may be chosen because they are widely used by specialists in one country, but may not be used by the same group of specialists in another country. Some comparison drugs may not be marketed in some of the countries where data are submitted. Another issue is when general practitioners use a standard drug that is different than that used by specialists for the same disease.

7. Ethical standards vary widely in clinical studies conducted between different countries. It may be impractical to conduct studies that will meet standards in all countries in terms of placebo, informed consent, Institutional Review Boards, and other issues.
8. National thought leaders who use a drug in one country may use it differently than in another country, based on differences in experience or opinion. It may not be easy for a core package of studies to accommodate these differences by designing multiple studies that explore different types of drug use in different countries.
9. If studies are performed at foreign locations that have less stringent monitoring than in the United States, serious issues that were either unknown by the monitors or inadequately addressed may arise in a study. Since most investigators are (rightfully) more oriented toward clinical results and helping their patients than they are to adhering to protocols, there may be a greater tendency to stray from the protocol in some foreign studies, unless monitoring is rigorous.
10. The language of medicine is not used the same way in different countries. This may lead to problems in combining data on patient diagnosis, measurement of effects, or adverse reactions from different countries.

Each of these situations may create pressures to use different clinical studies for each major dossier. The group of efficacy studies that support one dosing regimen may not generally be used to support others. Studies using one dosing regimen in one country may not be useful in another country where the dosing regimen differs. Studies performed with the formulation to be marketed in one country could not be used in countries where the final formulation differs, unless appropriate bioequivalence studies were conducted and yielded acceptable data. Additional considerations of these issues are listed in Table 13.11.

As part of the planning activities it may be prudent and possible to develop an international team of individuals who will assure intelligent, realistic, and imaginative plans to efficiently develop the drug. This step may occur without a need for utilizing any but a minimal core package of studies.

Mini-core Package

One alternative to a relatively complete core package of studies is to develop a small nucleus of studies, such as those for safety, pharmacokinetics,

TABLE 13.11. *Synopsis of arguments against the core package system*[a]

1. The core system may act to increase time and costs of drug development[b]
2. The core system is not useful for all countries (e.g., Japan)
3. The worldwide project team concept that is necessary to develop the core package system has various drawbacks[c]
4. If the company is foreign based it may be difficult for them to plan a development program that adequately meets U. S. standards
5. The absence of a systematic approach that has more apparent (or real) disorder may work to the advantage of larger companies. A highly organized and simplified system permits more competition to develop from smaller companies
6. When studies from one country are reanalyzed and reinterpreted in another, different interpretations may be drawn which tend to diminish or compromise the usefulness of the core package
7. Different philosophies of drug development in different countries may make it extremely difficult to reach consensus on (1) the studies to include in a core package, (2) how to design those studies, or (3) the order in which studies should be conducted

[a] See footnote to Table 13.10.

[b] The core system adds to pressures to increase the time and costs of drug development by raising standards all over the world. Many countries have a particular area where their requirements tend to be more stringent than in other countries (e.g., pharmacokinetic data in Scandinavia, geriatric data in England, pharmacy data in Belgium). If the core package attempts to meet all of these standards in all submissions there will probably be a major increase in both costs and time of drug development.

[c] See Table 13.10 for several examples.

and supportive Phase III efficacy studies that could be utilized as a mini-core package in most countries. Each country would add the major efficacy and/or other studies deemed necessary for registration. Nonetheless, even this alternative or a different type of mini-core package will require that dossiers be rewritten for most major countries in which the drug will be registered. By the time the core group of studies for each country are rewritten and reformatted, it may not have saved time over the traditional method of planning each country's submission independently, using as many studies from other locales as possible.

Conclusion

It is the author's opinion that careful planning of drug development to (1) obtain consensus on the strategy and approach, (2) seek input from marketing, (3) minimize duplication of efforts, (4) conduct studies at as high a standard as possible, (5) monitor all activities frequently, (6) maintain open communications, and (7) adjust the development program as necessary are among the most important factors in expediting registration of a new drug in multiple countries. The core package system should be developed to the extent that it expedites regulatory submissions worldwide. The appropriate size of the core package must be determined for each drug, but an extensive core package should be avoided in most situations.

There will probably never be complete congruence between the specific studies that must be conducted in the United States to obtain an NDA on a particular drug and those studies conducted outside the United States. Nonetheless there is some overlap, and certain studies conducted in foreign countries will meet the FDA's requirements.

MULTINATIONAL DRUG STUDIES

In addition to conducting various clinical studies in different countries as described above, it is also possible to conduct a single clinical study in multiple countries. There are occasions when conducting a multicenter study across national borders is a worthwhile idea. This idea is most practical when language, customs, culture, medical practice, and the processes of drug development are similar or comparable in each of the countries involved. If any of these factors differ, then it is usually not worthwhile to conduct multicenter studies that are also multinational. One exception is for certain extremely large multicenter studies where adequate resources are available to overcome the problems involved (e.g., the 71-center, extracranial/intracranial [EC/IC] bypass surgery study).

Even if the study is eventually successful, the efforts necessary to insure uniformity across national boundaries often outweigh the benefits obtained. A simple alternative is to break a single multinational study into separate national studies, each of which may be conducted at either a single site or multiple sites. Regulatory authorities are sometimes skeptical of data generated in a multicentered study when investigators in different countries are involved. There are a few instances when the multinational approach should be considered. One of those situations is for some studies conducted in both the United States and Canada. Factors concerned with coordination of multinational studies are listed in Table 13.12, and criteria to use in choosing a country in which to conduct a clinical study are listed in Table 13.13.

If there are compelling arguments to conduct a multinational study, then a prestudy roundtable meeting is essential. This session should review all aspects of the study and of collecting data. Methods to insure uniformity of diagnosis, treatment, and interpretation of terminology used in both the protocol and data collection forms should be discussed. A no-carbon data collection form can be prepared so that there is one language on the top sheet and English (or other language) on the second sheet. This process will assist in data editing and processing.

Conducting Studies in Developing Countries

A few considerations for conducting studies in foreign countries are discussed in Chapter 34 of *Guide to Clinical Studies and Developing Protocols* (Spilker, 1984). A number of additional considerations are presented below.

TABLE 13.12. *Coordinating multinational clinical studies*[a]

1. Establish the specific requirements of each country in terms of regulatory, patent, legal, ethical, political, social, marketing, and other perspectives
2. Determine if a multinational study is necessary or important and feasible to conduct, based on regulatory requirements and potential benefits of each prospective country that will participate
3. Develop a detailed integrated strategic plan that addresses these national considerations
4. Identify key personnel and assignment of responsibilities that minimizes duplication of effort. Many similar studies are often performed in multiple countries
5. Establish standards that protocols, data collection procedures, and statistical analyses must meet if the data are to be used in multiple countries. These are usually determined to be the standards of the strictest regulatory agency, provided that the efforts of achieving these standards are found to be cost effective
6. Provide reports of medical and other studies in a format from which local submission packages (dossiers) may be easily compiled
7. Plan Phase IV and marketing studies with the same thoroughness used to plan investigational studies
8. Consider using a central group to monitor clinical activities at each separate study site to help insure uniformity of data
9. Consider any changes in scientific, regulatory, financial, political, medical, ethical, and social aspects throughout the study (or studies) which may influence the study in any way
10. Meet on a periodic basis with the project manager and others to review and update the overall development plan
11. Communicate the revised plan, dates, and responsibilities to all relevant individuals

[a] These factors relate to a single study as well as to a series of multinational studies on one or more drugs. Almost all factors also relate to coordinating efforts of an international project group that does not have any multinational studies in their clinical plan. A multinational study refers to a single clinical study conducted in two or more countries. All multinational studies are multicentered, but not all multicentered studies are multinational.

TABLE 13.13. *Criteria to use in choosing a country for a clinical study*

1. Availability of suitable investigator(s)
2. Availability of an adequate number of suitable patients
3. Ability to conduct a study according to acceptable standards
4. Ability to monitor the study in the manner desired
5. Physical accessibility and convenience of the study site(s)
6. Cooperation, resources, expertise, and quality of local staff
7. Speed with which the study can be initiated and completed
8. Acceptability of previous studies conducted in that country by regulatory authorities in other countries
9. Manner in which the study fits worldwide drug development and registration plans
10. Projected impact on company's profitability in conducting the study in a specific country

TABLE 13.14. *Problems of collecting data on adverse reactions in developing countries*

1. Many patients are illiterate and unaware of the identity of drugs they are receiving
2. Many drugs which are available over-the-counter are only sold by prescription in other countries
3. Difficulties are involved in maintaining adequate patient care, especially in rural and overcrowded areas
4. Many physicians are overworked and do not have sufficient opportunities to report or study adverse reactions
5. Patients are often treated by multiple physicians with little or no continuity of patient care
6. Many patients have concurrent illnesses that complicate detection and evaluation of adverse reactions
7. People may have in their homes many potent and potentially dangerous drugs that they are willing to use, which decreases compliance with the prescribed regimen
8. Patients may be following local medical "folk" practices at the same time they are taking drugs developed in industrial countries
9. Difficulty of hiring and maintaining an adequately trained staff

If patients do not want to remain in a hospital for a study or if there are too few or inadequate hospital facilities, then it may be possible to:

1. Have patients leave the hospital during the day and return at night.
2. Have physicians travel to the patient's location to test patients and insure adequate compliance.
3. Enlist family members to give drugs, take measurements, or maintain a diary.
4. Schedule fewer patient visits, while lengthening the period between visits.
5. Shorten the duration of study treatment.

Other considerations relating to the planning and conduct of studies in underdeveloped countries include:

1. Definitions of diseases sometimes vary between countries. This is especially true of syndromes and conditions that are ill-defined.
2. Criteria of efficacy may vary greatly. Investigators in some countries may emphasize different endpoints that relate to pharmacological, clinical, or quality of life measurements.
3. Definitions of what is considered an adverse reaction, as well as judgments of its severity, may differ.
4. Collecting data on adverse reactions is often difficult (Table 13.14). Specialists may not be available to evaluate patients, provide consults, or use sophisticated testing methods.

Two other considerations that relate to the company which sponsors studies are: (1) resources may not be efficiently used if studies are duplicated unnecessarily in less developed countries; (2) the needs and goals of a company's local subsidiary may not match those of the central headquarters or those of an integrated international development program.

SELECTED ISSUES IN INTERNATIONAL DRUG DEVELOPMENT

Should One or More Countries Be Targeted for the Initial Registration?

Initial marketing of a new drug in countries with less stringent regulatory requirements serves to generate patient exposures while additional studies are conducted elsewhere. It also tends to provide some comfort to most regulatory authorities to know that a new drug they are evaluating is already marketed and patients are receiving the same drug elsewhere. Another positive aspect is that significant adverse reactions have a greater chance of being discovered at an earlier date. The probability of discovering new serious adverse reactions with a moderate frequency progressively diminishes as a drug is used more widely. This is a beneficial aspect of increasing patient exposures under monitored conditions.

What Role Should Marketing Play in Establishing Research and Development Goals?

Marketing should provide input into goal setting while not making decisions that control the direction of research and development departments. At some companies the marketing division identifies marketing needs and creates a business opportunity list of desirable research objectives. The question is whether marketing objectives control the areas in which research is conducted or whether research innovations provide marketing with drugs to sell and therapeutic opportunities to develop.

Ideally, marketing provides information to the research and development division at all stages of a project. That information assists in the decisions on management and direction of research, but without controlling the direction of that research. A prototype (ideal) package insert is used by some marketing groups at the initiation of a project to establish and link communications with clinicians inside the company. This technique may allow a project to be terminated relatively painlessly when the minimally acceptable clinical profile is not supported by data obtained.

Which Formulations Should Be Developed?

Each company attempts to balance the savings generated by having the least number of formulations developed with the needs, desires, and requirements of different countries and marketing groups. This is a highly complex issue. It is usually necessary and practical to develop several formulations of a single drug that is to be sold in several different countries. Technical and clinical development of multiple formulations may be conducted simultaneously, sequentially, or in an overlapping manner. Both cost and benefit should be evaluated for each dosage form and formulation that is considered for development.

Should Manufacturing Be Centralized or Diversified?

Despite numerous benefits that accrue as a result of centralizing the manufacture of a drug there are various reasons why this procedure is often impractical or impossible. For instance, (1) some countries require production to take place within their borders before a drug is allowed to be sold, (2) production facilities may be fully committed at one location and available at one or several other locations, (3) multiple formulations may make it impractical to produce all varieties of a drug at a single site, (4) cost savings and/or tax benefits may make local production attractive, (5) a final step in a synthesis may be the only part of the synthesis performed locally, (6) in event of a fire or other disaster at one site there will be another facility that can increase production to supply the affected markets, (7) special equipment (e.g., for manufacturing sterile products) may only be available at certain locations, and (8) there may be regulations preventing export of a finished product for sale in another country when the drug is not approved for sale in the country of manufacture. A related issue is whether all stability tests should be conducted in each of the multiple locales where a drug is made or whether they should be performed at a central site.

Are Statistical Approaches Applied Identically to All Studies Worldwide?

Just as standards of conducting clinical studies vary from country to country, so too do statistical techniques and standards. A worldwide consensus of approaches and methods to use can be developed by each company. A potential problem may arise when statisticians in two or more countries analyze and view data differently. This is a relatively common occurrence and may lead to different clinical interpretations of the same data.

One approach to minimize or prevent problems is to have the group that conducted the study derive the company-wide interpretation. This can only work if all relevant groups have an opportunity to review the data and results, plus have input into the methods chosen to analyze the data. This approach will sometimes fail, however, when different people are not able to reach agreement, or some regulatory authorities require new methods to be used or challenge interpretations presented. Thus, even a unanimous consensus by all company statisticians and academic statisticians on how to perform data analyses may not prevent regulatory authorities (with or without statistical training) from challenging the methods used.

Adverse Reactions

Many of the issues involving adverse reactions are compounded when reports from multiple countries are involved. In this brief section there is only space for indicating some of the complexities.

1. Medicine is practiced differently around the world and the type of physician or specialist who treats one kind of problem (e.g., skin problem) in one country may not be the type of physician or specialist who would treat patients with the same problem in another country. This means that the accuracy of diagnosis of the adverse reaction will vary depending on both the nature of the disease being diagnosed and the physician's training. In addition, adverse reactions are often identified differently in different countries. Thus, the reported incidence of a single adverse reaction in a country may be greatly over- or underreported when compared with another country. The difference may represent an artifact based solely on diagnostic factors. Some diagnoses blend into or overlap others, and the lack of an objective method of identifying many adverse reactions means that resulting data may be skewed in different ways. Achieving an accurate diagnosis is especially difficult for many syndromes (e.g., Stevens-Johnson Syndrome).
2. The more precisely an adverse reaction is defined and diagnosed, the lower its reported incidence is. But, different countries often use different methodologies in terms of processing and counting reports, in addition to differences in diagnosing reactions. All of these factors undoubtedly affect the incidence figures obtained.
3. Retrospective analyses of patient charts are fraught with problems in all countries, but when multiple countries are involved, the number of potential difficulties becomes much greater. One approach to this issue is to first establish criteria for the diagnosis. Second, design a data collection form and have medically knowledgeable individuals who are unaware of the study's objectives review patient charts. Finally, the completed data collection forms may be reviewed by a panel of experts, who rate degree of improvement or another endpoint without knowing which treatment group each patient was in. To evaluate the association of a drug with an adverse reaction, charts from patients who had the adverse reaction but were not taking the suspected drug should also be coded and examined. Any slides of biopsies, or any other documented evidence should also be reviewed in a blind manner.
4. Developing a unified interpretation of even a single adverse reaction from reports received from multiple countries is difficult. Some of the

reasons for this difficulty include differences in (1) allowable maximal doses (it is necessary to know the dose that each patient received), (2) medical practice (physicians may use the drug differently), (3) concomitant medications may be unknown or unreported and the adverse reaction may represent a drug–drug interaction, (4) excipients may differ for the "same" drug and might explain the adverse reaction, and (5) the source of the report (e.g., physician, patient, public health service nurse) may vary and affect its accuracy.

5. More than 10 countries currently require reporting of adverse reactions that have occurred in other countries. There are various definitions of adverse reactions used, various forms to use, and various timetables for filing reports in different countries. It is easy to imagine the administrative complexity that this is becoming for many pharmaceutical companies. Recent efforts by regulatory agencies, pharmaceutical companies, and trade associations are attempting to standardize reporting of adverse reactions between countries.
6. A number of national regulatory agencies (e.g., in Australia, Canada, England, Norway, Sweden, New Zealand) issue reports on adverse reactions caused by various drugs. The issue of causality assessment becomes more complex when a parent drug company receives these reports plus those of its subsidiaries in these and other countries. Assessments are not made using uniform criteria or applied in a uniform manner in all countries (or even within one country). For example, the assessment of the probability of causation may be made by the treating physician, drug manufacturer, and/or regulatory agency. Patients may be taking multiple drugs and the drug responsible for the adverse reaction may not be known or may not be identified on the report.
7. The issue of distortion of adverse reaction data is a major one. A company may attempt to minimize distortion between its subsidiaries and the central office, but assuring the quality of data at an earlier point (i.e., between physician and patient, or between physician and local company) is extremely difficult, if not impossible. Another problem is that of obtaining all information that is needed to adequately understand and interpret the clinical importance of the adverse reaction report.
8. The incidence of adverse reactions reported by physicians on a new drug (as opposed to the true incidence) goes through different periods. Most new drugs generate medical interest and attention to most of its adverse reactions. After an unusual type or frequency of an adverse reaction is reported, there is often a flurry of other reports on the same event. There may be overreporting during this period because physicians are alerted to the possible occurrence of the unusual or unexpected adverse reaction and may diagnose possible or questionable cases as definite examples of the adverse reaction. Physicians may also attribute these adverse reactions more readily to the drug than would

> otherwise have occurred. After a number of years, however, the incidence of almost all adverse reaction reports (except for possibly the most serious) generally fall below the expected rate. This occurs because many physicians have little or no interest in reporting well established adverse reactions. This leads to a period of underreporting adverse reactions.

Information on adverse reactions reported in package inserts is available in the *Physician's Desk Reference* in the United States. Comparable sources of information from other countries may be identified in *Drug Information Sources* (Revill, 1978). Various issues relating to the use of adverse reaction dictionaries are described in Chapter 4, United States reporting of adverse reactions are discussed in Chapter 21, and obtaining plus categorizing adverse reactions are covered in Chapter 6. Additional issues on international adverse reaction surveillance were presented at a Drug Information Association Workshop (Jones, 1985) and in a recent monograph (Inman, 1986). A review of international voluntary systems for reporting adverse reactions was presented by Griffin and Weber (1985, 1986).

14

Comparing Different Dosage Forms or Treatment Modalities

In some clinical situations it is important to compare two different modalities or dosage forms in the same study. For example, it may be relevant to ask whether radiation therapy or chemotherapy is a better treatment for patients with a certain type and stage of cancer. It may be important to compare medical and surgical treatment of unstable angina. In addition, there are many cases when a tablet is compared with another dosage form (e.g., cream, suppository, implant).

A few simple approaches for choosing methods to compare different dosage forms or modalities will be described. If the disease being evaluated is chronic and relatively stable, it may be suitable to use a crossover design. This design is often preferable to a parallel design because it requires fewer patients to demonstrate effects. There are various precautions, however, that must be considered before this design may be used, including the requirement that the patient's condition return to its original baseline between the two legs of the treatment (i.e., prior to the second treatment). Special care must be taken to prevent period or carryover effects from influencing data. A recent article by Dubey (1986) contains a description of some pertinent precautions.

Dosage Forms

Comparing two (or more) dosage forms often requires a placebo medication of each form. This is often impossible when different modalities are compared. Because of the many biases that will surround different dosage forms or modalities and the need for an objective evaluation, double-blind studies must almost always be performed. Patients are usually instructed to take or use both medications (e.g., tablet and suppository, capsule and cream) simultaneously, knowing that one, or perhaps both, is a placebo. The usual design is to utilize a three-arm study of (1) dosage form A, (2) dosage form B, and (3) placebo. Patients in the two-drug groups receive one test drug and a placebo of the other drug. Patients in the placebo group receive two placebo medications. Either a parallel or crossover design may be used.

If a suitable placebo cannot be used for ethical or practical reasons then one can consider either (1) a three-arm study with two doses of the study drug and an active drug as control or (2) a dose–response relationship for only one of the dosage forms. In the former design each patient receives one study drug and appropriate placebo(s) to keep the study double-blind, although no patient receives only placebo treatment.

If a suitable placebo can be made for dosage form A, but not dosage form B, it may still be possible to study both agents in a double-blind study. Conduct a dose–response study in one or more groups for dosage form B. All of these patients should receive the placebo for dosage form A. A separate group should receive the single dose of dosage form A and the lowest dose possible of dosage form B. This dose of dosage form B will have been chosen to be homeopathic (i.e., equivalent to a placebo) and should be insufficient to interact with the other dosage form.

Treatment Modalities

Although some treatment modalities may not be easily blinded in clinical studies, it is often possible to conduct a sham procedure (e.g., sham radiation treatment, sham insertion of a medical device) that may serve as an excellent "placebo." Thus, it may be possible in either a crossover or parallel design to initiate a double-blind study comparable to one of those proposed to evaluate two dosage forms. If both modalities cannot be compared in the same study it is important to evaluate each separately under double-blind conditions. In this situation of two separate studies it is preferable if each treatment modality is evaluated simultaneously at a single site by the same investigators. This will avoid the necessity of using historical data or data collected in a double-blind study conducted under other experimental conditions. Controlling studies with historical data is usually the least desirable approach.

Current standards used in designing studies vary for different modalities. Unfortunately, there are very different standards for introducing new drugs into medical practice and introducing other modalities, equipment, and techniques. Standards for new drugs are generally far higher than for other treatment modalities or for medical equipment. Challah and Mays (1986) describe this difference and illustrate that "Gastric freezing, high concentration oxygen for neonates, the use of hyperbaric oxygen in intensive care, and insulin coma for the treatment of schizophrenia are all examples of innovations introduced without evaluation and subsequently abandoned because they proved ineffective or unsafe." Clearly, it is in everyone's interest to utilize high standards before new nondrug modalities of treatment or diagnosis are accepted.

15

Planning Combination Drug Studies

Introduction • Relevant Questions to Address • Designing Clinical Studies to Evaluate Combination Drugs • Formulations

INTRODUCTION

Combination drugs consist of two or more separate active ingredients which are combined to improve the efficacy, safety, compliance, or another characteristic of the separate ingredients. In this discussion it will be assumed that the combination drug is scientifically and medically rational and has a clearly defined clinical objective. The drugs combined may each be of the same therapeutic class (e.g., two analgesics), of differing therapeutic classes (e.g., an antihistamine and a sympathomimetic decongestant), or where one agent is almost therapeutically inactive on its own for the indication but in combination potentiates the active drug (e.g., probenecid plus penicillin). Combinations of these objectives may be present in the same product, especially if three or more drugs are combined. Readers interested in detailed discussions on combination drugs are referred to monographs edited by Lasagna (1975) and by Mezey (1980).

The Food and Drug Administration (FDA) combination drug policy states that each active ingredient in the combination must contribute to the overall safety and/or efficacy of the combination. The exact wording of the regulations in 21CFR 300.50 states: "Two or more drugs may be combined in a single dosage form when each component makes a contribution to the claimed effects and the dosage of each component (amount, frequency, duration) is such that the combination is safe and effective for a significant patient population requiring such concurrent therapy as defined in the labeling for the drug."

RELEVANT QUESTIONS TO ADDRESS

1. Is there a patient population that needs or will significantly benefit from the combination?

TABLE 15.1. *Potential advantages of developing combination drugs*

1. We obtain an enhanced clinical effect by two (or more) drugs acting via different mechanisms (e.g., trimethoprim and a sulfonamide antibiotic for many infections, diuretic plus β-receptor antagonist in hypertension)
2. We improve the therapeutic ratio by utilizing a smaller dose of one or more drugs that avoids toxicity (i.e., decreases adverse reactions) (e.g., combination of L-DOPA and a DOPA decarboxylase inhibitor for treating patients with Parkinson's Disease)
3. Multiple clinical effects are achieved in a disease or syndrome where these activities are desired (e.g., various cough, cold, expectorant combinations)
4. We decrease the magnitude of peak-to-trough differences in physiological responses
5. We decrease the potential for drug abuse (e.g., naloxone plus pentazocine)
6. We increase the duration of effective treatment by combining an immediate-release form of one drug and a sustained-release form of another
7. We reduce the cost of drug treatment
8. We increase the convenience for oral dosing
9. We obtain a lower Drug Enforcement Administration (DEA) scheduling than for a single agent
10. We enhance patient compliance because there are fewer tablets or capsules to take
11. We give a controlled ratio of two drugs to patients[a]
12. We enhance ease of administration (e.g., multiple vaccines are sometimes given in a single injection)
13. We decrease vulnerability to competition from generic drugs (e.g., one of the drugs may be protected by patent, the technology of drug manufacture may be highly complex)
14. We allow for a more effective entry of a successful (or previously unsuccessful) drug into new markets

[a] This may also be a disadvantage.

2. If the combination drug is significantly better than placebo, is it necessary for each ingredient of the combination to also be better than placebo? The answer is "sometimes," which means that this question must be applied separately to each combination. It may be more relevant to ask whether the combination must be better than placebo. It is not always necessary for this comparison to be made. The combination, however, must have advantages over each of its individual constituents given alone.
3. If it is impossible or impractical to demonstrate that a combination is better than either one or both of the individual ingredients, is it possible to:
   a. Study multiple doses of the combination?
   b. Measure two or more different objective endpoints (parameters)?
   c. Use multiple study designs?
   d. Use multiple patient populations?
   e. Use less objective endpoints to measure relevant parameters (e.g., patient's clinical global impressions, quality of life measures)?

TABLE 15.2. *Potential disadvantages of developing combination drugs*

1. Physicians do not have adequate flexibility to adjust the dose of individual components
2. Cost of drug may be more for the patient than if each drug were prescribed separately
3. Combinations are sometimes prescribed by physicians as a "shotgun" approach to avoid careful diagnosis and/or therapy
4. Pharmacokinetics of the two drugs may be incompatible
5. Drug combination may be used inappropriately by physicians or patients
6. Physicians may be unaware of the identity of the specific drugs in combinations
7. Certain irrational combinations may be prepared
8. Technical difficulties of developing certain combinations may be insurmountable

4. If it is not possible to demonstrate greater efficacy for the combination product over one (or both) of the single agents, but the safety profile is better and/or the drug is better tolerated, can the drug be developed and marketed?
5. What is the importance of convenience as a factor for deciding to develop a combination drug?

TABLE 15.3. *Selected types of combination drugs*[a]

A. Both ingredients act on the same symptom, disease, or problem
   1. Two similar drugs of the same therapeutic class (e.g., two mild analgesics such as aspirin and acetaminophen; two diuretics with different, but complementary, mechanisms and sites of action, such as spironolactone and hydrochlorothiazide)
   2. Two drugs of the same therapeutic class, but of different potencies (e.g., aspirin and codeine)
B. Each ingredient acts on different symptoms, diseases, or problems
   1. Each contributes to the desired overall effect (e.g., triprolidine and pseudoephedrine)
C. Other type of combinations
   1. One active drug plus one adjuvant[b]
      a. To enhance absorption (e.g., aspirin plus sodium bicarbonate)
      b. To delay excretion (e.g., penicillin plus probenecid)
   2. One active drug plus a second drug to decrease an adverse reaction or potential for one
   3. One active drug plus a second drug to decrease abuse potential (e.g., pentazocine plus naloxone)
   4. Mixtures of drugs [e.g., multiple vaccines such as diphtheria–pertussis–tetanus (DPT)]
   5. One drug has an action that allows less of the other drug to be used (e.g., DOPA decarboxylase inhibitor and L-DOPA)

[a] All examples are of two-ingredient combinations. Three-or-more-component combinations could also be described.

[b] An adjuvant is an inactive agent on the primary symptoms treated which increases the effect of the other drug.

TABLE 15.4. *Criteria to be met for development of most combination drugs*[a]

1. Complete pharmaceutical compatability (e.g., no interactions between the chemicals)
2. Dosage of only one component in the combination should be critical (e.g., if two or more components were critical then numerous ratios of the fixed combination would be needed to have a practical combination)
3. The combination provides an effect that is not possible to achieve from either drug alone
4. Toxicity of the individual components is not synergistic nor potentiated
5. Frequency of administration of the two drugs is the same
6. A population exists that can use (or needs) the combination

[a] These criteria are not intended to reflect a policy of any regulatory agency or sponsor.

6. Which drugs should be combined and what is the scientific/medical basis for this?
7. How many different ratios of doses of the ingredients in a combination should be tested to evaluate the "ideal mix"?

Potential advantages and disadvantages of developing combination drugs are listed in Tables 15.1 and 15.2. Types of combination drugs are listed in Table 15.3; criteria to be met for most combination drugs are listed in Table 15.4.

DESIGNING CLINICAL STUDIES TO EVALUATE COMBINATION DRUGS

An initial step is to identify the optimal dose(s) of each drug to use in the combination drug. Holding the dose of one drug constant and then varying the other will probably provide information on the dose of the second drug to use. The study may be repeated, holding the dose of the opposite drug constant. Nonetheless, this method will not definitely identify the ideal combination of doses to use with even two ingredients. This may occur because the two studies described were both designed to demonstrate the best dose of the variable drug to use in relation to a fixed dose of the other drug. But, if a smaller (or larger) fixed dose had been used, then different results might have been obtained. This is especially true if one drug potentiates the effects of another. Because of the substantial knowledge that usually exists about at least one of the drugs when development of a combination product is considered, a small number of combination doses may usually be chosen on a rational basis. If the combination involves three (or more) drugs, then the number of possible dose combinations becomes extremely large and a definitive path to reaching the optimal combination is almost impossible to determine in advance of conducting studies. More "educated guesses" will generally have to be made in this situation.

Another approach to identifying doses to use in a combination is to utilize

TABLE 15.5. *Selected types of clinical results which demonstrate therapeutic superiority of a combination drug over its individual constituents*[a]

	Therapeutic value			
Scenario	Drug A	Drug B	Combination of drugs A and B	Placebo[b]
1	+ +[c]	0	+ + +	0 to +
2	0	+ +	+ + +	0 to +
3	+	+	+ +	0 to +
4	+	0 to +	+ +	0 to +
5	−	0	+ +	0 to +
6	−	+	+ +	0 to +

[a] Clinical superiority of a combination product may also be based on an improved safety profile (e.g., decreased severity or incidence of adverse reactions), improved pharmacokinetic considerations, or decreased abuse potential, compared with each component. In such cases the efficacy of the combination may not be enhanced over the efficacy of the individual components.

[b] A placebo arm in the study design is not mandatory for evaluating the components of a combination, although it is usually desirable.

[c] +, a positive therapeutic effect; + +, a stronger positive therapeutic effect; + + +, an even stronger positive therapeutic effect; −, a negative therapeutic effect; 0, no clinical effect.

multiple dose ranges for each drug. Patients in the first dosage group may receive from *X* to *Y* mg of drug A and from *V* to *W* mg of drug B (or placebo). A second group is given a larger dose and may receive from 2 to 4 times the dose given to the first group. A third group could receive an even larger dose. This study should provide data on which dose ranges were best (and least) tolerated and which ranges were most efficacious. Further studies could evaluate this issue in greater detail. Nonetheless, it is often only necessary to study one or two doses of one drug in a combination. A summary of some methods to demonstrate clinical superiority of a combination product are given in Table 15.5.

The classic study design to evaluate a combination drug uses a factorial design. The factorial design includes each active ingredient of the combination, the combination, and placebo. For a two-drug combination (drugs A and B), there would be four treatment groups and in a parallel study each patient would receive two medications: (1) placebos of drug A and drug B, (2) drug A plus placebo of drug B, (3) drug B plus placebo of A, or (4) drug A plus drug B. For a three-drug combination, eight groups are possible (the full combination, three combinations of two drugs each, three single ingredients, and placebo). Several examples of study designs useful for evaluating combination drugs are illustrated in Fig. 15.1.

In certain situations the effectiveness of one of the drugs in a combination is well established and it is then of interest to determine if its activity is

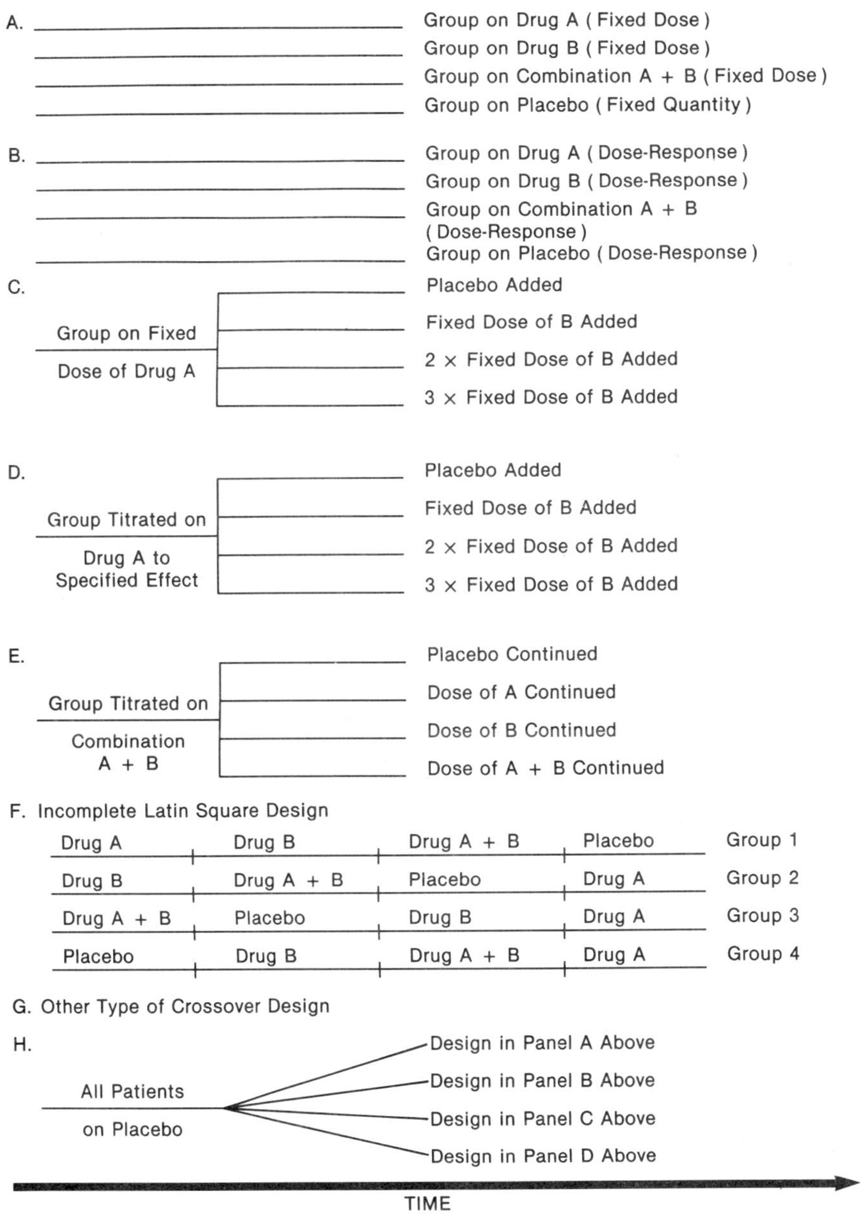

FIG. 15.1. Selected study designs to evaluate combination drugs. Many variations on these study designs are possible.

enhanced with a second drug. A semifactorial design could be considered where the effective drug is compared to the combination. In some ways this would be like testing a drug versus placebo, since the activity of the active drug is equivalent to a baseline. This design may be used to study a drug that potentiates another, but does not have any activity on its own (e.g., probenecid and penicillin).

FORMULATIONS

In developing a suitable tablet or capsule formulation of a combination drug product there are numerous problems that may be encountered. These are discussed under the headings of physical, chemical, and pharmacokinetic issues.

Physical Issues

Differences in bulk density, particle size, or particle shape between two drugs to be combined may cause problems during the mixing process from poor flow characteristics or particle segregation of the dry chemicals. This problem may result in poor content uniformity of the drugs in the dosage form. Poor compressibility of one or both components may produce soft, friable tablets. Hygroscopicity or eutectic formation between the components may cause the formulation to stick to the tablet punch, resulting in an unacceptable appearance, or cause chemical degradation. These problems may be minimized by careful sizing (sifting or milling) of the particles to prevent segregation; inclusion of a granulating step to minimize differences in physical characteristics or overcome compressibility problems; careful selection of ingredients such as compression aids, binders, lubricants, dispersants, and anti-adherents; or by inclusion of adsorbents to remove excess moisture.

How will capsules be filled to insure that each contains the precise amount of each ingredient? Capsules sold commercially are filled by machines and it is difficult to mix two large batches of powders sufficiently well in the correct ratio to insure that every capsule is filled with, for example, 75 mg of drug A and 25 mg of drug B. If small beads of one (or both) drugs are prepared, then mixtures may be made and adequate samples of the capsules may be taken to insure that they contain the correct weight of each compound. This same problem exists when tablets are compressed.

There are numerous excipients that have to be added to almost all chemicals to make a drug. Each excipient is carefully determined through many pharmaceutical tests. When two (or more) drugs are to be combined in a tablet then all of these procedures have to be conducted anew. There are many more difficulties in finding the ideal excipients for a combination than for a single drug. If all appropriate excipients are found, then the physical form of the drugs may differ from each other and may not be adequately homogeneous for tabletting. For example, one drug may be in the form of a light fluffy powder; the other, in a hard granular form. In order to compress the dry powder and form a single tablet the two drugs must be brought closer together in physical characteristics.

Chemical Issues

Chemical interactions between drugs may adversely affect the long-term stability of the combination. These problems may be overcome by addition of stabilizing agents (i.e., anti-oxidants), use of a more stable salt of the drug, or by a physical separation of the major components. For capsules, separation may be accomplished by inserting a tablet of one drug in a capsule followed by a powder of the second drug, or by filling pellets of each drug separately into a capsule. Further separation of components may be accomplished by applying a barrier coating to the tablet or pellets to be filled into capsules. Separation of components in a tablet dosage form may also be accomplished using bilayered or trilayered tablets, compression-coated tablets consisting of a core of one drug coated with a granulation of the second drug, or by microencapsulating one or both drugs prior to compression.

Because of all of the potential physical and chemical problems described above, innovative technical solutions to these issues have been sought. Several approaches involve development of a slow-release form. Slow-release forms may be created in many ways, including (1) creating pellets of a drug and coating them with a slowly dissolving polymer, or (2) coating an inert sugar granule with drug and then coating this with a slowly dissolving polymer.

Pharmacokinetic Issues

In addition to the physical and chemical problems which have been described, there may also be a large variety of pharmacokinetic issues to address. A combination of two drugs that makes rational scientific and medical sense may involve drugs with vastly different half-lives and durations of biological effects. This may prevent a combination drug from being developed if one ingredient had to be taken more frequently than the other and a suitable sustained-release form of that drug could not be prepared. The pharmacokinetics of the two may differ greatly in terms of absorption, distribution, metabolism, and excretion. An important point is that there should not be chemical or other interactions between the ingredients in a combination which affect pharmacokinetics in an unpredictable manner. The number of potentially important technical and clinical problems that may arise is almost limitless.

In conclusion, the successful development of combination products involves consideration of more variables and factors to be controlled than for a single drug. This makes the entire process of developing a combination product more time-consuming. There are often compromises that must be made (e.g., shorter product expiration dates). Production costs for combination drugs are usually greater than for single entity drugs, because of additional steps for granulating, microencapsulation, producing layered tablets, or other steps that must be incorporated into the manufacturing process.

The considerations in this chapter are for a single fixed dose combination of two or more active drugs. There are also drug "combinations" where two or more drugs are given as a mixture or are given sequentially. The study designs and many of the considerations of developing a single combination described are also applicable in these other situations.

Section III

Management of Multiple Clinical Studies

16

Management Styles, Staff, and Systems

Introduction • Management Styles • Management Staff • Staff Motivation and Morale • Considerations in Establishing and Maintaining Management Systems

INTRODUCTION

The innumerable issues and complexities that arise during the conduct of a single clinical study become exponentially more complex when multiple clinical studies must be managed. The term "multiple clinical studies" is used in the context of two or more separate and independent studies on one specific drug, or of several independent studies on each of two or more different drugs. In either of these situations it is important to develop systems and procedures that will assist in the orderly and efficient management of the myriad activities involved.

The chapters in this section present little information on the standard management techniques which are discussed in numerous textbooks and business or management courses and may be applied to almost any industry. The information included differs from most available material in two major ways. First, it minimizes theoretical discussions and emphasizes a practical, straightforward approach to management. Second, it is directed primarily at pharmaceutical companies and drug development, and only secondarily at academicians or medical device manufacturers, or others who conduct multiple clinical studies.

MANAGEMENT STYLES

Styles of management vary along several different spectrums, and no single style is universally best or most appropriate in each situation. The spectrums range from (1) authoritarian to democratic, (2) loose control to tight (rigid) control, (3) centralized to peripheralized, (4) matrix to line management, (5) ends oriented to means oriented, and (6) willingness to try the latest new management idea or fad to grudging acceptance of ideas only after

TABLE 16.1. *Styles of management*[a]

1. Rigid and authoritative, where one individual controls a group, determines most of the rules to be followed, and usually does not delegate real power or decision-making responsibility. This individual does not seek nor accept opinions from individuals willing to disagree or act independently
2. One individual runs a group, but delegates power and decision making appropriately (participative leadership)
3. One individual makes decisions, but only after consulting with others (consultative leadership)
4. A committee is established to make important decisions, as well as to monitor and review projects and issues. The committee follows highly formal monitoring and reporting procedures
5. A committee is established as above, but follows a loosely structured and flexible system for monitoring and reporting activities and for arriving at decisions
6. No formal systems are created. Managers depend on ad hoc meetings and discussions to solve problems and to provide a review of activities

[a] These styles are not mutually exclusive within a large organization, and several approaches are often observed to be used simultaneously. Most managers or small committees of about three to 12 people also exhibit different approaches in different situations.

they have been accepted by most other people. Appropriate management styles for an individual are based on the specific work environment, tradition of the institution, personality of the individual, and other factors. The most rapid movement of a project toward a goal usually occurs when a single authoritarian figure determines the goal and controls the resources allocated and the vigor with which the goal is pursued. On the other hand, a more conservative approach, which is usually adopted by most committees and institutions, is less likely to make a major error in going in a wrong direction for a long period without recognizing the error.

Individual companies often go through periods where they shift from one style to another. This may be a result of change in leadership or a desire to try something new. Different parts of an organization often utilize different and possibly even conflicting styles at the same time. Selected management styles are summarized in Table 16.1.

Different management styles emphasize a variety of approaches to overseeing a project's development. There are individuals who believe in emphasizing analytical tools and techniques in helping to make complex decisions. These techniques include quantitative methods described in management systems [e.g., Program Evaluation and Review Technique (PERT), critical path method]. Another group approaches management through consideration of the general functions that are conducted by most managers. These functions include planning, organizing, directing, reviewing, and controlling. Finally, some managers emphasize interpersonal relationships, since managers must complete a work assignment through the efforts of other people. Knowledge of group behavior, motivation, and other personal characteristics allow some managers to direct projects efficiently and effectively. Although multiple management styles may be used by the same person, each individual balances their use of these styles in different ways. One useful frame of reference for evaluating personal styles of behavior and management is presented by G. D. Bell in his book *The Achievers* (1973).

Another perspective on individual management styles focuses on styles of communication. Individuals usually develop preferences in the techniques they use for communication. These more or less include use of (1) personal notes sent to others, (2) telephone discussions, (3) short informal meetings generated as the manager walks around an area, (4) meetings of small informal groups, (5) more formal meetings, and (6) memoranda, as well as other methods of communication. When individuals are promoted or are given a new assignment they usually do not greatly alter their personal habits or style in the methods they use to communicate.

MANAGEMENT STAFF

Management staff involved with clinical studies includes numerous individuals whose responsibilities vary greatly. These individuals include:

1. Investigator(s)
2. Co-investigators and assistant investigators
3. Members of Institutional Review Boards (IRBs)
4. Professional consultants
5. Regulatory agency reviewers
6. Study coordinators
7. Study monitors
8. Monitoring committees and other staff
9. Project champions
10. Project managers
11. Supervisors of data processors and data entry operators
12. Statistical reviewers
13. Executives at the sponsoring institution
14. Contract organization staff and executives
15. Data analysis committees
16. Independent auditors of diagnoses, laboratory data, study conduct, or other aspects of a study
17. Independent review committee of study results and interpretation

Study personnel requirements vary from a single individual who performs every role from investigator to appointment clerk, to situations where large numbers of people with specific responsibilities are involved. This section describes several of the major management functions that are usually performed by different individuals. A subset of the staff positions listed above will be individually discussed. Their roles are summarized in Table 16.2.

TABLE 16.2. *Possible management roles within a clinical study*

Position or responsibility in a clinical study	Aspects of their managerial role
1. Receptionist	Schedules clinic visits and sends out (or telephones) reminders
2. Nurse	May be assigned duties of receptionist, nursing assistant, research coordinator, and/or assistant investigator
3. Research coordinator	Usually supervises data collection forms, schedules activities, dispenses drugs, and may assist or conduct other functions at the investigator's discretion
4. Assistant investigator[a]	Assists the principal investigator in managing the study, or may solely supervise the study. Usually conducts patient examinations and may sign data collection forms
5. Principal investigator[b]	Overall manager of study. Details of specific activities vary greatly between investigators. Often delegates many responsibilities to others
6. Clinical monitor[c]	Helps to plan and implement the study. Reviews conduct of the study, plus completeness and accuracy of data collection forms. Often monitors data processing, analysis, and report writing
7. Sponsor's medical representative	In charge of the particular study for the sponsor. May also act as study monitor
8. Project leader or manager	In charge of managing the development of the drug, medical device, or project for the sponsor
9. Medical department head	Academic (or sponsor's) department head, who has a formal or informal review function over the study
10. Executives of the sponsoring institution	Individuals who must approve and review the overall strategy and allocation of funds given the project and/or individual study
11. Institutional Review Board members[d]	Approve initiation of the study conducted at their institution and review its progress on a periodic basis. They must insure that appropriate ethical standards are maintained and may intervene in the management of a study
12. National regulatory agency	Usually reviews each protocol. Must approve the initiation of each study in some countries. Reacts to issues that arise and may intervene in the management of a study

[a] May be a resident or fellow.

[b] Usually an MD. Co-principal investigators may share this responsibility.

[c] For sponsored studies, one or more people from the sponsor and/or contract organization share this responsibility, or it may be conducted by a committee. This is performed by an individual at the study site for nonsponsored studies and for some sponsored studies as well.

[d] Known as the Ethics Committee in the United Kingdom.

Investigator(s)

From an organizational perspective the investigator is the central figure in a study. He or she is the focal point for contact with the patients, staff, IRB, professional advisors, assistants, and sponsor. Many investigators direct the conduct of the study through contact with each of these individuals or groups. Other investigators, however, deputize assistants or other staff (e.g., residents, fellows, study coordinator) to conduct the study. These investigators often limit their involvement to the use of their name on a protocol and the eventual publication. Between these two extremes are investigators who participate to varying degrees in the conduct of a study.

It is important for sponsors to identify the type and degree of personal involvement that an investigator is able and willing to accept in a study. Confirming the degree of the investigator's involvement is in the sponsor's interest, since an investigator may have been chosen for his/her special skills or talents. This often occurs in complex surgical studies where the investigator's assistants may not yet have mastered various techniques. The quality of a study may be seriously compromised if the investigator does not participate at a previously agreed on level.

In nonsponsored studies, an investigator may wish to minimize his/her own involvement and to delegate most or all parts of the study to assistants, residents, fellows, and/or others. In sponsored studies, a well-known investigator may not have the time (and possibly interest) to become involved personally with a study, yet has the facilities, staff, and patient population to conduct an excellent study. The degree to which the investigator is able to participate in a clinical study must be viewed individually, and an understanding must be reached as to the nature and necessary extent of the investigator's personal involvement.

Co- or Assistant Investigator

Two (or more) co-investigators equally share overall responsibility for a clinical study, although each may have their own spheres of responsibility and activity. Depending on the arrangements made for a study, a single co-investigator may have authority over the financial arrangements and allocation of funds. Reasons for utilizing co-investigators include (1) recognizing an already existing partnership, (2) recognizing an already existing collaboration, or (3) indicating that two or more individuals initiating a study are to be considered as equals in the venture.

Assistant investigators differ from co-investigators in that they are at least nominally directed by the investigator. An assistant investigator is empowered to sign data collection forms and to act for the investigator regarding administrative matters, if required.

Members of Institutional Review Boards

The functions of this group are briefly summarized in Chapter 22 of *Guide to Clinical Studies and Developing Protocols* (Spilker, 1984).

Professional Consultants

There are several types of consultants that may be utilized in a study. These include:

1. Consultant physicians who are requested on an ad hoc basis to evaluate and/or treat patients in a study for unforeseen events. These individuals are usually specialists in a specific discipline.
2. Consultant physicians or medical specialists who are requested to treat patients as part of the established clinical protocol.
3. Consultant specialists who are requested to assist in the diagnosis or evaluation of patients as part of the protocol (e.g., pathologists, electroencephalographers, individuals who conduct and interpret pulmonary function tests).
4. Consultants who review data and/or problems occurring in a study and make suggestions as to means of solving or addressing these issues.
5. Consultants who are asked to help plan a specific study, or the broad development of a single drug or nondrug project.
6. Consultant contract organizations that either act as intermediaries to place a sponsor's study at an appropriate site for its conduct or perform the study itself.
7. Lastly, there is a saying that anyone who calls himself (or herself) a consultant is one.

Regulatory Agency Reviewers

The roles of regulatory agency reviewers are briefly discussed in Chapter 21.

Study Coordinator

There are several other related titles for this function, such as research coordinator, site planner, clinical coordinator, administrative director, and so forth. The individual who is the study coordinator handles most of the administrative responsibilities of the study. Some of the tasks, such as scheduling appointments and sending out reminder cards to patients, may be delegated to another individual, if the size of the study and workload at the study site warrant. The study coordinator may also assist in conducting of the study. The specific responsibilities assigned, plus the types of assignments made by the investigator, depend on the abilities and training of the coordinator. The study coordinator may either devote 100% of his or her efforts to a single study or may be involved with many studies.

The study coordinator is usually the contact person who the sponsor deals with in most situations, both expected and unexpected. Data are usually reviewed for completeness and accuracy (i.e., to insure that they are quality assured) by the coordinator before the study monitor reviews them. Data may be entered on the data collection forms by the coordinator, who usually plays a pivotal role in insuring that the study is conducted as efficiently as possible.

Monitoring Committees

In large multicenter studies a separate committee is sometimes established to oversee the monitoring of the study. In some cases the monitoring function is subdivided and assigned to several committees. See Chapter 30 of *Guide to Clinical Studies and Developing Protocols* (Spilker, 1984).

Other Staff

Numerous other individuals may be involved in planning, conducting, and analyzing clinical studies, particularly sponsored studies. Many of these individuals are located at the sponsoring institution and include statisticians, pharmacokinetic specialists, data entry operators, data editors, medical writers, report editors, regulatory personnel, and so on.

Project Champion

An old adage is that jobs do not get done on their own and projects die when they are not being pushed. A champion of a project is considered particularly important by those who emphasize this viewpoint. There are strong proponents of the project champion concept who believe that this concept is essential, in order to optimize a project's overall progress.

In a management system where there is a project leader this individual usually acts as the project champion, although this is not always the case. The true project champion could be a senior executive, department chairman, or dean who is not even on the project team, but who encourages progress from "behind the scene." There are numerous articles and books that detail the ideal characteristics of project champions (e.g., entrepreneurial spirit, compulsiveness, workaholic nature, creativity) and indicate means through which potential champions may be identified and cultivated.

TABLE 16.3. *Selected factors used to evaluate project leaders/managers*

1. Interpersonal and communication skills, which facilitate interactions with many different people who have widely different backgrounds
2. Effective leadership of the project team as evidenced through motivation of others
3. Ability to concentrate on details and an overall perspective of the project being managed
4. Adequate self-confidence to seek help elsewhere when required, while still functioning independently and avoiding dependence on others
5. Organizational abilities to establish an effective monitoring system that observes each important area of the project for early signs of potential problems or other matters that require attention
6. Initiative and self-motivation to start activities without prompting, and perseverence to continue them to completion
7. Ability to plan, organize, and coordinate activities in a project. Ability to move the project toward its objectives in the most direct and efficient means practical
8. Taking necessary steps to keep activities as close to schedule as possible
9. Adjusting strategies and goals as appropriate and in a timely manner
10. Technical skills in area(s) of expertise
11. Ability to be imaginative in selecting the approaches taken
12. Using resources appropriately and only requesting resources necessary to meet objectives
13. Ability to write clearly and communicate effectively in reports
14. Ability to use sound judgment to make decisions and adjust priorities and plans as required
15. Ability to determine, in a timely manner, when the project should be terminated

Some of the major factors used to evaluate project champions/managers/leaders are presented in Table 16.3, and advantages of having projects led by champions are summarized in Table 18.4.

It is also possible for a project to have more than one champion. If this is the case, then one individual may be the primary champion and the other(s) will champion the project to a lesser degree. The primary champion is not necessarily the more senior person in the organization. When there are two or more champions for a project each champion will probably play different roles. There are also situations when a champion of a project in its early phases turns a project over to another individual to champion through its later phases.

When a senior individual has a "pet" idea that is not widely shared by individuals less senior in the organization, the senior person is often forced to become the champion. In some cases this person desires to adopt this role. It behooves the senior executive to be relatively certain about the importance and likely outcome of the project, since significant company resources are often expended with few of the checks and balances that are usually applied. For staff morale and sometimes even for the sponsor's economic vitality, it is generally important to apply the same standards to the boss's pet projects as to other projects.

TABLE 16.4. *Administrative functions to consider monitoring during a project's life*[a]

1. Tracking the status of the clinical data
2. Tracking the status of ongoing and completed nonclinical studies conducted by the sponsor, contractors, and others
3. Tracking both published and unpublished articles and reports
4. Tracking bulk chemicals and formulated drug supplies
5. Tracking funds that are committed and spent for both internal and external costs
6. Tracking the time and effort expended by various departments
7. Tracking the fate of all drug supplies sent to various sites
8. Tracking the status of competitive drugs under investigation
9. Tracking the market for which the drug is being targeted
10. Tracking trends in FDA reviews of similar drugs

[a] Forms may be created for each of these activities that are monitored.

Project Manager

One alternative to the project champion system is in having a project manager. This individual's primary professional objective is to guide a project through a maze of processes to a successful outcome. This individual usually controls (or manages) several projects at the same time. Proponents of this system claim that many of the emotional factors that often complicate the approach of the project champion do not concern the professional manager, since the project manager is not usually as emotionally involved in the project. Also, the project manager is often described as a professional administrator who is experienced in managing a project or projects and does not have to also contend with the specific discipline-related tasks that confront most champions. Proponents of the project manager approach also claim that a project champion is often a professional scientist, clinician, or other individual who is usually relatively unskilled in the administrative requirements for leading a project. Advantages of having teams led by professional project managers are summarized in Table 18.4. Some of the functions that a project manager must track (monitor) are listed in Table 16.4.

STAFF MOTIVATION AND MORALE

There is a wide spectrum in terms of the percentage of time that each investigator and his staff devote to any one study. This aspect often depends on, and in turn influences, their degree of interest, involvement, and motivation to conduct a study at the highest level. Unless some unexpected positive results occur, the high point of most people's interest in a study they are conducting usually occurs at or near the outset. This implies that if the investigator and/or staff members are lukewarm about conducting a study at the outset, the chances are great that their interest will rapidly decline after the study is initiated.

TABLE 16.5. *Selected areas in managing a project where great efficiencies may often be achieved*

A. Meetings
   1. Conduct well-organized and targeted meetings
   2. Terminate meetings when they are not productive
   3. Eliminate periodic or ad hoc meetings that are not necessary

B. Documents
   1. Eliminate unnecessary paperwork
   2. Eliminate unimportant periodic reports

C. Travel
   1. Cancel periodic business trips unless essential or expected to be productive
   2. Replace trips with telephone calls plus letters whenever possible

D. Allocation of time
   1. Evaluate whether one's time is spent on the most important issues and tasks that are pending
   2. Delegate matters that may be handled by others

An investigator and staff members with relatively little time invested in a study (e.g., below 10–20% of their workweek) often do not place the effort, enthusiasm, and emotional commitment in a study that is necessary to complete it in a timely manner. If a study is extremely long in duration (i.e., a number of years) or extends beyond the original plans (usually due to slower patient enrollment than anticipated), then the interest of the investigator and staff may be expected to wane. Improving the efficiency with which a project is managed also serves to improve morale. A number of areas in which efficiencies are often obtained are listed in Table 16.5.

To maintain motivation at a high level there are a number of techniques that a monitor (as well as the investigator) should consider. The most important is to discern at the outset what motivates the staff, primarily the investigator(s), and then to address their desires. Common sources of motivation include (1) professional recognition, (2) career advancement, (3) financial reward, (4) advancement of science, and (5) ability to more effectively treat a certain patient group. Motives often overlap, and several of these (plus others) may be present in any one individual.

Professional recognition may be stimulated by publications and by encouragement and travel funds to present data at professional meetings. Some sponsors assist investigators in preparing their posters, slides, or other materials. Career advancement may be stimulated through (1) publication, (2) public speaking at various meetings about important results, and (3) informing (directly or indirectly) the investigator's institution about the financial contribution that certain studies make to that institution. Financial considerations may be stimulated by providing bonuses for meeting target enrollments and by sponsoring trips to scientific meetings for the investigator and appropriate staff. Advancement of science is dependent on the importance of the study and the quality of the data. Treating one's patients in a study leads to its own rewards. Care must be used in offering financial bonuses to prevent any conflicts of interest or undesired influences on the study conduct (e.g., entering of inappropriate patients, excessive discontinuation of patients, sloppy study conduct). This practice cannot be generally endorsed. In some situations, however, it may be ethically acceptable.

CONSIDERATIONS IN ESTABLISHING AND MAINTAINING MANAGEMENT SYSTEMS

The choice of a suitable system of forms, reports, and meetings to review and manage multiple clinical studies and the personnel assigned to them depends on whether the clinical studies are to (1) be conducted on one drug by a single person or group, (2) involve one type of study (e.g., pharmacokinetic, Phase I, population survey) on many drugs, or (3) involve a variety of different types of studies on many different drugs. In many management situations all three of these types are followed, but by different individuals or groups within an institution. Questions to consider in implementing a management system are listed in Table 16.6, and issues relating to meetings and reports are discussed in Chapter 19.

In choosing the most appropriate management system(s) to oversee the planning, conduct, and analysis of multiple clinical studies there are several considerations that relate to the nature of the managing organization. Academic managers and clinical investigators often have different reporting relationships and pressure than do the government agencies which sometimes manage studies [e.g., National Institute of Neurological and Communicable Diseases (NINCDS) in their Antiepileptic Drug Development Program]. Both of these groups differ markedly in organizational structure and objectives compared with those of the pharmaceutical industry, which sponsors many clinical studies. Research-based companies within the pharmaceutical

TABLE 16.6. *Questions to consider in implementing a management system*

1. Are most people in agreement with the nature of the proposed system?
2. Do most people support the individual managers who will operate the system?
3. Have adequate descriptions of the system been written and distributed to relevant individuals?
4. Have adequate meetings been held with the staff to explain the system?
5. Has everyone had ample opportunity to raise questions and point out potential problems with the proposed system?
6. Has a pilot program of the system been tested in a group that is smaller than the entire group to be affected?
7. Should outside consultants review the system for possible flaws or potential problems?
8. Has the system been endorsed and approved by all of the relevant senior managers?
9. Have countermeasures and other mechanisms been developed for all the possible major exceptions and problems that have been anticipated?

industry which are developing drugs also differ from (1) contract companies that conduct studies or act as intermediaries to place and monitor studies and (2) other companies in the health area, such as manufacturers of equipment or medical devices.

Individual management systems used in academia, government, and industry may differ because of both general and specific variables. Each department, committee, or group of people in these three types of general organizations have different reporting responsibilities and groups with whom they interact. Some of these interactions necessitate the creation and use of certain types of management systems and preclude others. Secondly, each specific institution within each type of organization (i.e., academia, government, drug company, independent company) differs in size, goals, historical tradition, personnel, and resources, so that there will be major differences in the optimal systems that each institution develops. These factors have a major influence on the management system chosen, but in a few instances the type of institution will have a greater influence.

Several other factors which are independent of whether the institution is academic, governmental, or industrial, also influence management systems. For instance, some management systems are more appropriate to large institutions and other systems are more appropriate to smaller ones. Personalities of senior managers and traditional methods of management at some institutions often have the greatest influence on the choice of systems that are used. Some institutions use highly formal methods of managing projects, whereas others are quite informal. Although more formal methods are usually associated with large institutions and more informal methods are associated with smaller groups or institutions, there are numerous exceptions to this principle. An informal system can work well in a larger institution when people are trusted to be conscientious about performing their job well. This requires that the most senior manager have a great deal of trust in subordinates. In situations where this method works well, the most senior scientific manager is usually able to remain aware of most activities and is able to react quickly when decisions have to be made. There are not many strong, self-confident scientists who possess both the scientific and managerial skills necessary to make this approach work in a large company, government agency, or university. In small institutions with relatively few scientists it is much easier to make this style of management work effectively.

It is more common for large institutions to follow formal systems for managing projects and multiple clinical studies. These systems usually involve forming various committees and periodic reports to provide checks and balances to insure that each project is progressing at an appropriate pace and in the correct direction. The systems are intended to provide increasingly general summaries of the work, problems, and progress of the project as they are directed to progressively higher levels in the institution.

Individuals in management in academia, government, and industry all have

TABLE 16.7. *Issues that may be covered in a project summary for senior management*

1. Project name, number, therapeutic category
2. Drug generic name and trade name
3. Project leader or manager
4. Proposed initial indication(s)
5. Phase of current development
6. Background material and summary of the project's history
7. Milestone dates (e.g., project formation; IND submission; Phase I, II, III; NDA submission; product launch)[a]
8. Project costs (e.g., actual to-date, estimated total costs)
9. Major technical issues
10. Major clinical issues
11. General market background (e.g., market size in sales and prescriptions, growth trend, competitive environment and intensity, disease demographics, need for improved therapy)
12. Major marketing issues
13. Marketing considerations (e.g., final formulation, names of competitive products plus their sales and market share)
14. Patent status
15. Potential therapeutic and competitive advantages
16. Major production and manufacturing issues
17. Projected sales for first 3 years
18. Major uncertainties and questions to address
19. Potential indications
20. Significant changes since the previous report
21. Date of report

[a]IND, Notice of Claimed Investigational Exemption for a New Drug; NDA, New Drug Application.

to deal with questions of prioritization and allocation of resources (see Chapter 17). Other management issues at all institutions involve the coordination of multiple projects (see Chapter 18).

One means for senior managers to remain current with project status is to receive brief reports on a periodic basis. These reports should contain essential information on the project such as that listed in Table 16.7. The other major mechanism is for senior managers to receive briefings from the relevant senior manager, project manager, or another individual. Most institutions use both the techniques of reports and meetings to keep management informed. Every institution, department, and other group should periodically reassess whether their balance of meetings and reports is satisfactory for their needs and whether it may be improved. The quality and speed of senior managers' decision making and workers' productivity both suffer when there is an excessive amount or total lack of reports and meetings. Both formal and informal reviews by management should be used to facilitate progress on projects rather than impede it. It is clearly impossible to describe the appropriate blend of reviews, since this varies enormously between situations and institutions. The best management decisions can usually be reached when all information is available, all relevant people have given their opinions, all possible alternatives are known, and a thorough discussion has occurred among the relevant people.

A management style that emphasizes a strong leader is usually most effective when the environment of the organization is weak. The strong leader is best able to stimulate career growth, communications, and efficient work habits in this type of environment. In organizations with a positive climate, a team-oriented management style is more productive. It is unfortunate that as institution's environments change, the styles of the leaders do not often follow. Thus, many strong organizations become weakened, in time, by the very skills and management techniques that once made them strong. A related aspect is that when top managers retire they usually choose successors who most clearly resemble themselves, without adequate consideration of what style would best suit the institution in the years ahead.

17

Prioritization and Allocation of Resources

Types of Prioritization • Allocation of Resources

TYPES OF PRIORITIZATION

Prioritization of activities, projects, or studies is not required unless two or more activities are competing for the same resources. On the other hand, it is virtually impossible to plan, conduct, and analyze data from even a single clinical study without frequent need to prioritize various activities to help guide most people involved with the study. This necessity becomes much more critical when multiple clinical studies are considered. If no priorities are set within and between studies or projects one must deal individually with every issue and conflict of resources as they arise, and often one must reanalyze the same or similar decisions on several occasions. Even without establishing formal priorities in every study, *de facto* priorities exist.

Prioritization in its simplest form does not require documentation or special planning. It is performed by applying common sense to determine what activities should be done in which order. This simple approach to prioritization is usually not sufficient to handle large numbers of activities or potential activities that require resources and attention. A more formal approach to prioritization is to create lists to keep track and organize various activities. These lists may assign an order of priority to all items from 1 to *n*, or assign general classes of priorities, such as A, B, or C. Alternative techniques are to establish a "high" and "low" system and/or to describe functions that take priority over other functions (e.g., clinical activities take priority over technical development, which in turn takes priority over basic research), or to state that activities on marketed drugs have priority over activities on Phase III drugs, which in turn have priority over drugs in Phase II, and so on.

In addition to assigning priorities to different investigational and/or marketed drugs, there is an entire hierarchy of priorities. Above the level of individual drugs, certain groups of drugs, such as those in a specific therapeutic area may be given a high or low priority. Below the level of individual drugs, priorities may be assigned to certain studies, indications, dosage forms, routes of administration, etc. Within any of these categories certain activities will be given higher or lower priorities.

Criteria used to establish priorities often emphasize the potential medical and commercial value of the projects. Other criteria include (1) the availability of resources and expertise both within and outside the institution, (2) scientific value, (3) quantity and type of resources required to develop the drug, and (4) public health/political/regulatory issues surrounding the particular drug (or type of drug) being developed. For example, a new drug to treat a problem of importance to national health such as Acquired Immune Deficiency Syndrome (AIDS) will generally be given a higher priority by its sponsor than most other drugs.

Drugs being developed simultaneously may be assigned priorities such as A, B, or C, which designates their overall priority in the broadest context. Individual drug studies within each drug's development program may be assigned a numerical priority from 1 to *n*, or another type of priority may be used. The numerous priorities for the activities within each study may be identified with the same or different type of prioritizing system.

In most instances there will not be one individual, or even one group of individuals, that establishes each of these priorities. The broad type of drug development program described requires integration of many types of departments, individuals, and skills. Therefore, assigning priorities among different drugs when conflicts arise must be made by senior managers. It would be ideal if each individual could establish his or her own priorities for achieving objectives assigned by his or her immediate superior and fit these together with priorities of other individuals with a minimum of conflict. Unfortunately this does not usually occur, and conflicts frequently have to be resolved by others.

If there is a general agreement on drug development goals and the methods of operation to achieve those goals, then avoidance of a formal priority system is possible. The most important elements of a successful system for developing drugs are (1) a desire of the relevant people for it to work, (2) a clear statement and understanding of the objectives for each drug's development, and (3) periodic reviews to insure that activities are progressing appropriately and in the correct direction. Reviews are performed both by the individuals who supervise the system and by a person or group (e.g., matrix group) who is (are) different than the people who are responsible for conducting the work (e.g., line-function departments). Reevaluating relevant priorities, either formally or informally on a periodic basis is an important part of this review, as well as reviewing the strategies for the drug's development.

A corollary of this approach is that achieving harmony in a large organization often requires apparently conflicting priorities within various parts of the organization. As an example, assume that a corporation has placed its highest priority on developing and marketing three investigational drugs (drugs A, B, and C) and has assigned a low priority to three other drugs (drugs E, F, and G). Further, assume that drugs A, C, and E are close to having a New Drug Application (NDA) submitted, whereas drugs B, F, and G are in an early stage of development. Some departments are primarily active during the early part of a drug's development, whereas other departments are primarily involved as the drug gets closer to the market. Thus, the priorities within those departments whose activity is greatest during the early phases of a drug's development will be different (drug B will have the highest priority and drugs F and G will have high priority) than in those departments with responsibilities at the later points of development, where drugs A and C will have the highest priority and drug E will have high priority. The actual situation would have to include consideration of other factors as well, such as the technical ease of conducting the work, the skills of the staff, costs of development, availability of raw materials or drug to work with, and possibilities of contracting the work to others. In addition, some departments operate best with continuous input or flow of work, whereas others prefer job work where each job is actually a discrete bolus of work that may come every *X* months or weeks.

An actual case of drug development is usually more complex. Priorities at all levels are frequently changing because of (1) unexpected toxicities, (2) delays, (3) problems, (4) regulatory requests, (5) movements of personnel, (6) opportunities, or (7) other factors. It is partly for these reasons that formal systems of priorities are usually impractical except as a general guide. An elaborate and/or formal system that changes frequently requires more meetings and/or documents to confirm each change and rapid communication of changes throughout the relevant parts of the organization. Changes in an informal prioritization system are usually more easily communicated because of not requiring several steps to formalize and disseminate information.

Elaborate systems of prioritization may be developed which involve establishment of criteria and scores by which to judge the major competing elements (e.g., projects, studies) for resources. A range of possible scores is usually established for each criterion; the scores may be equal (e.g., a maximum of 5 points is assigned for each criterion) or weighted to reflect importance. Criteria that are scored should be those which impact on the decision of how best to allocate resources (e.g., time, efforts, money). Interrelationships between two or more criteria may or may not be considered. The goal of this type of exercise is to determine a numerical ranking of competing projects so that one may allocate resources either proportionally to their importance (assuming that this was the basis for the ranking) or to a project or projects at the top of the ranking. This approach is rarely ever useful for prioritizing investigational drugs because their status often changes rapidly. A summary of systems used to prioritize projects or activities is given in Table 17.1.

ALLOCATION OF RESOURCES

In allocating resources one may use any one, or combination, of various systems. The most simple approach is to give all required resources to the project that has top priority. Any remaining resources are then applied to the second priority project, and so forth, until all resources have been allocated. This approach may make sense in some situations, such as when a financially troubled company has one project that stands out above the others in terms of its commercial potential coupled with ease of development. In most situations, however, a company has many viable projects and focusing resources on a single project makes little sense.

Resources may be allocated by senior management with little input by department and section managers, or may result from joint discussions and decisions. The systems established by a group to allocate resources may be broadly based, narrow based, formal, informal, or nonexistent. In nonexistent systems, resources may be allocated to those champions and projects who make the loudest din or to those areas where crises occur, or may be

TABLE 17.1. *Systems to prioritize projects or activities*[a]

1. Do not establish any formal system for assigning priorities, instead, allow decisions on priorities to be made as they are required
2. Establish a priority sequence of 1 to *n* (for *n* activities)
3. Establish a classification of "A" (high priority), "B" (moderate priority), and "C" (low priority). Divide all projects or activities into one of these three (or other number) classes
4. Establish a two-tiered informal system of having "high" and "low" priority projects, possibly with a single project designated as a "top" priority
5. The priority system used may not be based on specific whole projects but on subparts (e.g., chemical development, analytical assays) of all or certain projects
6. Differentiate between marketed and investigational projects and establish separate systems or priorities for each group
7. Establish a two-tiered system. In the first tier, prioritize marketed drugs ahead of drugs with a pending NDA, which in turn come before Phase III drugs, which precede Phase II drugs, etc. The second tier refers to priorities made within each of these broad classes

[a]More flexible systems appear to work best in most situations within the pharmaceutical industry because of the frequent changes of drug status and the frequent modifications required in prioritizations.

TABLE 17.2. *Methods to temporarily expand capabilities of fixed resources*

1. Contract a facility to serve as a core laboratory to assay samples off site
2. Use outside contract groups to (1) obtain investigators, (2) monitor studies, (3) process data, (4) analyze results, and/or (5) prepare regulatory dossiers
3. Collaborate with government agencies interested in developing drugs (e.g., National Cancer Institute, National Institute of Neurological and Communicable Diseases)
4. Collaborate with United Nations organizations (e.g., World Health Organization) on development of drugs intended for Third World countries
5. Contract synthesis and/or evaluation of compounds to outside scientists or to contract laboratories
6. Conduct only a partial analysis of data to expedite decisions. Complete data analyses at a later date only for viable projects
7. Hire temporary employees to assist in handling a short-term excess of work
8. Reassign permanent employees to handle a specific issue or task for a limited period

based on a manager's whim, personal preference, or various nonrational bases.

It is sometimes necessary to increase resources for a short period to satisfactorily deal with a temporary need. Selected methods that may temporarily expand the capabilities of fixed resources are listed in Table 17.2.

Resources of time, effort, and money in terms of people, equipment, and other factors must often be apportioned to different projects. The intensity, duration, and quantity of resources are often allocated according to priorities. In an ideal world there would be a perfect correlation between allocations and priorities. In the real world, however, people do not often establish clear priorities because priorities are not all-or-none, but vary by degree and may change frequently. In addition, there are many cases when people do not reevaluate priorities as conditions change. People may also not pursue their most important priorities because of many reasons, including judgment errors or psychologically denying the correct priorities.

Individuals may be assigned to work on only one project so that each project has a certain number of unique individuals assigned to it. Alternatively, each individual may be assigned to various projects and their time must then be allocated according to priorities established either for or by that individual. Combination approaches are often used in industry and academia, where some individuals work only on one project and others work on several. The reasons for choosing between these approaches may be based on the specific department involved or on the methods used to allocate resources. Sample headings of tables used to summarize work-force allocations are given in Table 17.3.

The portion of total resources allocated to each project and to each study within individual projects should be periodically reviewed. This can be done at several levels within an organization or by the individual or group re-

TABLE 17.3. *Sample table headings to summarize work-force allocations to specific studies or activities*

A

Project number and protocol number	Title of study	Investigator name(s)	No. of patients	Current status	Name or initials of personnel	Percentage of time allocated for the period (*X* months)

B

Project activity	Current status	Name or initials of personnel	Percentage of time allocated for the period	Maximum total work force needed during the period

C

Project activity	Total work force allocated for the period (worker months/month)	Total worker months for the period	Senior level headcount assigned	Junior level headcount assigned

sponsible for the allocation of resources. Reviews may occur on either a fixed or variable time basis, or only when forced by a "crisis." If reviews occur on a fixed interval, that interval may either be tied to time (e.g., monthly, quarterly) or to the stage in a project's life [e.g., Notice of Claimed Investigational Exemption for a New Drug (IND) submission, Phase I, Phase II].

18

Coordination of Multiple Projects

Description of Projects and Project Groups • Matrix Organizational Structure • Central Coordinating Function • Training of Project Leaders/Managers • Instruction and/or Training of Investigators and Staff

DESCRIPTION OF PROJECTS AND PROJECT GROUPS

Within the pharmaceutical industry and a number of other health-care-related industries (e.g., medical device or equipment manufacturers), innovation and technology are primarily directed toward development of new products that will eventually be launched on the market. Conducting the myriad steps necessary to develop a new drug or product requires coordination of the input and substantial activities occurring in numerous departments.

Projects are defined differently in different pharmaceutical companies. In some companies, a project represents one potential drug no matter how many formulations, dosage forms, or indications are evaluated. In other companies, each dosage form, formulation, and indication studied is considered as a separate project. A second aspect of defining projects relates to the stage of development at which a project is formed. A project may be formed at any stage, from an early chemical lead to a drug that has demonstrated activity in Phase II evaluations. A third consideration relates to whether one or more than one chemical compound may be considered to be part of a single project. Thus, it is apparent that the number of projects existing at different companies can only be compared when each of the above factors is considered. The quality of a compound in terms of its potential medical and commercial value are probably the most important criteria in creating new projects. Companies use different standards in determining whether a compound should be developed as a drug with regard to these two criteria. The implementation of these standards also has a great influence on the number of projects that are present in a company at any one time.

To develop drugs efficiently, it is useful to bring together at least one member of each of the various departments that will be involved in the development. This usually occurs before a compound has been tested in humans. These members may be referred to as a team, product group, project team, project committee, or by another term. This group is usually given a certain level of autonomy plus limited authority by senior management to pursue the development of their project. The team meets to determine goals, set strategies, develop and revise plans, set priorities within their project, and solve problems. Their efforts are reviewed formally and/or informally by other groups or individuals at periodic intervals and/or on an ad hoc basis.

The authority of each of the project groups varies enormously between (and even within) companies as does the number of members. There is no ideal number of members on the project group. For most projects there will probably be anywhere from five to 20 members on the committee, although the precise number is highly dependent on various factors, including (1) tradition and practice of the corporation, (2) type of project involved, (3) current phase of development, (4) plans and goals of the project, and (5) constraints on resources due to the presence of other projects. A summary of the various alternative organizational structures that constitute a project team is given in Table 18.1.

The seniority and authority of the members of the project team varies between companies. Team members at many companies are those who lead the work within their own departments, but individuals may be appointed to the project team for other reasons. Some administratively oriented individuals (e.g., department heads) may also be members of a project team to act as a bridge between line management and the matrix management concept (see next section) or for other reasons. Service and support departments (e.g., statistics, data entry processors, metabolism, toxicology) may also be represented on the team at relevant stage(s) during the life of a project. At some companies the project team is composed entirely or almost entirely of more-senior staff (e.g., department heads). A description of international project teams is given in Chapter 13.

MATRIX ORGANIZATIONAL STRUCTURE

In the traditional system of management, generally referred to as "line function" or vertical management, individuals report through the "chain of command" to the top of the organization. This type of management is usually described as having a pyramid structure, because there are progressively fewer managers as one ascends the corporate ranks. A newer system of management that has become more widespread in recent years is called a "matrix organizational structure." This is usually described as a horizontal system.

TABLE 18.1. *Alternative organizations and characteristics of a project team*[a]

Alternative	Approach to completing work on project	Approach to developing a team	Responsibility for work	Project leadership	Coordination with limited authority	Coordination with full authority	Periodic and/or ad hoc review and control
A	Divide work into subprojects for functional departments	No team exists (pure functional organization)	Each functional manager or department head	None	Generally none	Department heads or functional leaders	Upper levels of management
B	Divide work into subprojects for functional departments	Functional managers appoint representative (pseudomatrix)	Each functional manager or department head	None, committee, or other	A member within each department	Department heads or functional leaders	Upper levels of management
C	Divide work into subprojects for functional departments	Functional managers appoint representative (matrix)	Each functional manager or department head	Project manager[b]	Project manager or individual from outside the departments	Department heads and project manager	Upper levels of management
D	Divide work into subprojects for functional departments	Functional managers appoint representative (matrix)	Department heads and project manager	Project manager[b]	Individual jointly appointed by functional and project managers	Project manager	Upper levels of management
E	Divide work into subprojects for functional departments	Functional managers assign personnel to joint a team full time (task force)	Project manager	Project manager[b]	Individual on team	Project manager	Upper levels of management
F	Core group exists to handle multiple disciplinary functions	Core group functions as a team (pure project)	Project manager	Project manager[b]	Individual on team	Project manager	Upper levels of management

[a]Many variations on these six alternatives are possible.
[b]Project managers may be champions or full-time professional managers.

In most instances the matrix system does not replace the more traditional hierarchical-oriented line management, but is superimposed on it. All individuals continue to report through the line-function organization, but many (possibly most) employees also have a second reporting responsibility. Those individuals report to a member of the project team or group. Each member of the project team reports to the leader of the project, and all project leaders report to a central coordinator of all projects who then reports up the pyramid (or directly) to the head of research and development.

The reporting relationships in the matrix system may be as formal as those of the line-function system or they may be quite informal. The optimal system for each corporation probably varies to some degree depending on the (1) historical traditions of the company, (2) personalities of the people doing the work, (3) nature of their projects, and (4) styles of management used in the line-function system. Other considerations (e.g., personalities of the senior managers) are also of importance in determining the optimal manner in which to establish the matrix system.

A matrix organization is often adopted for managing projects because it allows the company to (1) conduct a larger number of complex projects efficiently, (2) better allocate resources, (3) coordinate activities more easily between various groups, (4) facilitate communications between separate departments, (5) assist individuals (or a group) who have difficulty identifying important tasks of high priority, (6) provide intellectual stimulation to team members, and (7) remove some degree of the high emotional stakes in the outcome of studies supervised by line managers. Other benefits of this system are listed in Table 18.2. This approach requires management support to all levels in a company for it to operate effectively. If the managers do not want the matrix system to be successful it will not work.

TABLE 18.2. *Generally perceived benefits of the matrix system*

1. Improves management control. Provides an alternative to line management and is an easier means to monitor progress and current status on multiple projects. Helps resolve conflicts between project requirements and the functional roles of various departments
2. Improves flexibility of the system used to achieve NDAs
3. Improves visibility of more individuals to senior management
4. Improves cross-functional communication between different departments and groups working on a project
5. Provides a simple mechanism to solicit, receive, and use input from all relevant departments, groups, and functions
6. Applies expertise and resources flexibly and efficiently to multiple projects
7. Achieves project objectives more efficiently than without the matrix, since the entire project team usually operates as a group
8. Allows skilled professionals to work on multiple projects while working within their area of expertise
9. Allows the entire project portfolio to be easily viewed as a whole and may be more readily reviewed, modified, and/or directed

When problems arise within any section or department, the individuals involved must decide whether to pursue its resolution through line management or through the matrix system. Ideally, both avenues are open and there should be little or no friction or difficulties between the two when one system is used rather than the other.

This idealized view of two systems working in complete harmony is difficult to achieve in practice. An important consideration for some individuals in determining the system that should have priority in solving a problem relates to the system that is tied to promotions, salary adjustments, and other administrative matters. If each system's representative has equal input into these administrative matters, then a strong conflict is more likely to result as they each attempt to gain a superior position. If, however, one system is defined or created as having dominance then there is a better chance of achieving harmonious relationships in operations and facilitating solutions to problems. Within each of these spheres, certain problems and administrative matters will tend to become centered. Making these distinctions as clear as possible to all employees concerned with both systems is an important goal to pursue.

The case against the matrix system is that it dilutes authority and creates dual loyalties, especially when a formal reporting system is established on the same administrative level as line managers. This may lead to an undesirable competition between line managers and matrix managers. The matrix system requires greater interpersonal skills to operate effectively and is more time consuming to operate. Also, it is often difficult for project managers to accurately assess the contribution of each member of the team, since most of their work is performed within their line-function responsibilities.

Conflicts that occur between line and matrix managers are often over clearly defining the types of decisions that lie within each's purview. One approach toward resolution of complex situations when many people are involved is to clarify the major roles of the individuals involved in decision making. These roles include those of individuals who (1) have final approval, (2) should be consulted but who are without veto power, (3) may develop alternatives and provide analyses, (4) should be informed about decisions made, and (5) have responsibility for implementing a decision once it is made.

Scheduling Project Activities

Some of the most popular approaches currently used to schedule project activities are (1) milestones, (2) Gantt, and (3) PERT. Each of these will be briefly discussed.

Milestone Schedules

Milestones are the major time points and stages in a project's life. For projects involving drugs, these milestones usually include the time of (1) project formation, (2) Notice of Claimed Investigational Exemption for a New Drug (IND) filing, (3) Phase I (start, end), (4) Phase II (start, end), (5) Phase III (start), (6) New Drug Application (NDA) filing, (7) NDA approvable letter, (8) NDA approval letter, and (9) product launch.

Milestone schedules are rarely sufficient on their own to serve as an adequate project schedule. The milestone listings may summarize a great deal of information, avoid complexity, and present "the bottom line" for individuals to use as a measure to gauge progress. Both start and completion dates for a variety of activities may be listed. Although milestones are easy to prepare and review, they do not indicate interrelationships between activities or any details of the project plan.

Gantt Chart

A Gantt chart is a bar or line chart along an axis of time, often using a calendar. Figure 3.2 illustrates one example. This type of chart is easily understood and is therefore widely used. This type of chart may be modified in many ways, such as illustrating the time necessary to complete various parts of the task represented by one bar, through use of hatched lines, open spaces, or other markings. One of the drawbacks of this approach is that it is not suitable for most large and complex projects and its does not illustrate interactions between activities. As with the milestone charts, the Gantt chart may be used in conjunction with more complex schedules. In that situation, the Gantt chart may illustrate one or a few aspects of a larger project.

Program Evaluation and Review Technique (PERT)

PERT is more complex than the preceding two methods and illustrates the interdependence of many activities. The IND and NDA models shown in Figs. 18.1 and 18.2 are illustrations of the PERT technique. This network chart is usually accompanied by a listing of all of the separate activities shown. It is usually desirable to list activities for each individual group or department responsible for those activities. Those lists may then be used as a planning tool by those groups.

PERT, along with the closely related methodologies of Critical Path Method and Precedence Scheduling are network methods that illustrate and document how multiple processes may be followed in a project. This approach may consider the critical path, whereby those activities are indicated which are rate limiting. If activities noted as critical are delayed then the time for project completion will be delayed. Each event on a PERT chart may be considered as a milestone, albeit a minor one in most instances.

Whereas the Critical Path Method uses a single estimate of time required to complete an activity, the strict definition of PERT requires three time

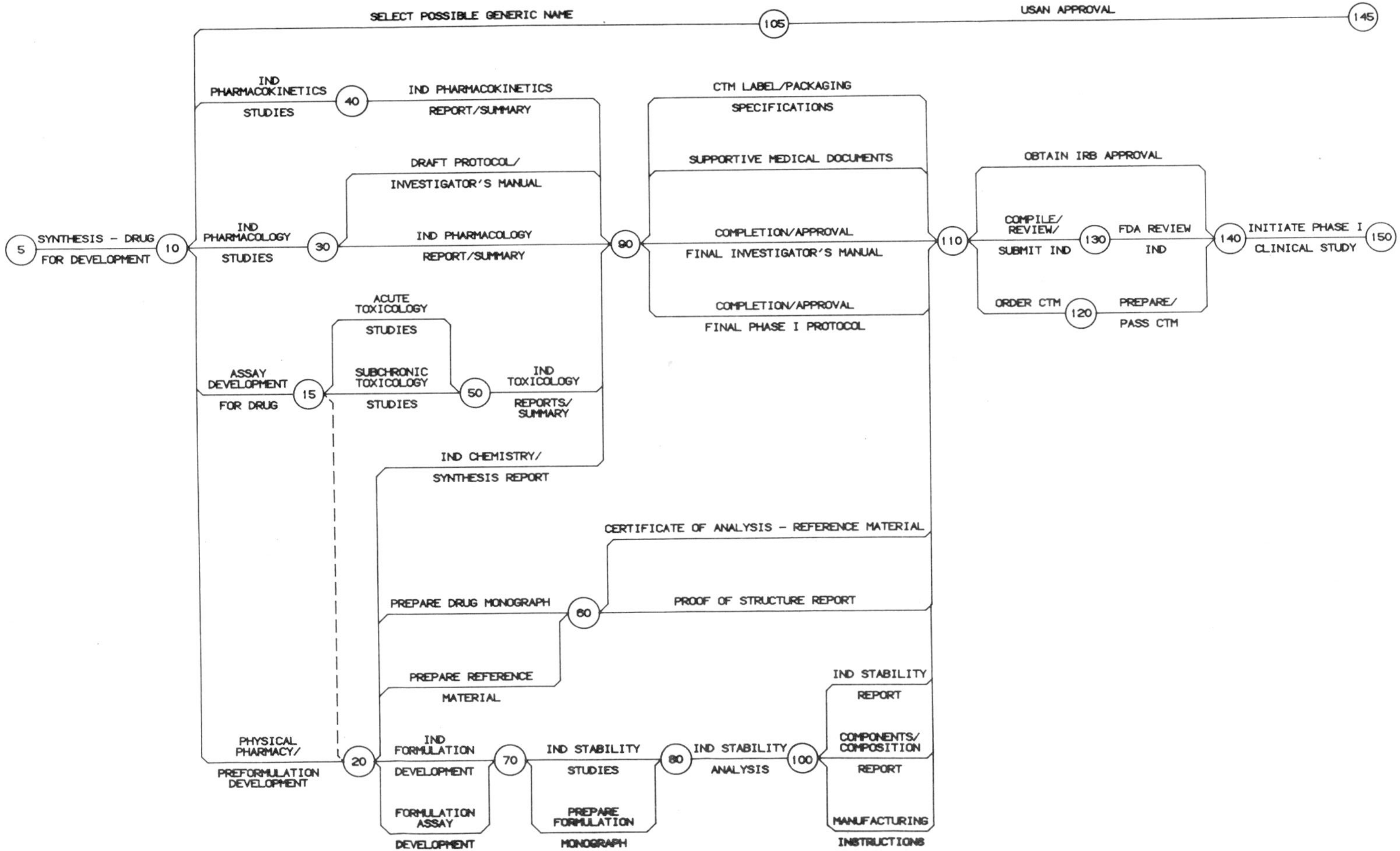

FIG. 18.1. Model of activities needed to submit an IND (PERT chart).

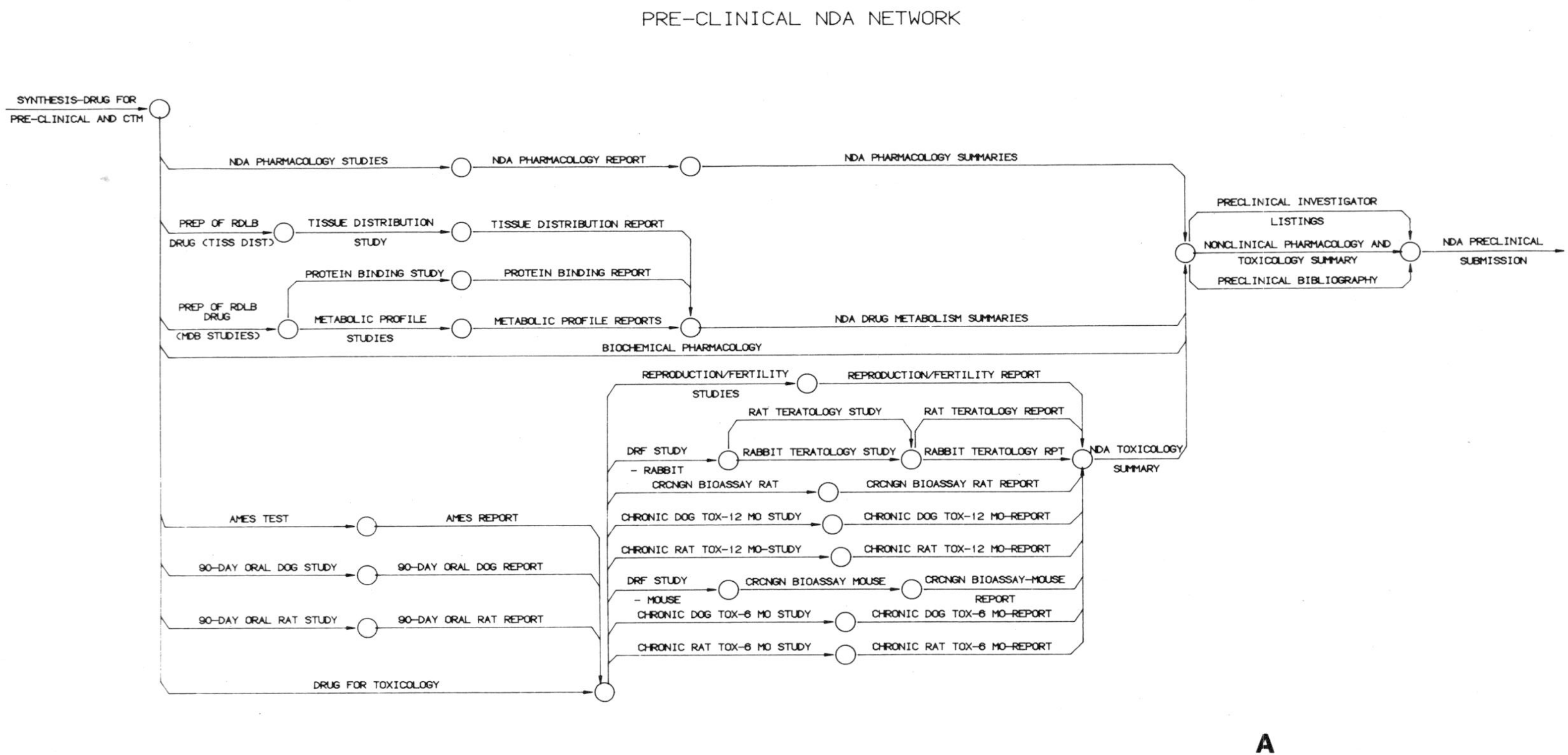

FIG. 18.2. Model of activities needed to submit an NDA (PERT chart). Panel A shows preclinical activities, Panel B shows clinical activities, and Panel C shows technical development activities. Abbreviations in Panel A are CTM = Clinical trial material, RDLB = radiolabeled, TISS DIST = tissue distribution, CRCNGN = Carcinogen, MO = month, DRF = dose range finding, and TOX = toxicology. In Panel B, new abbreviations are USAN = United States adopted names, PO = oral, and IV = intravenous.

CLINICAL NDA NETWORK

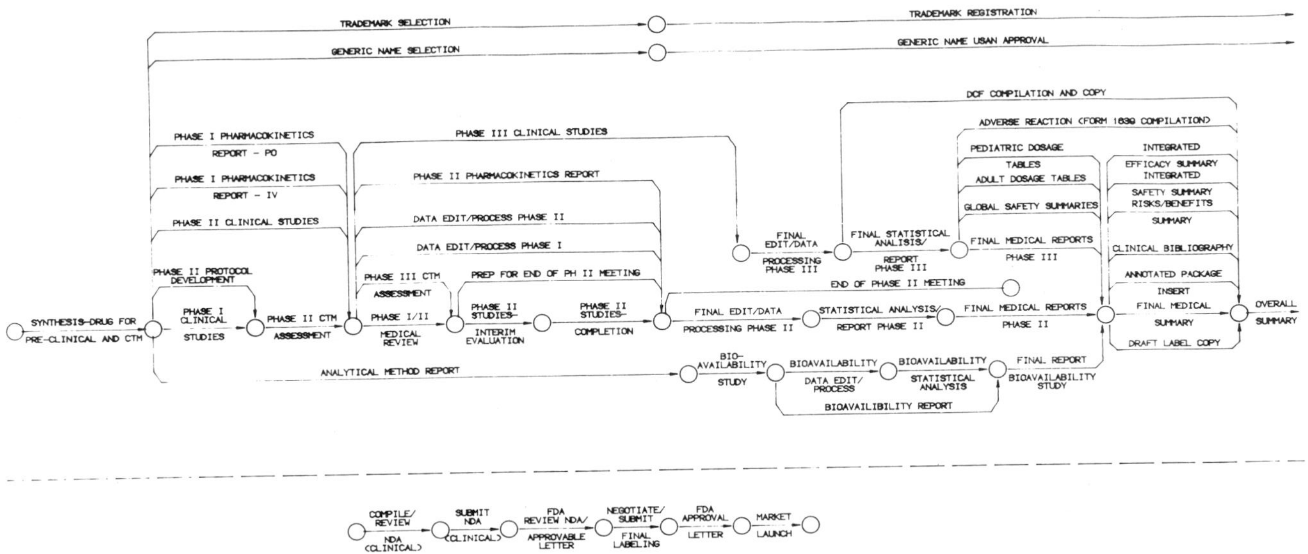

B

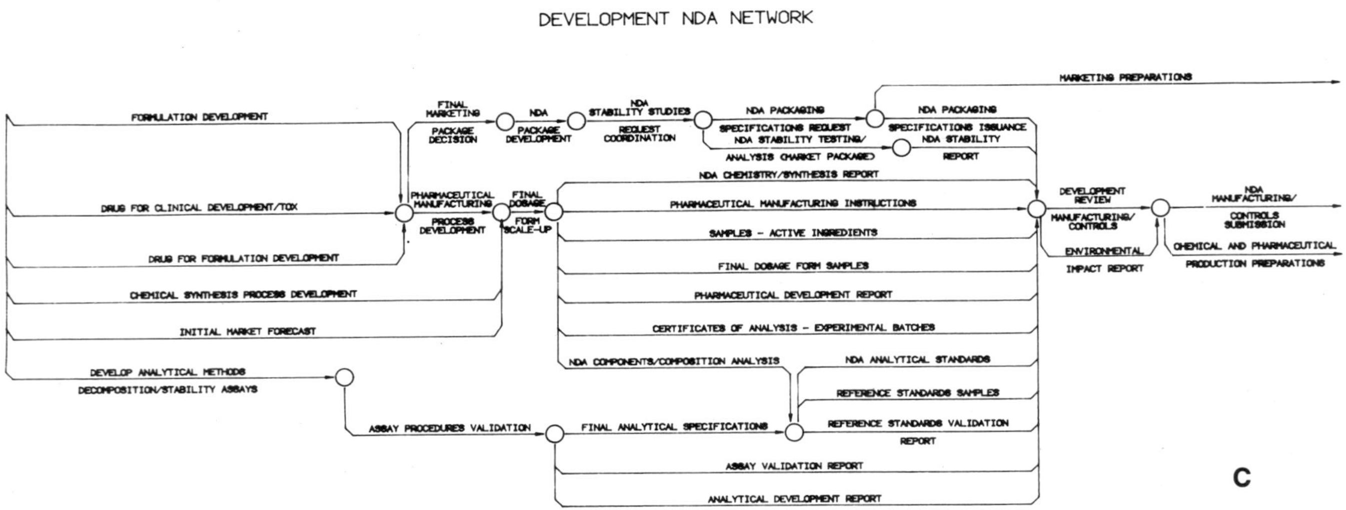

FIG. 18.2. *(Continued)*

estimates for each activity. These estimates are for the best case, worst case, and most likely case. These three estimates are then used to create a single time estimate, using a standard formula.

To use the PERT system it is necessary to have:

1. A well-defined set of activities that constitute a project. Usually 20 to several hundred events are listed.
2. Activities that are interrelated with other activities and conducted in a predetermined order.
3. The ability to designate which activities may be initiated and stopped independently of each other.
4. An indication of the time required to complete each activity or the probability that each activity will be successful.

Comparisons of the various techniques may be found in texts or reviews on project management (e.g., Cleland and King, 1983; Graham, 1985; Cori, 1985). It is usually most relevant to create PERT charts for drug projects for the IND, NDA, and launch milestones. These charts are not generally as useful at other times of a project's life, unless the sponsoring organization has implemented an ambitious overall cost and resource tracking and management system.

CENTRAL COORDINATING FUNCTION

It may be useful to establish a central coordinating function to assist in tracking and monitoring various activities within multiple projects. This is especially relevant if the multiple projects impinge on each other in terms of their need for resources and require central overall monitoring and administration. Some companies that have established this function utilize a single individual, but most larger companies have created a small group or department to fulfill this role. The size of the department varies between pharmaceutical companies, but is usually kept to a relatively small size of approximately three to 12 people. The role of this group in any company varies from simply consulting on planning to having a strong central management role in budgeting, expenditure review, global status reporting, and/or central control of investigational drug usage.

Coordination involves both planning activities that occur simultaneously in one or more departments and identifying those activities that occur sequentially. In a complex project such as developing a drug, both simultaneous and sequential processes must be planned. All of the activities within departments may be considered by creating a model that prepares a plan for each individual drug under development. The plans shown in Figs. 18.1 and 18.2 are generic ones and must be modified to include specific characteristics, requirements, and available resources for the particular investigational drug.

In theory, the plan developed for each particular project (e.g., Fig. 18.1) may be used as a road map. The plan outlines the route that each involved department will follow to reach the final goal. A drug rarely follows the original route without numerous modifications to the plan. There are two major types of reasons why the original plan is only an ideal route. The first reason is related to modifications that occur in the development plans of drug X itself. The second reason is that in most instances, the development project on a single drug is not the only major ongoing project, and demands for resources, priority, or other factors related to different projects often influence the development of drug X.

Plans for a drug's development are modified throughout the course of implementing and conducting the various activities. This occurs because only incomplete information for planning the entire development program is known at the outset of the project. As more and more technical and clinical information becomes available the plans for the regulatory submission usually become more clear. In addition, problems or significant issues invariably arise during the development of any drug which require modifications of the plans. Serious problems may cause the entire plan to be scraped, revised, or placed on hold. Numerous causes of a delay are possible. Many delays do not require major modification of the plan's logic and activities as much as they prolong the time necessary to carry out the activities in the plan. Selected procedures to follow in project management are shown in Table 18.3.

Personnel within the central coordination unit may act as planning consultants or as leaders or managers of the project teams. In certain instances these project managers are fully accountable for their projects, prepare reg-

TABLE 18.3. *Selected procedures to follow in project management*[a]

1. Define project objectives in terms of final tangible outputs
2. Develop a progressive breakdown of the project until manageable units of work (activities) are established
3. Establish a list of all activities required to achieve the project objectives
4. Establish a network, using all of the activities in a time sequence
5. Evaluate the network to establish early and late start and completion dates, plus the amount of slack time. Establish which activities constitute the critical path
6. Create a schedule that utilizes the network, availability of resources, priorities, and the calendar
7. Estimate the times to complete each activity. In some situations (e.g., with PERT techniques) an optimistic, pessimistic, and most likely estimate may be made
8. Assign responsibility for completing activities to appropriate individuals
9. Establish a method to monitor progress
10. Establish a method for management review and dealing with problems
11. Use milestones and other systems as needed to gauge progress and review activities
12. Revise network and schedule as necessary

[a] This list excludes financial aspects (e.g., costs, budgets) which must often be included.

ulatory (e.g., IND and NDA) summaries, and monitor details of their projects' activities. Most individuals who have this magnitude of responsibility can only manage a small number of projects (e.g., two or three).

The project team may also be led by a scientist or clinician. The choice of one or the other usually depends on the specific stage of a drug's development. This individual may or may not act as a project champion. He or she will have other (i.e., departmental) responsibilities in addition to managing the project. In this situation, personnel from the central coordination unit may act as an assistant to the project team leader or they may be restricted to a planning and coordination function. The project planner may then handle more projects. This number varies, but is often in the range of approximately six to 12 projects. Advantages of having project teams led by professional managers or by project champions are summarized in Table 18.4, and methods of assigning work among project planners are listed in Table 18.5.

TABLE 18.4. *Advantages of having project teams led by professional managers or by project champions*

A. Advantages of professional project managers	B. Advantages of project champions
1. Usually have a more even-handed and objective approach to all projects 2. Usually are more experienced with the methodologies used to develop drugs than project champions 3. Usually are more experienced with management methods 4. Less training is usually required in administrative methods and procedures 5. Can usually facilitate agreements between projects more easily 6. Improves the chance of choosing the most suitable individual to lead the project 7. They may be better leaders of a project than the champion(s) 8. Less chance of enthusiastic champions draining resources to a project prematurely (e.g., before efficacy is demonstrated) or to a less promising or less important project 9. Avoids problems that may develop when project leadership is given as a reward to an individual instead of giving it to the most appropriate person	1. Usually have more enthusiasm for their particular project. This generates a sense of excitement and a commitment to push the project forward 2. The process of utilizing project champions trains more individuals in managerial techniques 3. Provides more challenges to the most exceptional staff 4. Provides a goal for many potential champions to aspire to 5. Diversifies responsibilities within a company or organization

TABLE 18.5. *Assigning work among project planners*

1. Assign different therapeutic categories to each planner, who then becomes involved with all projects in that area
2. Rotate projects periodically among planners
3. Balance quantity of work independent of therapeutic area
4. Assign planners to specific departments or sections within departments
5. Assign different phases of clinical development to different planners
6. Assign different specialties (e.g., NDA preparation, IND preparation) to different planners

The training and background of leaders of coordination departments vary to a great degree, as does the training of the individuals within the departments. The department leaders usually, but not always, have a substantial background in science, but individuals with business, production, or other backgrounds have also been appointed to these positions. The orientation, attitudes, interpersonal skills, and managerial abilities of those people appears to be a more critical determinant of success in their role than their area(s) of previous training. The academic degrees achieved by these coordination heads also vary. If this individual has additional responsibilities in the organization, then the nature of these other tasks will greatly influence the background, training, and experience necessary for the coordinating position.

Members of coordination departments who perform various planning activities and monitor progress of these plans usually interact with all members of the project team. These planners also have a wide range of training and experience. A scientific background is highly desirable, and in some companies it is essential. Probably their most important attributes are interpersonal skills and attention to detail. If either of these skills is absent the abilities of these individuals to function effectively will be diminished. Experience with computers is becoming a more important part of success in these positions. Potential functions and issues to address for project planners are listed in Tables 18.6 and 18.7.

The field of project planning and coordination is a relatively young one in the pharmaceutical industry. Current activities within the Project Management Institute and the Pharmaceutical Manufacturer's Association demonstrate that the group of project planners is searching for a professional identity and also for an accepted role that allows professional career opportunities for growth and advancement. Preliminary efforts into certification, and acceptance as a profession by outside groups, have not been totally satisfactory to date, but efforts are continuing which will hopefully improve the professional image and career opportunities for project planners in the future.

TABLE 18.6. *Potential functions of project planners*

1. Develop a network chart(s) (e.g., PERT, Gantt) and schedule(s) for each project to help organize all activities necessary to complete the IND, NDA, or other goal
2. Monitor progress of all activities listed in the schedule to determine whether they remain "on time" and "on course"
3. Modify and/or expand the network and/or schedule as required to keep it current
4. Develop a network and schedule for the launch of either (1) a new drug or (2) an old drug with expanded indications, new dosage form, new formulation, or other modifications
5. Develop a network and schedule to plan and monitor Phase IV studies, toxicology, or studies within a specific department. Develop other plans as needed
6. Develop procedures and forms to monitor the flow of clinical, toxicological, or other data. Implement use of forms and monitor progress
7. Assist in the coordination between the group(s) representing the research and development function and marketing, production, financial, and/or foreign groups
8. Assist in interdepartmental communications to clarify and resolve issues
9. Follow the financial status of the project. If the company allots a certain sum to be used by each project, assist in the plans for its disbursement and monitor funds spent
10. Accompany project leaders to relevant meetings with regulatory personnel, senior managers, or other groups
11. Act as a secretary for the project at both official and unofficial meetings
12. Provide other assistance to the project leader as requested on an ad hoc basis (e.g., provide specific analyses, documentation, graphics, and/or other information on a project)
13. Facilitate meetings or actions that attempt to solve problems
14. Derive estimated times for completing disparate activities using a criterion of either optimistic, pessimistic, or realistic appraisals of time required[a]

[a] Estimates may include or exclude consideration of other currently active projects that may possibly (or definitely will) affect the schedule.

TABLE 18.7. *Selected issues for project planners to address*

1. Should planners passively accept dates that project members provide to devise a project schedule and network, or critically evaluate and question those dates to increase the speed of completing the project?
2. Should all departments submit work schedules and resource allocations to a central person or group? This might allow more rapid recognition of either underutilization or overcommitment of resources
3. Should planners closely monitor adherence to the schedules by all relevant groups?
4. Should estimated times to complete activities be based on the best possible, worst possible, or average times? Should other approaches be used to estimate time requirements?
5. How much effort should be expended in each project on strategies, PERT charts, and other planning activities? Is the amount of time and effort spent on these activities cost-effective?
6. If activities are falling behind schedule who should evaluate whether the reasons for the delay are legitimate and, more importantly, determine whether priorities must be adjusted?
7. Who has the responsibility for enforcing scheduled dates?

TRAINING OF PROJECT LEADERS/MANAGERS

Traditionally, project leaders receive most of their basic training while "on the job." Recently, some companies have created more formal systems to improve the quality of training. There is no single approach to training that meets everyone's needs, and a variety of programs are usually established. Some of the approaches that are used to train project leaders/managers are:

1. An experienced individual may be assigned to act as a tutor in an initial period and to act as a resource person in later stages. This experienced person may be another project leader, a project planner, or another type of individual.
2. An orientation program may be established for new project leaders. This may be organized such that interactive sessions are scheduled throughout a day, or it may be divided into separate sessions occurring over a period of weeks. The instructors are generally department and other senior individuals whose departments or functions will interact with project leaders. Experienced project leaders may also instruct the group on various issues that may arise during one's tenure as a project leader. It is usually best if these orientation sessions are limited to small groups, to facilitate discussion.
3. A periodic meeting of all project leaders may be conducted with (or without) senior management to provide an opportunity for discussing issues of mutual interest. Problems that exist in the project system may be discussed. The opportunity for interaction and problem solving is an essential part of this meeting. The format of the meeting should be chosen to allow this interaction to occur, and new formats may be tried from year to year. Retreats, work-dinner sessions, and small workshops are a few possible formats. Meetings between project leaders in research and development with product managers in marketing or production may also be useful.
4. A written guide or manual provides valuable information for project leaders to use as a reference. The guide may contain information along the lines of standard operating procedures, but should also contain background information on departments, their organization, and general means of performing functions that are of interest to the project leader. This type of guide rapidly goes out of date because many procedures change significantly or are replaced entirely. Thus, providing this guide in a loose-leaf binder with sectional tabs that serve as an index has advantages over creating a permanently bound version. The loose-leaf album allows new parts to be added or substituted for out-of-date material. The guide will then have a longer period of useful life.

A separate guide presenting information on regulatory issues may also be useful to prepare.

5. A mentor approach may be followed formally or informally, either as a substitute for point 1 above or as an additional technique. Most individuals are able to learn from the experience and wisdom of a mentor. This system usually achieves best results when it is implemented by project leaders informally on their own volition. It is uncertain whether formally establishing a mentor approach will achieve the same degree of success as providing encouragement to those interested in this approach.
6. Outside courses are being heavily promoted to the government, academicians, and the pharmaceutical industry. Some emphasize technical skills that the project leader may lack, whereas others focus on management and interpersonal skills. These courses are offering to fill a need that is usually not met in the training of scientists and professional managers who become project leaders.
7. A roundtable meeting of project leaders or managers may be conducted to discuss useful points and techniques they have learned which might be helpful for others to learn. Although every project teaches innumerable lessons about better ways to avoid and deal with problems, many of these relate to the highly specific nature and conditions of that project and the people involved. Nonetheless, many lessons are more generic and may be used by others.
8. Ad hoc seminars and meetings designed to train managers and/or improve their managerial knowledge have a role in improving skills, but are best viewed as supplemental material to the other parts of the training program.

Other educational opportunities for project leaders are to (1) tour man-

TABLE 18.8. *Techniques to use in training new investigators or staff*

1. Utilize lecture courses, seminars, and other types of formal verbal instruction
2. Provide video tapes of other investigators who are either interacting with, or examining patients. These tapes should illustrate points about patient diagnosis, treatment, identification of adverse reactions, or other aspects of the study
3. Make video tapes of the investigator-in-training with patients. Use these as a learning tool to help new investigators improve their techniques
4. Hold a roundtable discussion with the sponsor and/or other investigators, consultants, and staff. Review the protocol and other aspects of the study
5. Have the new investigator or staff work with an experienced investigator or study coordinator for a specified period
6. Have the new investigator or staff practice specific techniques or procedures with their colleagues
7. Monitor the site frequently to assess progress of the new staff

ufacturing facilities, (2) spend a day with a sales representative to obtain a better understanding of their role, (3) listen to prepared cassette programs, and (4) solve problem situations in a written or oral format that are based on previous company experiences. A number of qualities that are usually valuable for an effective project leader to possess are listed in Table 16.3.

INSTRUCTION AND/OR TRAINING OF INVESTIGATORS AND STAFF

In some clinical studies the requirements of the protocol may be complex or involve methods with which the investigator or staff are not familiar. Additionally, co-investigators or other staff often join a study already in progress, as a result of (1) staff turnover, (2) rotation of residents, (3) expansion of the study, or (4) other reasons. In all of these circumstances it is often important for the sponsor to review relevant information and/or techniques with the new investigator and/or staff. The sponsor usually has a clinical monitor serve this function, although it is possible for the project leader or others to coordinate and perform this role. Some of the techniques that may be used to assist in training new investigators or staff are listed in Table 18.8.

19

Use of Meetings, Documents, and Computers to Assist in Planning and Managing Drug Studies

Meetings • Documents • Computers

MEETINGS

Introduction

The types of meetings held to plan and manage projects vary, depending on the nature of the project, its needs, the personalities of the people involved, and the historical traditions and systems of the institution. A few general comments and principles are pertinent to mention.

Meetings are required at each relevant level within an organization to effectively handle project-related matters. These levels include section, department, interdepartment, and corporate (or institution) groups. The major factors in considering the nature of meetings relate to their (1) level within the organization, (2) time of scheduling, (3) objectives or goals, (4) degree of formality, and (5) size. After these points are considered, the relevant people who should attend that meeting are chosen.

Scheduling

Scheduling of meetings may be viewed in the context of (1) those scheduled at periodic intervals (e.g., once a month, three times a year), (2) those scheduled at variable intervals to coincide with project milestones or other events, or (3) ad hoc meetings called for specific reasons.

Purposes

General purposes or goals of meetings are to (1) establish objectives and plans, (2) deal effectively with and solve problems, (3) communicate information, (4) coordinate activities, (5) advise an individual or group, (6) discuss, review, and/or evaluate various aspects of a project, (7) formulate policy, (8) brainstorm, and (9) make decisions. Meetings may also deal with issues in a highly detailed technical manner. Meetings may include discussions of both technical and general issues when appropriate.

Principles

One of the most important principles of meetings is that the leader of the meeting should encounter "no surprises." This is the "golden rule" of meetings for many individuals. Individuals who will attend a meeting may have information to convey that is unknown and unexpected by the leader of the meeting. This information should be communicated to the leader as far ahead of the meeting as possible. The flow of meetings is often disrupted and meetings are sometimes unable to accomplish their purpose(s) when unexpected information is presented which significantly affects the topic or project. This information often achieves shock value, but is counterproductive to efficient management of a project. The practice of surprising people should be strongly discouraged by all project leaders and line managers. There should also be no surprises in who shows up at meetings.

Meetings that are called to solve a problem should initially define the specific nature and character of the problem. Preferably this should be done prior to the meeting, but it may be done at the meeting itself. A clear description of the problem to be discussed may be a simply stated matter or may require a great deal of time, discussion, and energy. It is often helpful if background material is prepared and distributed prior to the meeting to help expedite the discussion. A wise leader will have previously lobbied those who will attend the meeting. He will attempt to achieve their commitment to his point of view by persuading them to assist in planning and/or decision making. Involving others in a new idea or solution will increase their commitment to favor the idea or approach proposed. Doing this prior to a meeting will help insure its adoption and eventual success.

Types

Two basic types of meetings are held to review and evaluate progress, current status, future plans, and other aspects of a clinical study or project. The first is where the group that formulated the plan (or other information being considered) is reviewing and/or evaluating information that it has either directly generated or has had clear responsibility for generating. The second type of meeting is where a group is reviewing and/or evaluating various aspects of a project that it either did not create or directly request. This second type of review is often conducted by a senior management review group. In many situations there is an intermediate position where one or more of the people who helped formulate the plans are also members of a higher reviewing body, or where the more senior reviewing group has had some direct input into the plans.

Formality

The degree of formality of a meeting may not always be established in advance. There are situations where plans for one type of meeting are not carried through (for any of a number of possible reasons) and the meeting is treated either more or less formally than was anticipated or planned. In hindsight, the reasons for this disparity are often clear and should help in planning future meetings of a similar type.

Size

Various studies of a meeting's size illustrate that the type of interpersonal interactions change as the size of the group increases. Meetings tend to become more formal as their size increases. Meetings may be broadly categorized as small (5 or fewer people), medium (5–20 people), or large (20–50 people). When there are more than 50 people, one generally is in more of a lecture type of meeting where discussion becomes difficult. These numbers are not precise and in certain situations the boundaries may be quite different (either toward a larger or smaller number). The number of people invited to attend a meeting should be considered in the context of what type of discussions are desired and in relation to the approximate size of the group which is desired.

Technical Details

Technical details that must be planned for conducting a meeting also change markedly as the size of the meeting increases. Factors must be considered such as (1) voice enhancement with microphones, (2) suitable audiovisual displays, (3) introductions of people present, (4) ability to have informal interactions, and (5) a smooth flow and control of the meeting itself. A few issues to consider which may improve the conduct of meetings are listed in Table 19.1.

TABLE 19.1. *Questions to consider prior to a meeting which may improve its conduct and productivity*

A. Objectives
1. Is there a real need for the meeting?
2. Who should attend the meeting?
3. What outcomes of the meeting are desired?
4. What outcomes of the meeting are specifically not desired?

B. Decision making
1. Who should lead this meeting and control its flow?
2. What items will be on the agenda and in which order?
3. What methods will the group use to deal with each agenda item?
4. What processes will be used to reach decisions?
5. Who will make the final decision?
6. Will the meeting be allowed to continue past its scheduled conclusion? If so, by how much time?

C. Administrative matters
1. What type of meeting will be held?
2. When should the meeting be held?
3. Where would the best place be to hold the meeting?
4. What will be the length of the meeting and will there be breaks?
5. How should the chairs and tables be set up?
6. Who will keep notes/minutes of the meeting and how will these be reviewed and issued?
7. What equipment will be needed (e.g., flip chart, slide projector)?
8. What food/beverages will be available or served and at what times?
9. What documents should be distributed prior to and at the meeting?
10. What materials (e.g., pens, paper) should be available for participants?

Increasing Efficiency

To increase the efficiency of meetings it is often possible to (1) decrease their number by eliminating unnecessary ones or by combining two or more meetings, (2) use agendas, (3) use a time schedule, (4) decrease the number of participants, (5) limit discussion on each agenda item, and (6) assign activities for individuals to complete after the meeting. It is necessary to keep track of these latter assignments so that those people will report back to the group at a subsequent meeting or via a different mechanism. A highly readable account of how to run a meeting is presented by Jay (1976).

The arrangement of tables and chairs sometimes may encourage participation and discussion of the group or may serve as a barrier. For example, if everybody sits around a single table there appears to be better involvement and more active participation than when several sit in chairs behind or away from a table where the main focus of discussion takes place.

It is sometimes valuable to have an individual at the meeting who (1) summarizes discussions on a subject after it is clear that additional constructive comments have ceased, (2) brings the discussion back to the relevant topic if it wanders on a tangent for too long a period, (3) recommends taking up the next subject if too much time is spent on one topic, and (4) recommends that highly detailed issues be handled by a small group outside the larger meeting. This type of individual is often self-appointed, but a leader may easily encourage or discourage this type of behavior.

Concluding a Meeting

The final event of a meeting should be a summary by the leader. This insures that everyone leaves the meeting on the same "wavelength." Points to be pursued outside the meeting should be reviewed and these can also be put in the minutes.

Consultants Meetings

Two specific types of meetings are discussed in more detail because of their special nature to clinical issues. A meeting with consultants is discussed below, and a prestudy roundtable meeting is discussed in Chapter 34 of *Guide to Clinical Studies and Developing Protocols* (Spilker, 1984).

There are often occasions in the life of a project when it is valuable to bring a group of consultants together to discuss an important issue or problem. The two major occasions are: (1) the outset of a project when a general direction or emphasis is being charted and the strategies are being developed; (2) when an important problem has developed which will benefit from expert input into the decision that senior management has to make.

The group of consultants will be chosen from individuals who are (1) already acting as consultants to the sponsor, (2) other experts in the field, (3) thought leaders in the field, or (4) other individuals who may have a special contribution to offer, such as general practitioners. Consultants will provide suggestions and recommendations based on their own experiences and patients. The choice of specific consultants and their backgrounds will have a great influence on the type of advice they will offer. Consultants who understand the complexities of drug development have a marked advantage in many cases over other experts who do not. If only tertiary care experts from academic institutions are assembled, the sophisticated opinions and advice they offer may be totally inappropriate for a drug that will almost totally be used in primary care medicine. Another criterion for choosing consultants is based on identifying potential investigators to conduct future clinical studies. In addition to the type of consultants invited to a meeting, the advice they offer will be highly dependent on the specific questions posed and also how the questions are posed. Careful consideration should be given to this issue and to the communications with the consultants prior to the meeting.

A group of four to eight consultants are often assembled, plus members

TABLE 19.2. *Selected types of questions for expert consultants to consider regarding a clinical project*

1. Dosage forms to develop
2. Efficacy parameters to measure
3. Methods to measure efficacy parameters
4. Choice of patient population(s)[a]
5. Methods to recruit patients
6. Estimated rate of patient enrollment
7. Methods to identify an appropriate dosing regimen
8. Approaches to establish a safety profile
9. Choice of criteria to stop a study prematurely
10. Role of continuation studies
11. Priority of different indications and routes of administration
12. Choice of studies for Phases I, II, and III
13. Choice of criteria and measures to determine the benefit-to-risk ratio
14. Methods to diagnose patients
15. Choice of an active control drug

[a] This may include consideration of whether a placebo control group is ethically possible.

of the project team, senior managers, and individuals who are in charge of the project at a foreign subsidiary or parent company. This latter group (or individual) is extremely important to include in the discussions and decision-making process to facilitate international cooperation and acceptance of decisions reached.

The agenda for the meeting should allow time for (1) presentation of background, (2) statement of the issues, (3) discussion, and (4) recommendations. It may be useful to allot separate times for panel (i.e., consultant) discussion and discussion with the audience. Although the duration of the meeting may last from 1 hr to several days, it is usually impractical to have a meeting that lasts more than a single day. Almost all consultants are extremely busy and, with few exceptions, would prefer not to spend more time. A meeting that discusses an entire therapeutic area, however, may require several days. Selected types of questions for expert consultants to consider are listed in Table 19.2.

DOCUMENTS

Functions of Records

Although many people prefer to run projects without producing formal reports, there is a need for documentation in all projects. Many of the reasons why documentation is important relate to the functions that it serves. These functions include a need to:

1. Communicate and disseminate information among relevant individuals, some of whom may be many miles away.
2. Serve as a basis to discuss various issues or problems, where everyone concerned may read the same background material and statement of the issues.
3. Serve as a means for speculation about a point where input is requested.
4. Provide a blueprint of current and proposed plans and operational strategies to help allocate resources, assign priorities, and assign work responsibilities.
5. Seek response to a request or proposal.
6. Provide an archival document for future use, as an "institutional memory."
7. Provide a formal source of agreements, statements, commitments, and decisions made by individuals and by groups.

Types of Reports and Issues in Record Keeping

Various types of reports are generated. Almost any type of meeting may generate minutes, consensus agreements, points for action, or other information that may need to be documented. In addition, numerous reports are written independently of meetings. These reports include feasibility reports (see Chapter 1), project plans, project strategies (see Chapter 2), current status on one or more issues, issues to be resolved, plus many others.

In addition to reports there are many forms, lists, and schedules that will assist in the management of multiple clinical studies. Some of those are shown and/or described later in this chapter. A number of types of records that an investigator may adopt are listed in Table 19.3, and selected issues in record keeping are listed in Table 19.4.

Standard Operating Procedures

Standard operating procedures are intended to provide guidance for performing many of the activities needed to plan, conduct, and manage single or multiple clinical studies. This guidance reflects the policy of the institution in which the activities are conducted. Standard operating procedures are a useful guide in numerous activities, and a few selected areas are listed in Table 19.5. They are an important part of quality assurance activities necessary to insure that Good Laboratory Practices (GLPs), Good Manufacturing Practices (GMPs), and Good Clinical Practices (GCPs) are followed in developing a drug or medical device.

Standard operating procedures should only be established if they are going to be followed. A balance must be established between the ideal, practical, and actual case in using standard procedures in many situations. There

TABLE 19.3. *Types of record keeping that an investigator may adopt*[a]

A. Individual patient records for patients who are also part of a physician's clinical practice
   1. Maintain separate files of a patient's medical records and records for each drug study in which they participate. Place these files together under the patient's name
   2. Maintain separate files of a patient's medical records and records for each drug study in which they participate. Write "progress notes" for each clinic visit conducted as part of a drug study on the patient's permanent medical records. Place the two sets of records in separate files, one devoted to practice patients and the other to drug studies
   3. Cross-index all hospital records in a patient's medical record, with hospital number, dates of each admission, reasons for admission, and other pertinent data
   4. Cross-index all laboratory reports maintained in a drug study if the reports are not photocopied in the patient's permanent medical records
B. Individual patient records for patients who are also not part of a physician's clinical practice
   1. Duplicate basic information from the drug study record to a new file that is kept in the practice's permanent medical records
   2. Insert a form (or file) only with the patient's name in the clinical practice medical records. This serves as a cross-index to the data collection forms and drug study records
   3. Do not maintain any medical records for patients who are not part of an investigator's clinical practice, apart from the data collection forms and drug study files
C. Maintain one master set of all files, whether or not patients in a drug study are part of a physician's private practice[b]
   1. Order files by patient's last name, social security number, date of first visit, or using another system
   2. Files or file tabs may be color coded using a variety of methods to facilitate retrieval of information

[a] Some or all of the information collected may also be placed in a computer data base.
[b] Data collection forms will have to be maintained separately.

should not be a discrepancy between the official procedures and actual practice, because that establishes a situation that may potentially lead to legal complications. For instance, if established guidelines suggest one code of corporate behavior for adverse reactions reported to the company, but a different code is followed, then ethical and possibly legal problems may arise.

Standard operating procedures differ widely from company to company, and within a company they will change over time. This book will not attempt to provide specific procedures. It does contain, however, many factors to be discussed or considered when such procedures are developed.

Standardized Forms

Forms are often used to expedite dissemination of information about clinical studies and serve numerous other functions. Although forms may be

TABLE 19.4. *Selected issues to consider in record keeping*

A. Design and nature of the record
   1. Physical form of the record (e.g., hard copy, computer disk)
   2. Design of the forms used should be suitable to record data from the investigator's private practice and clinical studies
   3. Content of each form and changes in the format of the record form which may occur over time or be required to collect a different type or amount of data

B. Completing the form or record
   1. If different physicians treat the same patient include the physician's name on the record
   2. If different technicians test the same patient include their name on the record
   3. Determine who will be responsible for filling in and maintaining the records
   4. Insure legibility of the records
   5. Insure that an adequate amount of data is recorded
   6. Utilize black pens for all data recorded if a typewriter or computer is not used

C. Other issues
   1. Measuring quality of recorded observations and devising a mean to indicate this in the records
   2. Procedures to allow for patient follow-up
   3. Confidentiality of the data (e.g., sponsors should only receive pages with patient initials)
   4. Similarity of records in different institutions conducting a multicenter study (e.g., retrospective, prospective)
   5. Changes in studies tests and laboratory reference ranges over time (e.g., specific efficacy tests, equipment) may affect data placed in the same record
   6. Changes in patient diagnoses or severity of illness over time

created *de novo* for each clinical study or project of multiple studies, it is generally useful to have a number of standardized forms available for many projects. This also saves the time and effort that would otherwise be required to develop forms each time that they are desired or needed.

In some situations it may be possible to devise a modular approach to reports, using a series of standardized forms. Reports for many different purposes would be created by completing and combining a number of standardized forms. The purpose of this approach is to simplify report writing and the reviewing of multiple reports. There are numerous pros and cons to using multiple standardized forms for creating reports. In general, this approach is not recommended because it does not easily permit variations to allow for differences between drugs, exceptions, and special cases that frequently arise and do not fit the general pattern. If these variations were met by additional prose, then an entire prose report would often be preferable to multiple forms.

This section describes some types of forms that have been developed and illustrates a few examples. Selected forms used for manufacturing clinical

TABLE 19.5. *Representative types of standard operating procedures*

A. Related to study drug(s). How to:
  1. Request that drug be synthesized
  2. Request that drug be formulated into a specific dosage form
  3. Request that a finished dosage form of a drug be packaged for a clinical study and shipped to a study site
  4. Request points 1, 2, or 3 above from a facility in a different country, subsidiary, or parent company
  5. Return drug to the sponsor from a study site and have it destroyed
  6. Transport and store compounds
  7. Request that specific compounds be tested in specific (or general) tests
  8. Acquire clinical study drugs from other companies or from other parts of the same company
  9. Request for biological screening or advanced testing on a specific compound/drug
  10. Request that a new formulation of a drug be developed and placed on stability
  11. Complete laboratory notebooks as well as arrange for their storage, duplication, and safeguarding

B. Related to the study site and investigator. How to:
  1. Choose a study site
  2. Report on prestudy and periodic visits to a study site
  3. Report on a telephone conversation
  4. Request that money be sent to the investigator
  5. Request that data from a clinical study be entered in a computer and be quality assured
  6. Transmit data from the investigator's site to the sponsoring institution
  7. Correct data collection forms after they have been received by the sponsor

C. Related to the sponsor's institution. How to:
  1. Prepare a feasibility report and have it approved
  2. Prepare an investigator's brochure and have it approved
  3. Prepare a final statistical report and have it approved[a]
  4. Prepare a final medical report and have it approved[a]
  5. Prepare an annual report on a drug for the FDA and have it submitted
  6. Request changes in membership on a project team
  7. Request that reports be prepared for an IND or NDA[b]
  8. Change labeling on a marketed drug
  9. Report adverse reactions to the FDA[b]
  10. Communicate with the FDA and/or other regulatory agencies
  11. Set up a meeting with the FDA
  12. Register compound numbers for both internal and external use
  13. Review and approve protocols and amendments to protocols
  14. Request that plasma, urine, or other samples be assayed for drug levels or concentrations
  15. Request that data on a study be analyzed statistically
  16. Request that a new indication be considered for a drug's development
  17. Develop a new or modified standard operating procedure

[a] It may be desirable to prepare a joint statistical and medical report.

[b] IND, Notice of Claimed Investigational Exemption for a New Drug; NDA, New Drug Application; FDA, Food and Drug Administration.

supplies were recently published by Bettis (1985). A basic library of various schedules and forms used in managing previous clinical studies will simplify the creation of new forms. Forms should have prepunched holes if they are to be placed in loose-leaf binders. A description of a few basic forms follows.

Tracking Patients, Studies, Grants, and Data

Tables 19.6 and 19.7 and Figs. 19.1 to 19.5 illustrate some forms that may be used to keep track of patients, studies, grants, and the flow of data obtained in drug studies. Other forms were published by Frelick and Kyle (1984). Many of the forms used for these purposes may be entered in a computer and easily updated by the monitor or other staff.

Logsheet of Potential Patients Contacted About Study

Protocol Number ____________ Title ______________________________

____

Month: ____________ 19 _______

Date In Month	Number of Patients Contacted re: Study	Number of Patients Contacted But Not Screened	Number of Patients Screened
1	2	1	1
2	3	0	3
3	0	—	—
4	4	4	0
5	2	1	1
6	1	0	1
7	6	3	3
8	2	1	1
•	•	•	•
•	•	•	•
•	•	•	•
31	7	7	0
TOTAL =	N	X	Y

FIG. 19.1. Logsheet of potential patients contacted about a study and screened.

TABLE 19.6. *Sample table headings to monitor status of individual patients enrolled in long-term study protocols*

Site code or name	Patient no.	Pt's[a] start of drug (date)	Pt's end of drug (date)	Duration on drug to date	Current dose of drug	Length of time since last dose changed	No. of dose changes	Completed treatment (C) or dropped out (D)	Date when Pt will complete — months on drug	Comments

[a] Pt's, patient's.

TABLE 19.7. *Sample table headings to track clinical studies in Phases II and III*

A

Type of study[a]	Protocol no.	Purpose of study[b]	Number of patients	Start date	Actual end date	Data processing (due date)	Statistical report (due date)	Medical report (due date)	Manuscript[c]

B

Product	Study objective	Dose, route, frequency	Investigator and site	Monitors and staff	Start date	Target end date	Progress and comment about priorities and reasons for objective

C

Protocol no.	Number of patients	Number of treatments	Date of data cutoff for NDA[d]	Date of last DCF[d] entered	Date data base available	Date stat. report due	Stat. author	Date medical report due	Medical author	Date report to regulatory affairs

[a] This column may list the indication, general type of patients enrolled, and/or whether the study is evaluating pharmacokinetics or efficacy, or is being conducted for a specific purpose.
[b] To evaluate a specific indication, formulation, dose, or to provide support to marketing.
[c] The status may be either planned, in preparation, in press, or already published.
[d] NDA, New Drug Application; DCF, data collection form.

Logsheet of Potential Patients Disqualified at Screen

Protocol Number ______________ Title ______________________________ Month & Year ______________

Date in Month	Number of Patients Screened	Number of Patients Disqualified at Screen	Reasons for Disqualification of Patients at Screen[a]												
			1	2	3	4	5	6	7	8	9	10	11	12	Other:
1	2	1			✓										
2	4	0													
3	4	4					✓			✓		✓			✓ Pain resolved spontaneously ✓ Primarily due to anxiety
4	2	1													
5	0	0													
6	3	3					✓✓				✓				
7	6	1			✓										
8	1	0													
•	•	•													
•	•	•													
•	•	•													
31	11	7			✓		✓				✓		✓✓		✓✓ Pain in wrong location
TOTAL =	Y	Z	A	B	C	D	E	F	G	H	I	J	K	L	M

[a] 1 = Patients age or weight outside of inclusion criteria
2 = Previous medical history unacceptable
3 = Alcohol or drug abuse
4 = Recent surgery
5 = Insufficient severity of symptom
6 = Insufficient duration of symptom
7 = Presence of concomitant drug
8 = Previous participation in study
9 = Drug allergies
10 to 12 = Other defined reasons

FIG. 19.2. Logsheet of potential patients disqualified during screen and the reasons for their disqualification. A footnote may be used to describe patients disqualified for multiple reasons.

Logsheet of Potential Patients Entered in a Study

Protocol Number ______________

Title: ____

Week	Date	Number of Patients Screened	Number of Patients Passing Screen	Number of Patients Enrolled in Study	Reasons for Nonenrollment by Successfully Screened Patients					
					No Interest	Insufficient Inducements	Informed Consent Not Signed	Inadequate Time	Lives Too Far	Other (List)
1	Jan 14 - 20	17	12	10			1	1		
2	Jan 21 - 27	24	20	15	1	2	2			
3	Jan 28 - Feb 3	14	14	13		1				
4										
5										
6										
7										

FIG. 19.3. Logsheet of patients entered in a study and reasons for nonenrollment by successfully screened patients.

CURRENT STATUS OF CLINICAL STUDIES

DRUG[a] ______________________

Project No.: ______________ Prepared By: ______________ Current Status for 1. Planned Studies ______________

Date: ______________ Approved By: ______________ 2. Ongoing Studies ______________

Previous Update: ______________ 3. Completed Studies ______________

(Check 1 or more)

Type of Study (Indication, Route)	Blind (DB, SB, Open)	Purpose/ Objective	Phase No.	Study No.	Investigator Name(s)	City, Country	Monitors	Total Cost ($)	Start Date	Original End Date	Current End Date	Total No. of Patients To Be Enrolled	No. of Patients Enrolled	No. of Patients Completed
Atrial Fib.	DB	Efficacy	II	2125	Jones	Munich FRG	Smith, Taylor	16,525	Jan '86	Jan '87	Feb '87	45	24	12

Comments: ______________

[a]A separate form may be employed for planned, ongoing, and completed studies, or all three may be combined on one form.

FIG. 19.4. Tracking current status of clinical studies on a specific drug.

Schedules for Staff

Schedules may be developed for each staff member (e.g., physician, nurse, coordinator, receptionist, specialist). These schedules present a list of activities that must be performed on each patient at each visit or *in toto*. These lists may include dates and/or times when the scheduled activities are to be performed. Other staff activities in a study may also be scheduled (e.g., completion of data collection forms, discussion of results and issues, contacts with the sponsor).

Telephone Conversation Sheet

This form basically consists of a blank page with lines. A few lines at the top may be preprinted with headings such as date, time, drug, and study involved, as well as individual(s) on the telephone (see Fig. 19.6). If all forms used by one individual are for a single study or project, then some of the information on this form may be preprinted or stamped on the form.

The person completing the form should indicate the reason for the call as well as a synopsis of advice or information given. Any decisions reached or comments made that affect the study should be recorded. Forms of all con-

GRANT PAYMENTS ON A CLINICAL STUDY

Company Location: ______________________ Investigator's Name: ______________________

Drug Name: ______________________ Investigator's Address: ______________________

Protocol Number: ______________________

Grant Number: ______________________

Total Amount of Grant ($): ______________________

Checks Are Made Payable To: ______________________

Agreed On Payment Schedule: ______________________

Address To Which Payments Are Sent: ______________________

(If different than investigator's address) ______________________

Payment Number	Date Check Requested	Date Check Received	Person Requesting Check	Work Being Paid For	Check Number	Type of Currency	Amount of Payment (US $)	Exchange Rate	Date of Check	Amount of Check	Total (US $)	Balance (US $)

FIG. 19.5. Tracking grant payments on a clinical study.

versations should be copied (if carbonless paper was not used to create copies) and placed in both permanent and study record files. Some companies send a copy of all telephone reports to the investigator as well.

Patient Screening Forms

Many studies have data collection forms that are used as soon as a patient has been enrolled in a clinical study. It is often useful to have a special form that can be used for patients who are undergoing various procedures in the screening phase of a study. If a patient either does not "pass" the screen or passes but does not agree to sign the informed consent and enter the study, a set of data collection forms will not have had to be used and the patient will not have been assigned a study patient number. Unless there is a specific reason to retain these forms on patients who are not entered in a study, they may be discarded after the study is completed.

The patient screening form should indicate the patient's name, address, telephone number at work and home, source of referral, and a checklist of the inclusion and exclusion criteria. The disposition of the patient must be indicated (i.e., the patient either entered or did not enter the study). A form to be used for telephone interviews should be a condensed version of the

Telephone Conversation Report

Project: ______________________

Study No: ______________________

Investigator: ______________________

Spoke To: ______________________

Date & Time: ______________________

Reason for Call: ______________________

Important Points: ______________________

Action to be Taken: ______________________

Place top copy in the study file and the other copy in the telephone log.

Send copies to: ______________________

Signature: ______________________

FIG. 19.6. Telephone conversation report form.

inclusion criteria. Telephone interviews are usually used as a preliminary screen to decrease the number of potential enrollees to those most likely to be suitable for enrollment.

Patients entering a clinic or place where screening occurs usually go through a carefully planned series of steps culminating in their agreement to participate in a study. It is usually unwise and unnecessary to have anyone undergo an expensive test (e.g., electroencephalogram, CAT scan) prior to insuring that they meet other parts of the entrance criteria. The reasons why patients fail the inclusion criteria are usually important to record so that trends or important factors may be determined. A form for this is shown in Fig. 19.2. The number and reasons of patients who pass the screen but decline to enter the study because of the information in the informed consent or for other reasons may also be collected (Fig. 19.3).

Data Update

At some point prior to a patient's visit it is usually valuable if one member of the clinical study team is assigned to review the patient's data collection forms for completeness and accuracy. A separate single-page form could be completed and attached to the front of each chart which would indicate the points that had to be completed or answered by relevant people prior to, or at the time of, the patient's next visit. These points include: (1) adding any missing data that are now available, (2) noting any abnormal laboratory, adverse reactions, or other data that have to be followed up at the upcoming visit, (3) having signatures put in all relevant places, (4) raising questions that should be asked at the upcoming visit, or (5) providing information that will enable the next visit to run more efficiently and be more productive. Some of these points may be handled by the monitor if the investigator and staff do not complete this function.

Other standard forms may be prepared at the study site which will complement those prepared by the sponsor. These forms will provide the investigator and staff with a straightforward means of implementing the study with the least number of difficulties.

Study Files

There are numerous ways to organize files on multiple clinical studies. It is important for investigators as well as sponsors to adopt a single or primary method for organizational consistency within their project of multiple studies. This practice will help in the rapid retrieval of information as well as in case of an audit from a regulatory agency. A workable hierarchy should be used. Two examples are:

1. Project name and number/Specific indication/Protocol number/Study site number/Patient number.
2. IND number/Site number/Study number/Patient number.

A more complete type of file organization for investigators is shown in Table 19.8.

Study Visit Log and Report

At each study site and sponsor's location it is generally important to maintain a log for documenting each visit by (1) representatives from the sponsor, (2) FDA personnel, (3) consultants, (4) contract group representatives, or (5) other individuals regarding the study. This log should contain (1) name, (2) date, (3) purpose of visit, and (4) comments. Reports of periodic visits by study monitors for their own records and the sponsor's official files are

TABLE 19.8. *Possible organization of an investigator's files on a clinical study*

A. Regulatory documents
   1. Curriculum vitae of investigator or co-investigators
   2. Signed copy of the study protocol
   3. IRB[a] approval to conduct the study
   4. Copy of informed consent and pregnancy waiver
   5. Copy of data collection forms
   6. Copy of laboratory certification
   7. Copy of all correspondence with regulatory groups

B. Study documents
   1. Financial records and correspondence
   2. Forms regarding drug shipments to and from the site and disposition of drug to patients
   3. Visits by monitors (e.g., reports, correspondence, study log)
   4. General correspondence
   5. Study reports (e.g., statistical, medical)
   6. Publication(s)

C. Patient records
   1. Signed informed consents
   2. Completed or current data collection forms
   3. Medical records relating to the study
   4. Laboratory and other reports

[a] IRB, Institutional Review Board.

generally prepared as separate documents. Figure 19.7 shows one typical form that may be used for this purpose.

Contents and Monitor's Review of Data Collection Forms

A short table of contents for all pages of the data collection form can be prepared. Either insert one copy in front of each patient's "book" of data collection forms or prepare a single copy for the investigator and staff to use for all patients. Monitors may also use a different form (Fig. 19.8), which lists the general contents of data collection forms to point out items that the investigator has to complete, modify, or change.

Doctor's Medical Chart on Patients in a Study

In addition to the data collection form, the physician must also maintain independent medical records on each patient in the study who is also in his private practice. Some physicians maintain separate patient charts on all patients in a study in addition to data collection forms. This patient chart record should include the following:

Periodic Site Visit Report

Project: ______________________________

Product or drug: ______________________

Study no: ____________________________

Investigator: _________________________

Date of visit: _________________________

Conducted by: ________________________

Personnel with whom visit was conducted: ______________________________

Purpose of visit: ____

Number of data collection forms edited: _______________________________

Data collection forms returned to sponsor: _____________________________

DCF errors found that were not corrected by the staff during the visit: __________

____

____

Protocol violations (if any): _____________________________________

____

Items to receive from site: _______________________________________

____

Items to send to site: ____

____

Other follow-up: ____

____

Is a more detailed report of this visit available? ____ Yes ____ No. If yes, doc. no.______

Comments:

Signature and date: _________________________________

Copies to: ____

FIG. 19.7. Periodic site-visit report form for study monitor to complete.

1. A list of each patient visit that was part of the study, including the date.
2. A typical office visit note may be written.
3. A rubber stamp may be used to refer to the study record for additional details.
4. A statement could be added that the patient's study record is part of this medical chart.

Data Collection Form Checklist

Study No. ________ Patient No. ________ Monitor Initials ________ Date ________

Part of DCF	Page No.	Specific Questions
Admission Criteria		
Medical History		
Physical Exam		
Electrocardiogram		
Blood Chemistry		
Hematology		
Dosage Record		
Pill Count		
Adverse Reactions		
Clinical Global Impression		
Etc.		

FIG. 19.8. DCF = data collection form. Data collection form checklist for use in monitoring. A copy of this form may be attached to the front of data collection forms that have questions to address.

Other Forms

Many other forms are used in most clinical studies, including forms for monitors to choose investigators (Fig. 19.9), transmit drugs to sites (Fig. 19.10), return drugs from sites, plus forms used for various other purposes.

COMPUTERS

The rapid and enormous expansion of computer use in drug development over the past few years has made them an integral part of many, if not most, clinical studies. Their role will undoubtedly continue to grow, although the exact pace and nature of future uses are not certain.

Areas of Use

Selected areas where computers may assist in the conduct of clinical studies are given in Table 19.9. This table illustrates many applications related to the acquisition and processing of data. Functions that are not listed in this table relate to the involvement of computers in many efficacy tests that

Form for Evaluation of Potential Investigator

Name of Potential Investigator ____________________

Address and Telephone No. ____________________

Protocol Name and Number ____________________

Drug Name and Phase (I to IV) ____________________

Reviewer Who Made the Visit ____________________

Date of This Report ____________ Date of Visit ____________

People Visited and Title ____________________

Final Recommendation

Definitely Use Site ____

Use Site if Necessary ____

Definitely Do Not Use Site ____

Consider Only If ____________________

____

Specific Rating and Comments:

(Rate from 1 [Unacceptable] to 10 [Top in Field or Acceptable]; NA = Not Applicable)

		Comments
1. Investigator's qualifications and previous experience	____	________
2. Investigator's interest in the study	____	________
3. Investigator's time availability for the study	____	________
4. Adequacy of support staff(list names and positions)	____	________
5. Adequacy of physical facilities and security	____	________
6. Adequacy of laboratories and pharmacy	____	________
7. Patient population — numbers (how was it determined?)	____	________
8. Patient population — quality for study (same as above)	____	________
9. Cost of the study (proposed budget)	____	________

10. Additional comments ____________________

____

____

____

Prepared by ____________________
(Signature)

FIG. 19.9. Form for evaluation of potential investigators.

are conducted, plus areas of administration such as making appointments and billing patients for services rendered. Although relatively few studies *require* the use of computers for their conduct, it is clear that computers possess an incredible potential to expand the abilities of the people who are involved in all parts of a clinical study. Improvements in data collection

Shipment of Study Materials to Site

Drug Name and Protocol Number: ______________________

Investigator's Name and Location: ______________________

Name of Contact and Telephone Number: ______________________

Item	Sent (Date)	Received (Date)	Comment
Final Protocol			
Drug			
Drug (Second Shipment)			
Drug (Third Shipment)			
Data Collection Forms (DCFs)			
DCFs (Second Shipment)			
Plasma Sample Tubes			
Plasma Tube Labels			
Plasma Forms to Accompany Samples			
Box for Shipping Plasma Samples			
Pharmacist's Book			
Investigator's Log			
Other ______________			
Other ______________			
Other ______________			
Other ______________			

FIG. 19.10. Form for shipment of study materials to a study site. It may also be desirable to identify the batch and lot numbers of drug sent.

through use of a computer system in oncology studies are described by Kent et al. (1985).

Measuring Clinical Parameters

Some efficacy parameters may only be measured with the use of computers. For example, the computer is essential to obtain evoked responses, and thus this efficacy parameter is impossible to measure or obtain without computers. Various types of radiological imaging (e.g., computerized tomography, positron emission tomography) also require computers.

TABLE 19.9. *Selected areas where computers may assist in the conduct and management of clinical studies*

A. Prestudy
   1. To develop PERT[a] charts and schedule of activities for planning the conduct of a project and monitoring its progress
   2. To provide randomization codes
   3. To assist in preparing drug information labels that are applied to containers
   4. To weigh capsules automatically after their manufacture and insure correct weight

B. During study
   1. To develop various graphs illustrating progress of individual projects or of an entire program
   2. To enter data from data collection forms
   3. To obtain data online or direct from distant sites of clinical investigation
   4. To obtain data online or direct from distant laboratories
   5. To develop data bases and monitor study progress
   6. To communicate between sites using electronic mail
   7. To monitor current status of some or all patients
   8. To track and plan drug supplies, patient enrollment, and other aspects of the study

C. Poststudy
   1. To compile data and compare doubly entered data
   2. To analyze data from clinical studies
   3. To analyze plasma and other biological samples with analytical equipment connected to a computer
   4. To track completion and receipt of data collection forms

D. Throughout study program
   1. As word processors in preparing protocols and other documentation
   2. Maintain current status of ongoing and completed clinical studies
   3. Follow grants, payment records, travel records, expense items, contract laboratories, and publications

[a] PERT, Program Evaluation and Review Technique.

Handling Data

The computer has expanded the abilities of individuals to handle data and to conduct analyses that previously were impossible or extremely arduous. Nonetheless, the essential core of most clinical studies continues to be the interaction of physician and patient. Computers should be viewed as important aids to assist the investigator and/or others involved with the study, rather than being an integral part of the study's conduct.

Integration of Computers

The integration of numerous types of computers is being carried on today to create wider networks and increased functions. This includes the use of computers in remote data entry and retrieval (Yu, 1986), which will undoubtedly become more common practice in the future. Numerous uses of an integrated computer system are described by Bleich et al. (1985) for a teaching hospital (Boston's Beth Israel Hospital). Although this system is not spccifically designed to conduct clinical studies it is clear that this system may be used to assist such studies in many ways.

Electronic Searches of Data Bases

A final use of computers which has become indispensible to many clinicians and scientists is in the search of electronic data bases for information regarding medical literature, patient treatment, and many other areas. This enormously diverse area has recently been summarized by Williams (1985).

20

Monitoring of Multiple Clinical Studies

Introduction • Stereotyped Styles of Monitoring • Monitoring Strategy • Monitoring Large Multicenter Studies • Relationships Between Monitors and Investigators • Improving a Poor Performer or Study • Games Investigators Play

INTRODUCTION

Definitions

Monitoring is a general term that is used in many different contexts in the pharmaceutical industry. The word is used both as a verb and as a noun. As a verb it means to watch, observe, or check, especially relating to a clinical study. It also means to keep track of, regulate, or control. As a noun, the word relates to individuals who are employed by a company and who monitor, i.e., oversee the planning, initiation, conduct, and data processing of clinical studies. These individuals also confirm that the execution of each step follows agreed-on plans. This chapter is primarily concerned with this latter type of monitoring. Many of the other uses of the term monitoring are listed in Table 20.1 and are discussed in other parts of this book.

Functions

Clinical monitors have a wide variety of backgrounds in terms of both their disciplines of training and their experience of clinical medicine. Although many monitors perform similar functions they do so at highly different levels of expertise. Broad functions of general monitors include participation in most or all of the following activities: (1) planning studies, (2) writing protocols, (3) initiating studies, (4) assessing the conduct of studies, (5) assisting in their termination, (6) assisting in data editing and analysis, and (7) assisting in data interpretation and extrapolation.

More specific functions of medical monitors during the conduct of a clinical study may include (1) observing what is being done, (2) assessing or

TABLE 20.1. *Selected types of monitoring conducted in the pharmaceutical industry*

1. Monitor clinical studies (i.e., the primary subject of this chapter)
2. Monitor preclinical studies conducted at facilities outside the company (e.g., toxicological or specialized studies)
3. Monitor data processing or statistical analyses being conducted at facilities outside the company
4. Monitor the status of, and progress on, projects at several levels within a company[a]
5. Monitor potential and/or actual conflicts between projects in terms of priorities, problems that arise, or need for resources
6. Monitor the coordination between activities conducted at different sites and/or in different countries
7. Monitor the implementation of a divisional, departmental, sectional, or other strategy to conduct research and/or develop drugs
8. Monitor the quality of research being conducted
9. Monitor the quality of clinical data during the study[b]
10. Monitor the quality of clinical data on the data collection forms after the study is completed but prior to its statistical analysis
11. Monitor the quality of drugs produced (i.e., quality assurance)
12. Monitor the financial projections for new and upcoming drugs to reach a New Drug Application (NDA) status or other milestone
13. Monitor the costs of clinical studies

[a] See Fig. 3.2.
[b] A separate quality assurance group may perform this role.

evaluating the quality of the study's conduct, (3) comparing the quality to preset standards, (4) discussing results with the groups being monitored as well as with other monitors and supervisors, and (5) proposing improvements to be made in the study or proposing solutions to problems. Other specific functions are listed in Table 36.67 of *Guide to Clinical Studies and Developing Protocols* (Spilker, 1984).

STEREOTYPED STYLES OF MONITORING

The most important aspect relating to monitoring and choice of investigators is attitude or style. Two extreme attitudes may be characterized with stereotypes as either "old-fashioned" or "modern".

Old-Fashioned Style

In the old-fashioned style the investigator is usually seen as a highly respected individual (almost always in academia) who is doing the sponsor a great favor by his willingness to conduct a study. "His" is used in the sense of "grand old man", before the time when many women were permitted to enter the academic hierarchy. Even if the investigator was a virtually unknown clinician, the relationship with the sponsor was characterized as the investigator's "doing a favor" for the sponsor. Therefore, the monitor was never allowed to seriously question the investigator's decisions, comments, actions, or inactions. Little money was usually paid to the investigator to conduct the study, and the investigator usually wrote the protocol without assistance from the sponsor. This protocol usually consisted of only a few pages.

When the study was completed, the investigator often performed the statistical analyses, interpreted the data, and then had the sponsor prepare the publication on which only the investigator's name appeared. As a result of this relationship, the sponsor had little or no leverage to exert on the investigator's activities. The sponsor could only hope that the study would be conducted at a high standard, and was thankful if and when data were received. The data received rarely met the sponsor's expectations in either quality or quantity. If the investigator did not adhere to agreed-on patient entry rates or other commitments, the sponsor had little choice but to allow the study to drag on, hoping that it would eventually be turned around and become productive. This miracle rarely occurred.

The monitor in the above scenario has a menial role and probably runs errands instead of acting in the role of a professional colleague. The extreme case occurs when development of an entire drug program is turned over to an investigator. In this situation, the investigator is asked to evaluate the drug in a number of studies. After these studies are completed, the investigator is requested to inform the sponsor of his opinion about whether the drug is worth developing further and whether a regulatory submission should be prepared. Protocols are generally prepared by the investigator and may be sent as a courtesy to the sponsor, who waits for a number of years while the investigator evaluates the new drug. This stereotype is somewhat exaggerated to make a point, and hopefully does not occur any more to this degree. Nonetheless, elements of this style still persist.

Modern Style

The modern stereotype is a situation where the monitor interviews a number of potential investigators who each have excellent reputations. The monitor chooses which investigator will conduct a study, based on the investigator's demonstration that he/she can conduct the study most efficiently and effectively. The protocol, often written by the monitor, has appropriate input from both the investigator(s) and sponsor. The investigator chosen is expected to adhere to the highest standards of clinical practice and maintain open communications and a sense of collaboration with the sponsor and monitor. The monitor is treated like an integral part of the clinical team by the investigator, and their relationship is based on mutual respect. The monitor's opinion on relevant issues is sought, carefully listened to, and evaluated. The investigator is paid a fair market value for conducting the study. Through frank and open communications the monitor may exert pressure on investigators if their performance slackens or commitments are not achieved.

Although both of these patterns are idealized and represent extremes, the real world of the pharmaceutical industry has been gradually moving from the former pattern toward the more modern one. It is clear that companies in some countries tend to operate more closely to one style or the other. In addition, there are various idiosyncrasies that tend to characterize the monitor–investigator relationship in certain countries and for certain rules of the game that are generally followed.

MONITORING STRATEGY

In developing an overall monitoring strategy for a study it is essential to determine the answers to several questions, including: (1) What will be monitored? (2) How will it be monitored? (3) Who will monitor it? The answer to the question of *what* to monitor depends on the functions of the particular monitor(s). The most usual answer to this question includes the (1) facilities, (2) study, (3) investigator and staff, and (4) data. The question of *how* to monitor is answered differently for each study and for each monitor. Important principles are discussed throughout this chapter and in *Guide to Clinical Studies and Developing Protocols* (Spilker, 1984). The question of *who* will monitor is generally an obvious one, but includes consideration of the sponsor(s), contract groups (if relevant), numbers and functions of each monitor, and blinding of relevant monitors. This latter issue is discussed later in this section. Monitors include individuals with various backgrounds and experience, ranging from college graduates to Ph.D.s, to M.D.s, and to medical specialists who monitor one aspect of a study (e.g., pathologists, radiologists).

Monitors are members of the team that is developing a drug (or device), whose primary responsibility is to work constructively with investigators and staff to insure that each study achieves the highest possible standards of conduct. An ideal standard of performance should not be used by monitors in judging a study's conduct or in judging the staff, since that approach invariably leads to frustration and disappointment for the monitor. Nor should a lax or laissez-faire approach be adopted by the monitor. Learning the appropriate balance between these two extremes requires experience, knowledge, and tact. Questions that arise in this regard should be posed to more experienced monitors. The appropriate style and intensity of monitoring differs in different therapeutic fields of medicine, and appropriate standards for one study in a specific field will sometimes be totally inappropriate for another study in the same field. The feeling of a joint effort and common interests between the monitor and investigator plus staff should be developed and maintained. This can partially be achieved by the monitor's understanding the investigator's true motivation for participating in a study. These factors are discussed later in this chapter.

Most clinical monitors are not police officers who must crack the whip to correct problems. When problems arise a graded approach should generally be used by the monitor. Minimal actions should be initially tried because they may solve the problem. Progressively stronger actions may be taken, if necessary. The study may be terminated if other approaches, including telephone calls, visits, or letters from senior management, are unsuccessful in improving a problem situation.

Intensity of Monitoring

All studies have to be monitored with diligence and attention to detail. Certain clinical studies must be monitored more closely than most others to insure that there are few problems/issues which could compromise the integrity and validity of the data obtained.

Monitoring Studies of Short Duration

A general principle is for medical monitors to remain at a site for the duration of a study if it is only scheduled to last a few days. If a study is of special importance to the sponsor then it is advisable for a monitor(s) to remain at the study site for up to 2 (or even more) weeks.

Monitoring Critically Important Studies

The intensity of monitoring should generally increase as the importance of a study increases. The investigator's motivation, interests, and priorities may markedly differ from those of the sponsor, and even what the investigator views as the scientific objectives of the study may differ. What may be a critical study for the sponsor might be a minor fund-raising exercise for the investigator. In some occasions the opposite situation occurs especially if an investigator contacts a sponsor for supplies of an investigational drug to conduct a study of primary interest to the investigator. This type of study is usually monitored less assiduously than a study initiated by a sponsor. Other studies are of equal interest to the investigator and sponsor.

Phase III Studies

The intensity of monitoring some Phase III studies is usually relaxed as compared with Phase II studies. This is because the profile of a drug's activity is better defined in Phase III and many of the precautions and procedures necessary for the investigator to follow are better understood. Moreover, many Phase III studies are not as tightly designed and controlled as well-controlled Phase II studies.

Methods of Monitoring

Monitoring by telephone may initially appear to be a convenient technique. Nonetheless, excessive reliance on the telephone may lead to a false sense of security in regard to a study's progress. A trip to the study site may provide unexpected surprises. One possible exception to this principle would occur if data are being transmitted directly from the site to the sponsor and the telephone calls are made to discuss details of the data. Monitors should be prepared to challenge any investigator whenever data seem strange, unexpected, too perfect, or unclear.

If a significant problem occurs at a site, it may be relevant for the monitor to write a letter that is frank, but diplomatic. If the desired result is not achieved, a second letter may be more strongly worded. This is important to do, because inaction usually allows a poor situation to deteriorate and diminishes the possibility of exerting appropriate control over the study if an important issue arises at a later date. The monitor may establish a regular as opposed to ad hoc system of placing telephone calls to the study site, especially during the early phases of a clinical study. If this is done then the site should be informed of this approach and a mutually agreed-upon time should be arranged.

The frequency of monitoring visits should be considered prior to initiating a study, but may easily be adjusted during the study. In general, more frequent visits are made at the start of a long-term study and fewer visits toward the end. The exact frequency should depend on (1) rate of patient entry, (2) time elapsed since last visit, (3) problems observed during the previous visit, and (4) problems reported since the last visit. Visits should therefore rarely be made on a fixed frequency (e.g., every 6 weeks) throughout a long-term study. Monitors are often present at the initiation of a study and often return after a few patients are enrolled to insure that the study is being conducted according to the protocol.

Monitors who interact with investigators should be blind. Inform investigators and the staff at all sites if monitors are blind to patient randomization. This may prevent misunderstandings that may arise if an investigator is interpreting reactions and comments of the monitor, believing the monitor is aware of the patient's treatment. If there are multiple monitors and only some are kept blind, it should be those who interact most closely with the investigator who remain blind. Types of monitoring methods are listed in Tables 20.2 to 20.4. Sample formats of tables to follow activities on multiple studies are shown in Table 20.5.

TABLE 20.2. *Types of monitoring methods utilized to oversee multiple projects*

1. Forms are completed by the investigator, research coordinator, or another individual at each study site on a periodic basis. Completed forms are sent to a single individual or group at the sponsoring or monitoring institution
2. Project leaders or managers prepare written reports on a periodic basis
3. Telephone calls, correspondence, and formal and informal meetings are used between the monitor and study-site personnel. These may occur on an ad hoc and/or scheduled basis to review status of the study
4. Transmit data electronically from the study site to the sponsor or to an intermediate contract group that has organized and is monitoring the study for the sponsor. Data are either sent on-line or transmitted at a later time
5. Monitoring groups are established which are independent of the sponsor and investigator
6. Each study is periodically spot-checked, as opposed to monitoring all aspects of every study
7. Every aspect of a study is monitored as thoroughly as possible[a]

[a] Many specific aspects are listed in Table 20.3.

Monitoring is a continuous process. If problems develop in this study, such as if there are more dropouts than expected, the monitor must attempt to solve the problem. A number of possible interpretations are described in Table 20.6. After the correct one(s) are identified for the problem, a systematic approach to improving the situation must be developed.

Training of Monitors Who Are Untrained in Clinical Medicine

Many medical monitors at pharmaceutical companies are not trained in clinical medicine. Allowing interested monitors to personally go through the screening and possibly some testing procedures used in a study will provide them with a better understanding of the study. This practice will also help a monitor better appreciate various issues and problems from the investigator's perspective.

Monitors should be encouraged to attend relevant professional meetings, courses, and seminars to improve their medical knowledge and skills in interpreting data. Discussions with more-senior monitors will provide important education and professional development. Some companies offer internal training courses for their monitors and provide appropriate educational materials (see Cocchetto, 1986).

Remote Data Entry

This concept involves workers at an investigator's site entering clinical data into a computer and periodically (e.g., daily, weekly) transmitting data to the sponsor's site. Variations on this flow of data are possible, such as having data initially sent to a central site or consultant's office prior to being sent to a sponsor.

TABLE 20.3. *Aspects to monitor in a large group of clinical studies*

A. General data on each study
   1. Protocol number and name
   2. Name, address, and telephone numbers of investigator and relevant staff members
   3. Total number of patients to be enrolled and number actually enrolled
   4. Number of data collection forms completed at the investigator's site
   5. Number of data collection forms received by sponsor
   6. Disposition and status of data collection forms
   7. Dates of initiation and completion of patient evaluation; dates of other milestones

B. Log of patients[a]
   1. Potential patients contacted about a study
   2. Potential patients discontinued at screen
   3. Patients entered
   4. Patients prematurely discontinued during study
   5. Patients completing study

C. Log of monitoring site visits[b]
   1. Date of visit
   2. Names of monitors and staff members involved
   3. Important points covered and decisions reached
   4. Reference to a trip report (maintained at the sponsoring institution)

D. Status and projected dates of reports (e.g., generated, planned, or in progress)
   1. Statistical reports
   2. Medical reports (e.g., by investigators, by sponsors)
   3. Other reports

E. Outcomes of studies
   1. Brief synopsis of conclusions

F. Plans for overall program of studies
   1. List status of all studies (e.g., planned, ongoing, completed) and list actual or estimated dates of milestones
   2. Status of clinical protocols

G. Problem or "red flag" areas
   1. Follow details of safety or efficacy parameters in an open label study that are of particular interest or concern

H. Availability of materials for studies to monitor
   1. Bulk chemical available
   2. Needs of various departments for bulk chemical
   3. Bulk formulated drug available
   4. Finished drug available (e.g., number of tablets, capsules)
   5. Schedule for packaging of drugs
   6. Dates that drug is needed by investigators

[a] See Figs. 19.1–19.3.
[b] This log is maintained at the investigator's site until after the study is complete, when it is sent to the sponsor for storage. A periodic site visit form is shown in Fig. 19.7.

The purpose of remote data entry is to increase the speed and efficiency with which data may be processed and analyzed. The computer assists the data entry operator by questioning inappropriate entries of data. Other advantages are that missing data may be easily flagged by the computer. The computer program may provide feedback if all entry criteria are not met, if visit dates are not entered in correct order, and if other preset criteria are not met. Simple calculations may be used both at the investigator's site and at the sponsor's site to maintain current information on total patient enrollment, trends in laboratory data, and other parameters of interest which do not affect the study's blind.

TABLE 20.4. *Some potential problems to look for in monitoring clinical studies*

A. Concerning patient enrollment and randomization
   1. Ineligible patients allowed to enter study
   2. Patients being enrolled more than once
   3. Patients assigned to treatment groups incorrectly
   4. Slow rate of patient enrollment

B. Concerning data collection forms
   1. Incomplete data collection forms (e.g., missing data or signatures)
   2. Errors in completing data collection forms (e.g., inconsistent data)
   3. Illegible data collection forms
   4. Vague or questionable entries

C. Concerning patient abnormalities
   1. Abnormalities in laboratory values, including unusual values recorded
   2. Trend toward abnormality in laboratory values
   3. Unreported severe adverse reactions
   4. Trends in the occurrence or nature of adverse reactions
   5. Any other abnormalities reported

D. Concerning study conduct
   1. Patients who are not compliant
   2. Lack of adequate efficacy noted when all patients are receiving active drug[a]
   3. Efficacy noted in all patients on drug, no efficacy noted for those on placebo; or other evidence that makes data appear too perfect
   4. Patients not examined by investigators, staff, or others who should have examined them
   5. Data or reports not being returned from outside groups as rapidly as desired and/or required (e.g., X-ray reports, pathology reports, pulmonary function studies)
   6. Scheduled tests not always conducted
   7. Tests incompletely conducted on some or all patients
   8. Unauthorized interim data analyses being conducted
   9. Errors in dispensing of drug or in returning unused drug
   10. Evidence that study blind has been broken
   11. Problems in storage of drug (e.g., lack of refrigeration, lack of security)
   12. Study not conducted according to good clinical practices

[a] In studies where this is permissable (e.g., open-label studies).

One of the major technical issues in remote data entry between countries involves telecommunications. Three potential problems or issues are:

1. The same modems are not legally able to be used in all countries (e.g., United States and West Germany).
2. The quality of local telephone companies and their lines vary greatly within some countries and between countries.
3. There may be multiple vendors responsible for hardware maintenance in some countries.

Geographical Location of Corporate Monitors

All monitors may be based at the sponsor's central location and may travel to and from the various study sites. Some sponsors utilize sales represen-

TABLE 20.5. *Sample table formats used to monitor activities on multiple clinical studies conducted at various sites*

A

Drug or product	Indication or formulation	Study doses, route, frequency	Study sites	Principal investigator	Sponsor monitor(s)	Estimated start date (* = started)	Estimated end date (* = ended)	Current status and comments

B

Study number	Principal investigator	Site location(s)	Study objectives	Total no. of patients planned	No. of patients entered	Comments

TABLE 20.6. *Possible interpretations of the situation where "many" voluntary patient withdrawals occur at a single study site*

1. Poor physician–patient relationship
2. Lack of incentives for investigator to try to keep patients in the study[a]
3. Lack of incentives for patients to remain in the study[a]
4. Incentives are present for investigator not to keep patients in the study
5. Some attribute of the site or protocol is not conducive to a successful study
6. Study drug is escalated too slowly, which yields an insufficient clinical response
7. Patients escalated too rapidly on drug, which yields excessive toxicity
8. A specific factor is affecting the study, which must be detected through careful monitoring
9. Study drug is not effective at the dose and/or conditions studied
10. Study drug is too toxic at the dose and/or conditions studied

[a] Includes both medical and nonmedical incentives.

tatives and/or other individuals scattered throughout the country to monitor sites located in reasonable proximity to their homes. Various combinations of these approaches are also possible. When a study is sponsored by two different companies, a parent company and a foreign subsidiary, or by two subsidiaries of a single sponsor, monitoring is often performed by individuals from both groups.

In certain situations, a monitoring representative from a third country or group may be present. For example, when monitors of a subsidiary initiate a study in a different country than that in which the main organization's headquarters are located, monitors may come from the parent, host, and subsidiary countries. There are also occasions when monitors of a contract organization accompany monitors from a sponsor on a monitoring trip.

Travel

Monitors often travel a great deal to and from various study sites. It is usually necessary to balance taking fewer long trips versus more frequent shorter trips. Each situation differs, but most monitors attempt to cluster sites which are relatively nearby (or on a circle route) and which are to be visited in a single trip. Long trips rarely last for more than 10 days for most monitors. A few practical considerations for travelers are listed in Table 20.7.

Training of New Staff at the Study Site

In most studies of "long" duration there will be a need at different times to train new staff members who join the study. Planning is required to develop appropriate means to do this efficiently. One useful method is to have

TABLE 20.7. *Practical considerations for travelers*

A. Prior to a trip
  1. Copy the relevant airline, bus, ferry, or other schedule(s) that will allow for alternate arrangements to be made if changes are required en route or prior to return
  2. Consider an alternative plan if planes or other modes of transportation are delayed or canceled[a]
  3. Obtain maps of the area(s) to be visited
  4. Reserve all transportation and hotels as far in advance as possible
  5. Reserve hotel with guaranteed late arrival and become familiar with cancellation terms. Request an upper floor, lower floor, or room with a specific view (if desired)
  6. Make arrangements for anticipated business and nonbusiness activities
  7. Reserve restaurants long in advance for important business meetings. It is often desirable to call the chef to discuss the menu, especially if everyone will be having the same meal
  8. Obtain currency for each country to be visited for international travel. Consider obtaining traveler's checks issued in a foreign currency (or currencies)
  9. Set up as many business meetings as possible in advance and confirm each within 3 days of leaving
  10. Prepare a list of (1) activities and questions to cover at each appointment and (2) points to cover at each meeting
  11. Bring a copy of all relevant addresses and telephone numbers
  12. Bring credit cards, including a telephone card
  13. Take sufficient traveler's checks in suitable denominations
  14. Evaluate the total cost and convenience of a car rental versus using taxis or other transportation. Make arrangements that provide for the most efficient, cost-effective, and reasonable use of one's time
  15. Prepack a small suitcase with as many needed items as possible, to be ready to take on a trip. Travel as lightly as possible
  16. Maintain a list of additional items needed for a warm and cold climate to add to the prepacked suitcase prior to leaving
  17. Check the weather forecast of the place(s) to be visited
  18. Put a change of underwear and socks in one's briefcase in case one's luggage is delayed or lost
  19. Consider membership in one or more airline lounges

B. En route
  1. Do not check luggage at an airport unless necessary
  2. Avoid scheduling airplane changes in cities where bad weather may cause delays (e.g., generally attempt to change airplanes in a southern city in the United States during the winter)
  3. Understand passengers' rights on public carriers (e.g., regarding smoking or nonsmoking sections)[b]
  4. Remove shoes on long airplane flights and carry lightweight slippers
  5. Bring a variety of work and reading material to suit one's mood at the time
  6. Allow ample time to reach each destination, thereby preventing most travel delays from affecting one's schedule
  7. Do not plan a tight schedule at airports or on the ground unless necessary. This is especially relevant for international travel
  8. If taxis are difficult to find at the airport terminal consider sharing one, renting a car, or taking a bus
  9. Use express services provided by many automobile rental companies

(*continued*)

TABLE 20.7. *(Continued)*

C. At the destination
   1. Request a hotel room with specific view or facing a specific direction if not done in advance. Insure that the room is not next to an elevator or in a particularly noisy location (e.g., immediately above a ballroom)
   2. Obtain directions to your meeting(s) or activities in advance, including information on where to park or how to obtain taxis for the return trip to the hotel
   3. Reserve seats for entertainment, restaurants, theater, or other activities as early in your stay as possible
   4. Allow extra time to get to appointments or an airport if the trip will be made during "rush hour" in a city. Ask hotel or other personnel about the length of delay to expect and possible solutions
   5. Reserve a taxi in advance (if possible) whenever needed
   6. Consider express check-out from hotels
   7. Consider rapid return procedures for rented automobiles

[a] Delays of one air carrier to a destination because of weather problems does not necessarily mean that all other air carriers to the same destination are also delayed.
[b] Obtain *Fly Rights—A Guide to Air Travel in the U.S.* from the Civil Aeronautics Board, Washington, D.C. 20428.

the investigator, coordinator, or other staff member spend appropriate time (generally 1 day to a week) with a counterpart at another study site. Another possibility is for the monitor and/or other individuals from the sponsor or another study site (e.g., research coordinator) to spend time (at the study site) directly training the new person and reviewing the study with them. Whatever plan is adopted, it should not generally consist of merely allowing the person to gain their own "on the job training." A training manual may be considered as an adjunct in special cases, such as large multicenter studies. Flow charts should be included which illustrate how to change dosages when adverse reactions occur or the drug is not sufficiently effective, plus how to perform various other modifications which may be necessary. But this or other types of guide will never be sufficient to provide adequate training on their own. Insure that only the final version of the protocol is present at the site, plus any appendices if relevant.

Items to Monitor

Important items to monitor in a single study were discusssed in Chapter 36 of *Guide to Clinical Studies and Developing Protocols* (Spilker, 1984). The present section indicates important aspects to monitor in multiple clinical studies conducted on a single project or drug. A few additional aspects of a single study which may be evaluated will be described.

Monitoring of a single study is primarily concerned with insuring that the study is well-conducted and that all data are collected as efficiently and accurately as possible. Monitoring of multiple studies conducted on a single drug is generally concerned with tracking progress, identifying causes of delays, allocating resources, and managing the project. Individuals who monitor single studies may or may not be the same people who monitor progress on a group of studies. Monitoring is also performed at a more senior level in a corporation through formal and/or informal review and other mechanisms. Reports of each monitoring trip should be documented. This may be done with a note to the file plus completion of a log book or by completing a preprinted form (see Fig. 19.5 for an example), which is then distributed and stored. Many of the administrative functions of monitoring may be managed with a computer.

To identify all of the important points to monitor on multiple clinical studies or on multiple projects, it is necessary to determine the objectives of monitoring. There is certainly a balance between monitoring too little and too much. Once the objectives are listed the appropriate items to monitor should become more clear. These may be discussed with colleagues and supervisors to confirm that the list chosen is appropriate.

Monitors at the sponsor's site may better prepare for their site visit by concentrating on the issues raised, rather than seeking issues to identify through a time-consuming review of the data collection forms at the site. It is also possible for the monitor and investigator to conduct some of these discussions by telephone.

Forms to Use in Monitoring

Each sponsor develops forms which are appropriately suited to the needs of the particular project and procedures in the sponsoring organization. Either of these factors may be the major one in determining the exact makeup of the forms used. Forms are presented in Figs. 19.1 to 19.8 and Table 20.5 to illustrate a few samples that may assist in the design of forms for related purposes. Since the organizational makeup of sponsors as well as their "standard operating procedures" differ to such a great degree, it is not possible to describe in a generic way how these forms should flow between individuals, groups, or departments.

Individuals sometimes make up and use their own systems and forms to keep track of and monitor activities and status of studies. Their forms may reflect those of their sponsor, or they may be highly individualistic. The forms may be handwritten on scratch paper, printed, or kept on a computer disk. These forms are usually the major means an individual uses to keep abreast of what he/she believes to be the most important items to monitor.

MONITORING LARGE MULTICENTER STUDIES

Monitoring large multicenter studies presents special problems to insure intersite consistency. This is usually addressed by having many specialized monitoring groups, such as those illustrated in Fig. 30.15 of *Guide to Clinical Studies and Developing Protocols* (Spilker, 1984). Separate groups of monitors may be utilized to confirm diagnoses (e.g., through examination of pathology reports), observe treatment, and evaluate follow-up. Groups may be established based on modality (e.g., radiation, surgery, clinical oncology, pathology in certain cancer studies), function, and therapeutic discipline (e.g., neurology or ophthalmological examinations) to monitor data collection and/or data analysis. It is clear that it may also be necessary to have one or more overall monitors whose function is to monitor the specialized monitors. Well-developed quality assurance programs have been used to monitor many large clinical studies (e.g., Glicksman et al., 1980).

When specialized monitoring groups are utilized they may be based at each study center and have responsibility only for that site. Alternatively, each specialized monitoring group may periodically visit each center. A third alternative is to use both approaches to monitoring and to have some specialized monitoring groups located at each site while other groups travel to the various sites of a large study.

RELATIONSHIPS BETWEEN MONITORS AND INVESTIGATORS

It is always important to be considerate of the study investigators and all of their staff who assist and often have major roles in a study. For example, it is wise to learn the names of the staff and something about their interests. It is also important to discuss relevant aspects of the study and the drug's development program with them. This often helps maintain cooperation, enthusiasm, and high study standards. It is recommended to take the staff out for lunch and/or to provide other reasonable and appropriate benefits (e.g., snacks) at appropriate times.

Situations often arise during the career of a clinical monitor when the relationship with an investigator ceases to be solely concerned with, and limited to, business. This usually refers to development of a friendship (no other types of relationships will be considered). Furthermore, the motives for developing a friendship are assumed to be totally honorable and without any ulterior motives on the part of either individual.

In developing a relationship with an investigator (or possibly with a member of the investigator's staff) there are a number of questions for the monitor to consider. These include:

1. Can a satisfactory distinction be made between the professional and personal relationship to allow the professional relationship to continue in an appropriate manner?
2. Could the personal relationship potentially compromise the abilities of the monitor to act professionally with the investigator?
3. What is the potential for the personal friendship to compromise the

conduct of the study and compromise the professional career of the monitor?
4. What is the potential for the relationship to evolve beyond its present scope in a manner that is not presently desired?
5. Is it possible to define the limits of the relationship which the monitor considers acceptable?
6. Is it relevant to discuss this relationship with more-experienced monitors or others at the sponsor's site?

Each situation will differ and there is clearly no single approach that is always appropriate. There are ways, however, of socializing as professionals that promote a cordial friendship while maintaining an appropriate and positive business relationship. No monitor should either encourage or participate in a greater friendship or social involvement than is considered appropriate and reasonable.

IMPROVING A POOR PERFORMER OR STUDY

Monitors may perceive that the quality of an investigator's performance in a clinical study has either diminished over a period of time, or else has never achieved an acceptable or agreed-on standard. In approaching this issue there are several stages to follow. The first is to identify the precise area or areas in which the investigator's performance is deficient. This may relate only to a single aspect of the study (e.g., low patient enrollment). Alternatively, the problem may be more widespread and involve the investigator's overall motivation and morale, or his overall performance of the study. The seriousness of the problem must then be assessed.

After the problem areas and its degree of seriousness are identified, it is essential to discover the reasons for the problem. This may not be simple or straightforward, but usually should be attempted. The major reasons for the problem(s) may be unrelated to the study or to anything that a monitor may be able to affect (e.g., personal problems of the investigator, the study site has moved to new quarters, students who are the major source of patient enrollment are on vacation). There may be many reasons that directly relate to the problem and may be affected by the monitor. These problems include those relating to the conduct of the study (e.g., if the investigator overestimated the number of suitable patients available). The reason(s) per se usually do not provide the solution, but often allow an approach to be found which may be used to reach a solution.

A few common problems that may often be solved are:

1. Incentives offered patients are inadequate to encourage or convince them to enroll in the study.
2. The protocol is too demanding of a patient's time or efforts in performing tests.

3. The protocol is too demanding of an investigator's time or efforts.
4. Staff available at the investigator's site is inadequate in number, training, or other factor to effectively handle the patient load.
5. Patient visits are scheduled at inconvenient times of day or on weekends.
6. A schedule of patient activities is established which is too demanding (e.g., having patients go from one location to another for tests or examinations versus having professional staff visit patients at a central location).

Another aspect of problem situations at an investigator's site relates primarily to multicenter studies. It must be ascertained whether the problem is isolated to one site or is a common problem at all or most sites. The situation is markedly different if nine of 10 investigators in a single study at different sites are performing well or if nine of these 10 investigators are performing poorly. This balance may also indicate whether the primary problem is related to the specific investigator and location or to more general problems with the protocol or all sites. If each of the nine investigators are performing poorly for the same reason(s), this usually means that immediate attention is required to help the study.

In seeking a solution to a protocol-related problem, consideration must be given to how the protocol may be modified while not compromising the value of data obtained. If the problem relates to conditions at the investigator's site, then possible alternatives should be considered and discussed. If the protocol is too complex to be easily followed, then steps must be taken to create flow charts, diagrams, and other aids to explain each step or factor in a sufficient and clear manner, or else certain parts of the protocol must be modified. If too many patients are dropping out because of adverse reactions then consideration must be given to steps such as eliminating the top dose of the study drug. When the source of the problem lies outside the ability of the monitor or sponsor to affect or modify, then a decision of whether to terminate the study must be considered.

If the problem is believed to be primarily focused on the investigator's motivation as opposed to the protocol or other areas, then it is extremely important to understand the reasons why the investigator is conducting the study. Reasons often vary widely between different investigators, even among those who are participating in an identical multicenter study. Common motives involve (1) professional recognition resulting from being associated with an exciting new drug or special study, (2) career enhancement, (3) scientific interest, (4) financial rewards as part of a professional drug testing business, (5) financial rewards to obtain funds to support other research, (6) greater ability to treat one's patients, (7) obtaining medical or scientific equipment, and (8) doing a personal favor for, or returning a favor to, someone at the sponsor or another site. Numerous other motives exist which may be the investigator's primary reasons for conducting a study.

Once the investigator's motivation is understood it is possible to determine ways to help solve the problem and also benefit the investigator. This could be in the form of a *quid pro quo*. The monitor should try to make the investigator share a stake in the study outcome and the problem's resolution. Enlist the help of others, if necessary, to solve the problem.

When the investigator's primary motives relate to financial considerations it does not imply that the sponsor should merely increase the study budget to improve the investigator's motivation. This may only offer a short-lived stimulus to the investigator. A number of other approaches may be more effective. Providing assistance to the investigator by paying for a full-time (or part-time) research coordinator, nurse, or other individual to help with the study may cause a dramatic improvement in the study's conduct and the investigator's motivation. Paying for patient meals and transportation, or for previously unanticipated actual study costs, is generally acceptable.

Paying a bonus to investigators to complete a study by a certain deadline or to enroll a certain number of patients within a specified time is considered by some sponsors and investigators to be unethical. This practice places often-strong monetary incentives on rapidly enrolling patients. An investigator may thus be influenced to enroll a patient who would otherwise not be enrolled. Thus, the bonus may have an undesired effect on increasing risks that patients are exposed to in a study, and may have an adverse impact on the investigator's adhering to "good clinical practices."

An alternative to a bonus payment which is more acceptable, from an ethical perspective, is to pay investigators different per-patient sums for completed patients who meet a defined standard, as opposed to patients who do not meet the defined standard(s). These standards may be established in terms of duration of treatment (e.g., investigators get paid more for patients who remain in the study for a given number of weeks or months than for those who remain in the study for a shorter period) or in terms of quality of data (e.g., investigators are paid a different rate for patients whose data collection forms are complete or meet certain criteria than for patients whose data collection forms have more than a preset minimum of missing or erroneous data).

One of the most difficult roles for a monitor is to help maintain motivation at study sites during a long-term study, or during a study of short duration which is conducted over a long time period needed to enroll a sufficient number of patients. Knowledge of the positive attributes of a drug, the potential value of the study, motivation of the investigator, and potential problems that might arise in the study will assist a monitor in both preventing and solving problem situations.

GAMES INVESTIGATORS PLAY

Some of the common types of "games" are listed in Table 20.8. Many others could be included. The primary reason for listing these is to provide

TABLE 20.8. *Games investigators play*

A. Prior to the study they may
   1. Overestimate the number of available patients who will enter the study. This is an example of "Lasagna's Law"[a]
   2. Assure the monitor that they will conduct the study themselves and then spend less time than agreed to or have assistants conduct the entire study
   3. Indicate they are definitely able to conduct the study, whereas they know their health is inadequate for the task
   4. Exaggerate their technical skills in studies where their skills are important (e.g., surgery using medical devices, using sophisticated equipment)
   5. Place pressure on the sponsor to modify the protocol in a way that benefits the investigator
   6. Provide too optimistic a date for study completion
   7. Indicate they have adequate staff to conduct the study when they actually do not have staff available

B. At the time of study initiation they may
   1. Delay starting the study
   2. Not obtain IRB[b] approval on the agreed schedule
   3. Include additional parts or tests in a study because of personal interest, but which are not written in the protocol and are not approved by their IRB
   4. Share drug supply with preclinical scientists

C. Regarding patients entered in the study, they may
   1. Enter hard-core nonresponders despite requests not to do so
   2. Enter patients whose disease severity is too mild
   3. Enter patients (or volunteers) with a history of alcohol or drug abuse who are believed or known to be unreliable
   4. Enter patients and start treatment before the patients' screen or baseline laboratory values are returned. It is important to have these values in order to confirm that they are acceptable
   5. Enter the same patient two (or more) times in the same study
   6. Enter the same patient in two (or more) different studies being conducted simultaneously by the investigator

D. Regarding randomization they may
   1. Assign patients to treatment based on their own biases
   2. Takes bottles of drug from a box haphazardly, rather than randomizing patients according to the code provided

E. During the study they may
   1. Complete some or all tests on patients scheduled for one visit at a later date and fill in the data collection form under the original date
   2. Replace a departing staff member but not adequately train the new individual
   3. Change laboratories used to analyze samples without informing the sponsor
   4. Increase or decrease drug doses inappropriately
   5. Fail to notify the sponsor about a serious adverse reaction or drug overdose
   6. Enter patients after the date used for cutoff of new patient entry
   7. Indicate additional costs which were not discussed prior to the study, although they were known or could have been anticipated
   8. Initiate studies for other sponsors that slows or affects the original study
   9. Not communicate with the sponsor as they agreed

F. After the study they may
   1. Prepare and/or submit a publication without adhering to an agreed-on review and discussion procedure with the sponsor
   2. Analyze data independently of the sponsor in violation of an agreement
   3. Not complete reports by agreed-on dates
   4. Not prepare reports that adequately describe results

[a] See Figure 32.16 in *Guide to Clinical Studies and Developing Protocols* (Spilker, 1984). Overestimating the number of available patients is usually inadvertent, but may be done purposely to obtain the sponsor's agreement to conduct the study.

[b] IRB, Institutional Review Board.

monitors with a sample list of undesirable situations that may be prevented or corrected. The major approach to solving most of these issues is to discuss them openly and frankly with the investigator. Reasons why these practices are undesirable and/or unacceptable must be given in a manner that does not criticize the investigator or staff. The monitor and investigator should aim to reach agreement on a course of action that is acceptable to both.

When monitors discuss or negotiate the contents of a protocol with an investigator, or discuss the conduct of a study, it is important to remember that each investigator has different needs and desires. Even assuming that an investigator does not have a "hidden agenda," there are numerous shortcuts, ploys, or actual protocol violations that investigators may introduce (or attempt to introduce) into the study. It is the monitor's responsibility to keep the study moving forward on as high a level as possible and to prevent undesirable or unacceptable variations from occurring in a study. These deviations often arise from the investigator's lack of awareness of the importance and need to adhere strictly to a protocol. Deviations also arise from the investigator's busy schedule and desire to expedite patient treatment and care. Situations of actual deceit or fraud are not considered as "games investigators play."

21

Interactions of Regulatory Departments, Regulatory Agencies, and Medical Departments

Introduction • Major Types of Regulatory Submissions • Components and Strategies of Regulatory Submissions • Types of Interactions Between Clinical Departments, Regulatory Departments, and Regulatory Agencies • Regulatory Issues and Problems • Selected Regulations and Guidelines

INTRODUCTION

Regulatory submissions (and approvals) play a major role in the livelihood and survival of a company. This chapter briefly describes the major types of regulatory submissions and how they are generally planned and compiled. It also discusses the types of interactions that occur between regulatory affairs departments in drug companies, regulatory agencies, and medical departments. Many activities conducted within a pharmaceutical corporation are either directly or indirectly targeted toward an eventual filing of a regulatory submission.

Academicians who conduct unsponsored clinical studies (with or without active participation of a pharmaceutical company) usually have few interactions with a regulatory agency or department. There are some situations, however, where academicians may interact with a regulatory group either at their own institution, with an agency at the national level, or with a pharmaceutical company. Common interactions of these types will be described.

Organization of the Food and Drug Administration (FDA)

Figure 21.1 gives us (1) a perspective of the FDA organization in the Department of Health and Human Services, one of the major cabinets in the U.S. Government, and (2) a description of the various offices of the

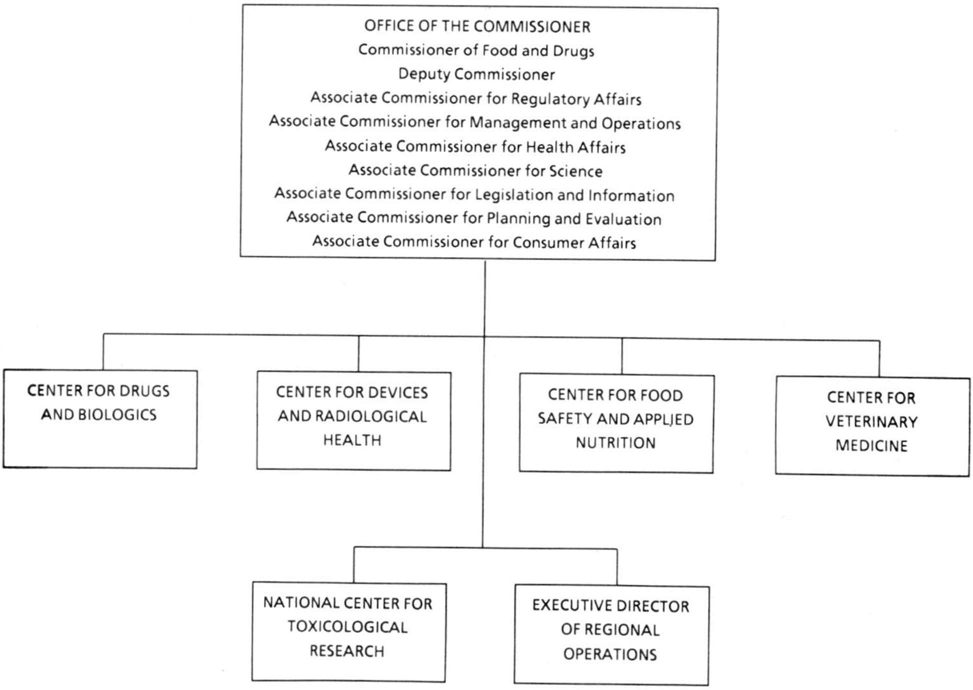

FIG. 21.1. Organization of the FDA.

FDA. A more detailed organization of the Center for Drugs and Biologics is shown in Fig. 21.2. This figure shows the component parts of both the Office of Drug Research and Review (ODRR) and the Office of Biologics Research and Review (OBRR).

MAJOR TYPES OF REGULATORY SUBMISSIONS

There are many different types of regulatory submissions made by multinational companies to regulatory agencies throughout the world. A few of the most important submissions in the United States and the United Kingdom will be indicated.

United States

IND. This abbreviation stands for Notice of Claimed Investigational Exemption for a New Drug (Form FDA 1571). It is the document that allows initial clinical testing of a new drug or a new dosage form of an already marketed or investigational drug. INDs are not approved, but may be dis-

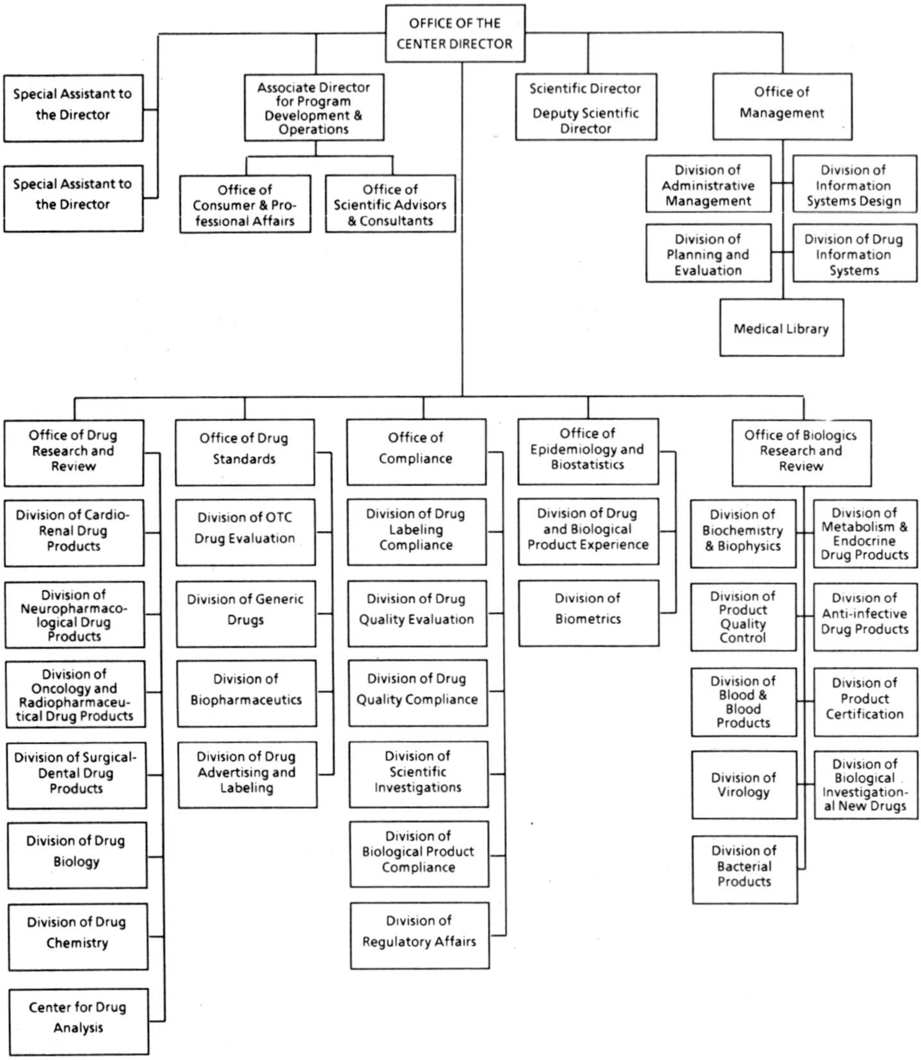

FIG. 21.2. Organization of the Center for Drugs and Biologics within the FDA.

approved for good cause. Clinical testing may begin 30 days after filing the IND, unless the FDA places the IND on hold or raises questions that must be answered prior to initiation of studies. The 30-day delay requirement may be waived by the FDA if the sponsor demonstrates a good reason for a waiver. Preclinical testing of the investigational compound usually takes from 2 to 4 years prior to submission of the IND application. The contents of an IND application are outlined in the forms required, as shown in the

TABLE 21.1. *Contents of the overall summary of an NDA*[a]

1. Proposed text of product labeling, with annotations to the information in the summary and technical sections
2. The drug's pharmacologic class, scientific rationale, intended use, and potential clinical benefits
3. The drug's marketing history, if any, outside the United States
4. A summary of the chemistry, manufacturing, and controls section
5. A summary of the nonclinical pharmacology and toxicology section
6. A summary of the human pharmacokinetics and bioavailability section
7. A summary of the microbiology section (required only for antiinfective drugs)
8. A summary of the clinical data section including statistical analyses
9. A concluding discussion of benefit/risk considerations, proposed additional studies, and postmarketing surveillance plans

[a] Based on the 1985 "NDA rewrite."

Appendix (Figs. A.1, A.2, A.3 and Table A.3). The section in the Code of Federal Regulations (CFR) that provides regulatory guidance is 21 CFR 312.

IND Amendment. Filed for any change in protocol, drug strength, investigator, or other aspects of a study or drug development program.

NDA. This abbreviation stands for New Drug Application (Form FDA 356h). This application requests approval by the FDA to market a drug for the indications specified in the application. It is usually submitted to the FDA at the end of Phase III studies after most major investigational studies have been completed and the sponsor is satisfied that all requirements for safety and efficacy have been met. In some circumstances, such as when a drug will be used to treat a rare disease, or a serious disease for which no satisfactory treatment is available, the NDA may be submitted at the end of Phase II studies. The contents of the NDA summary according to the 1985 "NDA rewrite" are shown in Table 21.1, and the general contents are shown in Table A.1 in the Appendix. Form FDA-356h is shown in Fig. A.4. The section in the CFR that provides regulatory guidance is 21 CFR 314. The FDA rates new chemical entities (NCEs) as A, B, or C. Type A represents important therapeutic gains, Type B represents modest therapeutic gains, and Type C represents those with little or no therapeutic gain. These categories are described in more detail later in this chapter.

NDA Amendment. An applicant may submit an amendment to an application that has been filed but not yet approved. An amendment may contain either significant new data from a previously unreported study or detailed new analysis of previously submitted data. A major amendment may extend the review period of the NDA (see 21 CFR 314.60 for more details).

NDA Supplement. A supplement to an approved application is required for any significant changes in the conditions described in the NDA. It is

TABLE 21.2. *Contents of annual reports of marketed products submitted to the FDA*[a]

1. Summary of data affecting safety, effectiveness, or labeling
2. Amount of drug distributed during the preceding year
3. Samples of labeling
4. Changes in chemistry, manufacturing, and control, including reports of experiences, investigations, studies, or tests involving chemical, physical, or other properties of the drug. Changes made during the year which did not require prior FDA approval
5. Nonclinical study reports of unpublished data and summaries of published reports of toxicological and *in vitro* studies
6. Current status of postmarketing studies conducted by the sponsor or on their behalf
7. Published clinical studies of the drug[b]
8. Summaries of unpublished clinical studies that have been completed

[a] Annual reports are submitted within 60 days of the anniversary date of approval of the application using form FDA 2252.
[b] See Trombitas and Simpson (1986).

usually required for substantive modifications (e.g., in labeling, packaging, manufacturing methods, chemical synthesis). Certain minor changes are permitted without submitting a Supplement to an NDA (SNDA) (see 21 CFR 314.70 for more details). Supplements may only be filed by the holder(s) of the original NDA.

Abbreviated NDA. Approval of this application is required prior to the sale of drug products that already meet the statutory standards for safety and effectiveness. It is usually reserved for duplicates and drug products previously approved under a full NDA and has become the standard for requesting approval of generic drug products (see 21 CFR 314.55 for more details).

Annual Report. Drug companies must submit an annual report on every investigational and marketed drug to the FDA. The contents of the annual report for marketed products are listed in Table 21.2 (see 21 CFR 314.81 for more information). Other records and reports to be submitted to the FDA are detailed in 21 CFR 310.300, 310.302, and 310.303.

Premarket Notification (*510k*). A notice to the FDA, Center for Devices and Radiological Health, of the intent to market a medical device of Class I [those subject to only the general controls of the Food, Drug, and Cosmetic (FD&C) Act] or II (those that are or will be subject to a performance standard in accordance with the FD&C Act).

Investigational Device Exemption (*IDE*). A research permit to allow an unapproved medical device to be tested on humans to evaluate safety and efficacy.

Premarket Approval Application (*PMA*). A permit to allow the sale of a

TABLE 21.3. *Selected differences between regulatory agencies for drugs in the United States and United Kingdom*

United States	United Kingdom
1. Companies have some access to decision makers during the review period	1. Companies have less access to decision makers during the review period
2. The same reviewer(s) will review all or most applications on one type of drug	2. Reviewers are assigned applications to review in sequence. It is uncertain who will be the reviewer of a specific application
3. A public advisory committee usually meets to provide a recommendation to the FDA for Class A or B drugs[a]	3. Nothing comparable
4. Appeal process is possible by a sponsor for a rejected application	4. Either a written or oral appeal is possible by a sponsor
5. A fishbowl atmosphere is sometimes present with many observers, which slows speed of approval	5. A more closed environment is present

[a] See text for definitions.

Class III medical device. This application is usually filed after completion of clinical trials that assure safety and effectiveness of the device or that establish an acceptable performance standard.

United Kingdom

There are several major differences between drug regulations and regulatory agencies in the United States and the United Kingdom. One important difference is that clinical studies conducted in normal volunteers do not require government approval in the United Kingdom, whereas the FDA requires submission of a full IND. Some other differences in the drug review process for the FDA and the Department of Health and Social Security (DHSS) in the United Kingdom are listed in Table 21.3.

CTX (*Exemption to a Clinical Trial Certificate*). This application is submitted to the regulatory authorities after initial clinical studies have been performed in normal volunteers. There is no requirement for volunteer studies to have been carried out before application is made for a CTX. In fact, it would not always be ethical to conduct volunteer studies with a new drug, but any volunteer studies conducted must be reported in the CTX. After approval of this application, drug studies may be conducted in patients with the disease or problem for which the drug is intended. This is approximately equivalent to pilot Phase II studies in the United States. A summary of the regulatory dossier submitted to the European Economic Community countries is shown in Table A.2 in the Appendix. If initial clinical studies are to be performed in patients with the disease or condition for which the product is to be indicated, the DHSS requires a CTC.

CTC (*Clinical Trial Certificate*). Application to conduct studies (in patients) that are more extensive than those conducted under a CTX. This is approximately equivalent to regulatory approval to conduct late Phase II and all of Phase III studies in the United States. The CTC contains more data than a CTX. The licensing authority might request a CTC for a new drug if they had initially considered a CTX and did not wish to approve it without more complete data and obtaining a second opinion from the Committee on Safety of Medicines (CSM). CTX applications are not reviewed by the CSM but are judged solely by the full-time professional Secretariat of the Medicines Division (within the DHSS). Thus, the Secretariat can only get the opinion of the CSM by asking for a full CTC application.

PLA (*Product License Application*). Application to obtain approval to market a new drug. There are three major sections to this application: clinical, preclinical, and pharmaceutical.

Comparing Drugs and Biologicals

Drug approvals are governed by the FD&C Act of 1938 plus amendments passed since that time. Biological products are governed by a different law, the Public Health Service Act of 1944 (58 Stat 682).

Separate registration documents are submitted to the FDA for each of these two types of product. NDAs are submitted for drugs to the ODRR, and PLAs are submitted for biological products to the OBRR. Anyone, whether sponsor, distributor, or manufacturer of a drug, may submit an NDA, but only a manufacturer of a biological product may submit the PLA. A PLA in the United States thus differs from a PLA in most other countries, because in other countries a PLA is submitted for either a drug or biological product.

Estimating the Date When a Regulatory Application Will Be Submitted

There are various ways that a sponsor may estimate the future date at which a project should complete Phase III and an NDA or other dossier will be submitted to a regulatory agency for review. In the early life of a project, before the compound has been tested in humans and also during Phase I studies, most drugs are in a "guess stage." At this time, approximate estimates are made which are based on past events (approval of drugs in the same therapeutic class), resources devoted to study the drug, and future expectations of a project's progress.

In late Phase II and early Phase III a drug enters a period that may be labeled as the "forward stage" for estimating dates. During this period the remaining clinical and development program is planned and dates are estimated at which each step will be completed. Based on an optimistic, but realistic, plan of which studies may be conducted simultaneously and which must be conducted sequentially, plus estimating resources available and potential conflicts with other projects, an estimated date for submission of the regulatory application is determined. This means that all steps are identified, their time requirements are estimated, and a total time is derived from adding up the critical paths or control points.

During Phase III a drug enters a different period of study which may be labeled as the "backward stage" for estimating dates. This means that a realistic target date is established for regulatory submission based on many factors, including those listed above. This date is used as a starting point, and plans are established by working backwards from that date to set all of the other dates for required activities to be completed. This process is meant to apply more pressure to complete activities than usually exists in the forward stage. A reasonable time to set a backward-oriented date is when the regulatory submission is about 1½ to 2 years in the future.

Personnel participating on a project will generally realize if a date given for completion of a regulatory submission is too ambitious. Instead of serving to spur activities and enthusiasm of the staff with a large amount of resources moving in a common direction, it will either lead to (1) sloppy and incomplete work that was rushed to meet the deadline or (2) setting an unrealistic target date that will backfire and people will build resentment and/or ignore the dates completely. In the first case, the submission's flaws will eventually be uncovered and will probably require more time and effort to undo and correct any problems that might have been created, whereas in the second case, people may lose faith in the plan and any value it has for the project.

The above techniques for estimating dates are not used by all sponsors and probably are not useful for all projects. They are described as methods that may be used in appropriate situations.

COMPONENTS AND STRATEGIES OF REGULATORY SUBMISSIONS

Components

This section briefly discusses the components of the IND and NDA submissions in the United States. Early preclinical work is sometimes targeted toward an IND even before a formal commitment is made to advance a compound to human clinical studies. An example of this approach is noted when a pharmacological or toxicological evaluation of one or more compounds is conducted according to Good Laboratory Practices standards relatively early in a compound's life. The data obtained are available for inclusion in the IND submission if the compound advances to that stage. All other biological and chemical data and reports on the compound should also be suitable for inclusion in the IND.

Once a decision is reached to advance the compound toward an IND, a plan should be developed which lists all of the activities needed to meet the requirements of the IND. A generic model of the identity and flow of activities required for an IND is shown in Fig. 18.1. This model or chart must be modified for each specific drug since the characteristics of each product differ and special requirements may be necessary for inclusion. Modifications of the original plan must be periodically made to allow for time delays, new routes that must be followed to prepare the IND, and/or additional steps that must be added.

The NDA model plan (Fig. 18.2) is much more complex than the IND model plan. This plan may be established at any point after the IND is filed (or even before), but many of the necessary steps will not be identified until sometime during Phase II. At that point a fairly accurate understanding of the drug's clinical activity is usually achieved and the clinical program required for the NDA may be assembled with a reasonable chance of knowing which studies must be conducted prior to submitting the NDA. Phase II determines which indication(s) may be included in the NDA. The technical development of most drugs also cannot be planned with great certainty prior to Phase II. Technical development issues include items such as route of synthesis and manufacturing, final formulation, dosage strength, packaging, and so forth.

Regulatory Strategies of a Sponsor

There are a number of general strategies that most pharmaceutical companies follow in attempting to improve the rate at which their submissions are processed by regulatory agencies. Probably the single most important factor relates to the overall quality of the submission. Documents that are well organized, well written, read easily, are internally consistent, and do not contain major omissions tend to be processed more rapidly than those submissions that are carelessly assembled and sent to a regulatory agency. Reviewers are understandably exasperated when pages are missing or misnumbered, the text or tables are illegible or difficult to understand, or important descriptions are incomplete. The overall quality of a submission also refers to the standards with which studies are conducted. This is evidenced by the study design, completeness of data, and other characteristics. Poorly conducted studies will probably initiate a more thorough review of all data and more inspections of participating investigators and thus, greater delays in processing a submission. Tables 21.4 and 21.5 list the most common de-

TABLE 21.4. *Summary of deficiencies found through FDA-conducted routine inspections of clinical data at investigator's sites*[a]

Most common deficiencies	No. of deficiencies (%)[b]
Inadequate informed consent form	489 (48)
Inadequate drug accountability	338 (33)
Nonadherence to protocol	235 (23)
Inaccurate records	189 (19)
Records not available	39 (4)
Failure to keep IRB informed	52 (5)
Other deficiencies	137 (14)
Total	1,479

[a] Sloboda and Currier (1985). Data obtained from 1,012 routine audit inspections conducted between June 1979 and January 1984. This sample constitutes all of the routine audits conducted, with the exception of a few which were not evaluable.
[b] The percent refers to the number of inspections.

ficiencies and their severity found by FDA auditors in their inspections at investigator's sites, and Table 21.6 lists the results of routine data audits at sponsor's sites. It is important to present any problems with a study or submission "up front" and discuss it openly. Trying to bury problems in a submission will only raise the ire and suspicions of a reviewer.

Some sponsors routinely attempt to obtain regulatory approval through submission of what they believe to be the minimal amount of data necessary to demonstrate safety and efficacy of a new drug. Other sponsors utilize as much data as they can muster to support their application. One major dif-

TABLE 21.5. *Summary of severity of deficiencies found through FDA-conducted routine data audit inspections*[a]

Results of routine data audits	No. of audits (%)
No action required	165 (16)
Voluntary action indicated for Categories I, II[b]	727 (72)
Voluntary action indicated for Category III[c]	66 (7)
"For cause" audit initiated[d]	54 (5)
Total	1,012

[a] Inspections conducted at the investigator's sites are those described in Table 21.4.
[b] Categories are defined by the FDA. Violations in categories I and II are minor and do not warrant any FDA action.
[c] FDA communicates with the site and requests a response.
[d] An in-depth follow-up inspection is conducted on the study in question plus on other studies conducted by that investigator.

TABLE 21.6. *Summary of FDA inspections of sponsors since June 1977*[a]

	No. of sponsors	Percent of sponsors
1. Sponsors with whom no significant deviations from current or proposed regulations were noted	151	67
2. Sponsors with whom significant deviations were noted	74	33
Total	225[b]	100%
3. Common deficiencies	**No. of deficiencies**	**Percent of all inspections**
Failure to maintain adequate records of drug accountability	47	21
Absence of standard monitoring procedures	42	19
Failure to establish adequacy of laboratory facilities used by clinical investigator	37	16
Failure to review patient records	33	15
Failure to assure IRB approval	29	13
Failure to document monitoring visits	24	11
Failure to visit study site before and during clinical study	15	7

[a] This table was provided by the Division of Scientific Investigations of the FDA's Center for Drugs and Biologics. It is current as of March 1, 1986.

[b] This number includes some reinspections. Note that percentages have been rounded off to the nearest whole number.

ference between these two approaches lies in the amount of foreign data submitted. If a drug is marketed in at least one foreign country, then data should be available to support its use in the United States. Even if pivotal well-controlled data are not obtained outside the United States (generally a positive point in an American appplication), data from clinical studies or postmarketing surveillance efforts in foreign countries provide additional information, which may influence the regulatory review, especially if the foreign data are of a high quality.

If multiple submissions are anticipated on a single drug for different dosage forms and indications, then a strategy is needed to obtain approval on the most important applications in the most timely matter. This may entail temporarily delaying submission of an application for a relatively minor dosage form until favorable regulatory action has occurred on a more medically and commercially important submission, even if the former application was prepared first. If both applications are submitted simultaneously there is a possibility that regulatory reviewers will process the less important one first, or that they will process both together and not issue a regulatory decision until both can be approved or rejected. Also, if the drug represents a major therapeutic breakthrough and a minor dosage form is approved, it will probably decrease pressure to approve the drug which might be exerted on the regulatory agency from sources outside the sponsor (e.g., investigators, medical community, patients, Congress). It is important to hold a pre-NDA meeting(s) with the FDA reviewer(s) and to learn (insofar as possible) whether a simultaneous or sequential review of the applications will occur.

Some sponsors believe that maintaining close contact with regulatory agencies (whenever possible) assists in a rapid and efficient review, whereas other companies follow the opposite approach. The author has not noticed evidence where one general approach yields uniformly better results for a sponsor. It is probably preferable to use both approaches. The choice of the appropriate response should depend on the particular individuals the sponsor is dealing with at the regulatory agency and on the nature and importance of the regulatory submissions involved.

Meetings with regulatory authorities to discuss clinical plans, problems, contents of submissions, and other issues provide a valuable basis for developing a submission of the quality and format that will be most acceptable to the individuals who will have to review and approve the application. It is important for both the sponsor and regulatory agency to strive for agreement in the approach to be used for regulatory submissions. Effective use of these meetings to define an appropriate development path is an important strategy for many sponsors. Unfortunately, there is a relatively high turnover of staff at the FDA and new reviewers are not bound by any agreements reached by their predecessors about a particular drug.

Some sponsors prefer informal meetings at the FDA to identify preferable approaches to follow in drug development. The types of meetings possible are described in the next section. At meetings with the FDA, company representatives usually make proposals or ask for FDA responses to specific questions. Open-ended questions (e.g., What do you suggest we should do?) are not posed, because answers given may place a company in an extremely difficult position.

TYPES OF INTERACTIONS BETWEEN CLINICAL DEPARTMENTS, REGULATORY DEPARTMENTS, AND REGULATORY AGENCIES

Representative types of specific interactions that occur between clinical departments, regulatory departments, and regulatory agencies are briefly described. In most situations the flow of information and interactions are between a sponsor's clinical and regulatory departments and also between a sponsor's regulatory departments and various regulatory agencies. It is uncommon for most clinical departments and regulatory agencies to interact without representatives of a regulatory department present, or without their initial input. Individuals in most regulatory agencies prefer dealing on each major submission through a single company representative for more formal

TABLE 21.7. *Types of interactions between clinical and regulatory departments in the pharmaceutical industry*

A. Interactions initiated by the clinical department
   1. Request for information or clarification about regulatory requirements, laws, practices, or company procedures
   2. Submission of data and reports as part of a regulatory application
   3. Request to schedule a meeting with a regulatory agency
   4. Submission of data and reports as part of a request for a meeting with a regulatory agency
   5. Request to obtain information, guidance, or an advisory opinion from a regulatory agency
   6. Request for an interpretation of a regulation, guideline, or legal action
B. Interactions initiated by the regulatory department
   1. Request for information solicited by the regulatory department and/or government regulatory agency
   2. Provide information obtained from a regulatory agency
   3. Provide information and/or advice about regulatory issues, opinions, problems, or commentary
C. Interactions initiated by either department
   1. Discussions of regulatory strategies and procedures to be followed either in response to a regulatory agency request or independent of a regulatory agency
   2. Regulatory assistance in planning and/or compiling a regulatory submission

actions. Regulatory reviewers will occasionally contact their counterparts in industry to discuss various issues or questions that may be easily resolved.

A number of common types of interactions that occur between clinical and regulatory departments within a pharmaceutical company are listed in Table 21.7. This table is organized to illustrate those interactions that are usually initiated by the clinical department, by the regulatory department, or by either department.

Table 21.8 illustrates various types of interactions that occur between regulatory departments in a pharmaceutical corporation and a government regulatory agency. Many other types of interactions are not described, because they have less relevance for investigational drugs.

Meetings

There are many reasons why requesting meetings with the FDA to discuss development plans and issues is beneficial to a drug sponsor. Various types of meetings are listed in Table 21.9. A few circumstances where it is desirable to have a pre-IND meeting with the FDA are listed in Table 21.10. In setting up meetings between the FDA and a sponsor it is important to agree on which individuals should be present and the major points on the agenda. This allows each side to bring the most appropriate people and information, which improves the possibility of agreement. Table 21.11 lists additional considerations for initiating and preparing for a formal meeting with FDA

TABLE 21.8. *Types of interactions between regulatory departments in the drug industry and government regulatory agencies*[a]

A. Formal meetings[b]
B. Informal meetings may be held on occasion, to discuss problems or issues
C. Information transmittal from a pharmaceutical company to a regulatory agency
   1. Company submits and requests approval of regulatory submissions of various types (e.g., NDA)
   2. Company submits regulatory documents (e.g., IND)
   3. Company informs a regulatory agency about modifications covered by an existing regulatory submission (e.g., additional protocols to be conducted under an IND)
   4. Company provides data on adverse reactions according to statute, provides annual reports on open INDs, and provides other required documentation
   5. Company provides data and other information in response to regulatory requests
   6. Company requests clarifications and responses to specific questions
   7. Company provides responses pertaining to proposed new regulations or changes in existing regulations
D. Information transmittal from a regulatory agency to a pharmaceutical company
   1. Responses are provided to company requests for (1) approval of various submissions, (2) formal meetings, (3) information on specific questions
   2. Statements are made to companies about (1) violations of the FD&C Act, (2) minor problems, or (3) potential problems
   3. Responses are made about actual or potential issues or problems relating to one of the company's drugs
   4. Questions are posed about one of the company's drugs

[a] These interactions are primarily those concerned with new drug development.
[b] See examples listed in Table 21.9.

TABLE 21.9. *Types of meetings held with regulatory authorities*

1. Prior to submittal of application to evaluate an investigational drug in humans. The purpose of this meeting is to discuss the nature of the application and possibly the clinical approach and plan to be followed ("pre-IND meeting")
2. Any time that a problem or situation arises when regulatory input would be useful
3. At the conclusion of Phase II studies ("end-of-Phase II meeting")[a]
4. To discuss overall or specific aspects of the drug development strategy, plans, or protocols at any time during the drug's investigation
5. To discuss contents to be included in the NDA and the format for its organization, prior to submittal of the application for drug approval ("pre-NDA meeting")[a]
6. At the time of NDA submittal to review its contents and organization
7. Between the time of NDA submittal and NDA approval, to address issues that arise[b]
8. To discuss final labeling after an "approvable letter" has been received ("labeling conference")[a]

[a] These are the types of meetings that are most frequently held.
[a] Meetings, conference calls, and correspondence between the FDA and the sponsor usually occurs with greatest frequency during this period.

TABLE 21.10. *Selected circumstances where it is desirable to have a pre-IND meeting with the FDA*

1. When the IND will consist mainly of foreign data
2. When an unorthodox approach will be followed in the initial clinical study (or studies)
3. When there is an unusual aspect of the IND application which should be discussed or explained (e.g., amount of data of a certain type, unusual metabolism, toxicology profile, mechanism of action)
4. When apparently conflicting data are presented on an important issue
5. When data are included which are expected to raise serious questions
6. When input from the FDA is desired relative to proposed clinical studies
7. To discuss a waiver of the 30-day review period

personnel. Some of the points that may be discussed at an end-of-Phase II conference are in Table 21.12. Following meetings of company representatives with the FDA (Table 21.8) a summary of the meeting may be sent to the FDA by the company. A reply is requested if their understanding of the discussion differed from that which is presented in the letter, or to confirm that the FDA's minutes of the meeting are in agreement with the company's minutes.

Adverse Reactions

Information on serious adverse reactions reach a sponsor from many sources and trigger responses that often include interactions between various departments of the sponsor and regulatory agencies. Figure 21.3 illustrates some of the activities and interactions that often occur as various groups become involved in the implications and flow of information about serious adverse reactions. This chart does not consider the various processes in-

TABLE 21.11. *Considerations for initiating and preparing for a formal meeting with FDA personnel*

1. Contact the FDA's Consumer Safety Officer (CSO) by letter or telephone to propose a meeting and outline the purpose as clearly as possible
2. Discuss the attendees but do not attempt to determine who the government should have at the meeting
3. Submit a proposed agenda and any other information requested by the CSO
4. Provide sufficient background material to the FDA prior to the meeting
5. Bring only those individuals who will contribute to the meeting
6. Rehearse relevant portions of the company's presentation
7. Consider questions which the FDA or others at the meeting might pose
8. Be totally clear about relevant FDA procedures and regulations
9. Remain courteous at all times, even if provoked. Do not embarrass FDA staff
10. Refer to FDA Bureau of Drug's Guide BD 4800.3-81-11, issued May 29, 1981, for additional information on meetings with the FDA

TABLE 21.12. *Points that may be discussed at an end-of-Phase II conference with the FDA*

1. Adequacy of safety and efficacy data from Phase I and II studies for the desired indications
2. Reasonableness of proceeding with Phase III studies from a safety perspective. This includes consideration of animal toxicology data
3. Adequacy of Phase III study designs and possible specific protocols
4. Completeness of preclinical studies
5. Relative completeness of the manufacturing and controls data for the current stage of the drug
6. Discussion about the adequacy of current data and proposed studies for the NDA
7. Discussion about Phase III plans
8. Discussion on specific topics of interest or particular problems
9. Discussion on the drug's pharmacokinetic profile
10. Discussion about the intended dosage of the new drug
11. Discussion of the proposed format and organization for the NDA

volved in diagnosing and treating the adverse reaction, evaluating its severity, or assessing its relation to drug intake. This chart includes consideration of adverse reactions that reach the drug company via clinical studies, postmarketing surveillance, or voluntary reporting systems. Numerous variations of this scheme are possible and depend on the particular circumstances of the adverse reaction, company, and country (or countries) involved. Some of the major categories of adverse reactions and reporting requirements are shown in Table 21.13. The FDA's interpretation of postmarketing adverse reaction requirements is presented by Sills et al. (1986).

TABLE 21.13. *Reporting of spontaneous adverse reactions by sponsors to the FDA*[a]

Nature of adverse reaction	Action to be taken	Mechanism to use	Time frame
Serious and unlabeled[b]	Submit 15-day report and follow-up	FDA 1639 form	15 days
Serious and labeled	Submit data periodically	FDA 1639 form and tabulation	Periodically
Serious and labeled	Detect if there is an increased frequency	Narrative	15 days
Nonserious	Submit data periodically	FDA 1639 form and tabulation	Periodically

[a] This table relates to those adverse reactions that occur in the United States and come to the attention of sponsors. Spontaneous adverse reactions reported by physicians to the FDA are often considered as a measure of concern by the physician about the drug and/or adverse reaction observed.

[b] The terms "labeled" and "unlabeled" refer to whether the specific adverse reaction has been identified in the package insert.

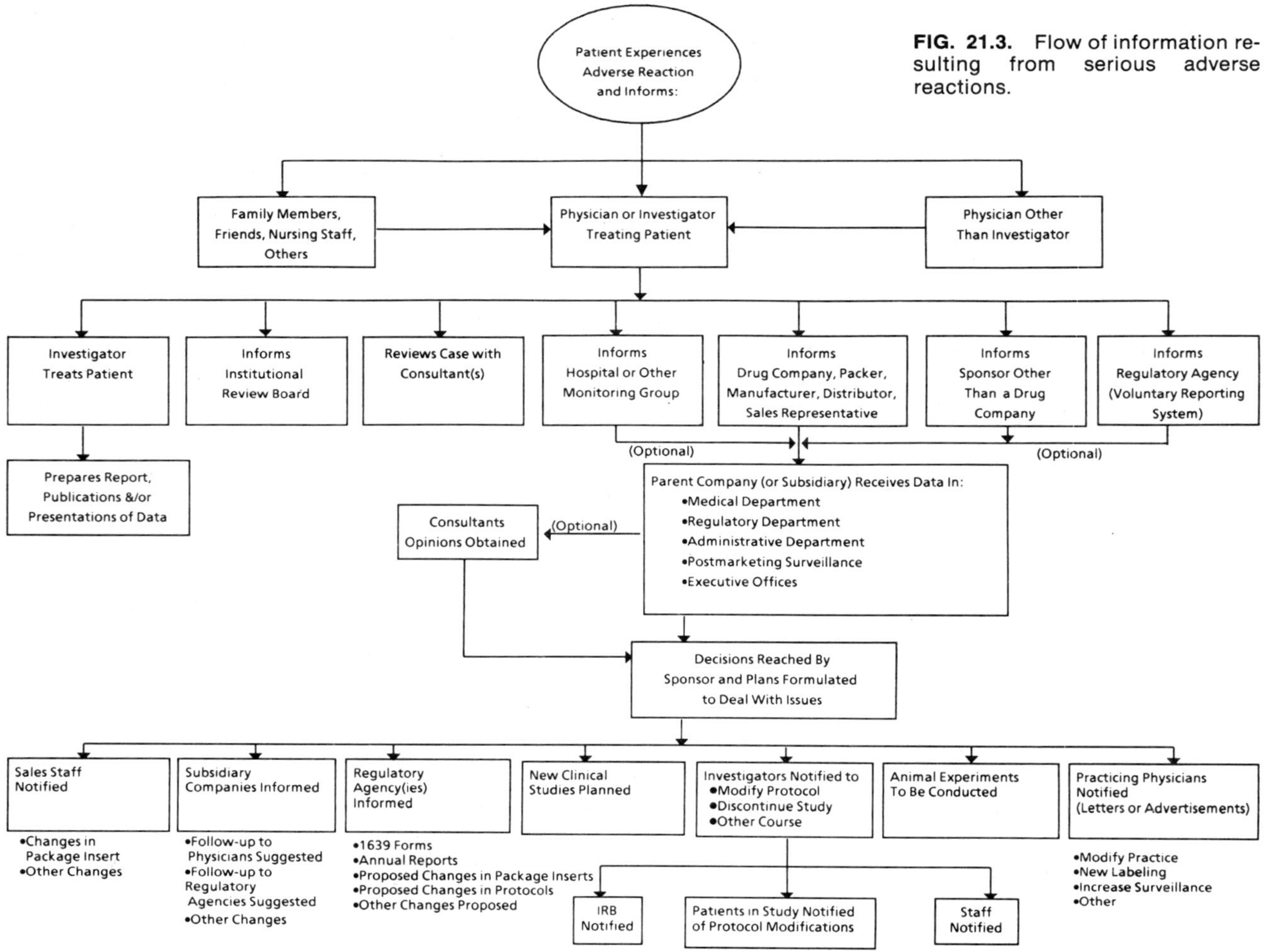

FIG. 21.3. Flow of information resulting from serious adverse reactions.

DEPARTMENT OF HEALTH HUMAN SERVICES
PUBLIC HEALTH SERVICE
FOOD AND DRUG ADMINISTRATION (HFN-730)
ROCKVILLE, MD 20857

ADVERSE REACTION REPORT
(Drugs and Biologics)

Form Approved: OMB No. 0910-0001
Expiration Date; May 31, 1986.

FDA CONTROL NO.

ACCESSION NO.

I. REACTION INFORMATION

1. PATIENT ID/INITIALS *(In Confidence)*

2. AGE YRS.

3. SEX

4.-6. REACTION ONSET — MO. | DA. | YR.

8.-12. CHECK ALL APPROPRIATE TO REACTION
- ☐ DIED DUE TO REACTION
- ☐ TREATED WITH Rx DRUG
- ☐ RESULTED IN, OR PROLONGED, INPATIENT HOSPITALIZATION
- ☐ RESULTED IN SEVERE OR PERMANENT DISABILITY
- ☐ NONE OF THE ABOVE

7. DESCRIBE REACTION(S) *(Underline single most important clinical event or reaction term)*

13. RELEVANT TESTS/LABORATORY DATA

II. SUSPECT DRUG(S) INFORMATION

14. SUSPECT DRUG(S) *(Give manufacturer and lot no. for vaccines/biologics)*

15. DAILY DOSE

16. ROUTE OF ADMINISTRATION

17. INDICATION(S) FOR USE

18. THERAPY DATES *(From/To)*

19. THERAPY DURATION

20. DID REACTION ABATE AFTER STOPPING DRUG? ☐ YES ☐ NO ☐ NA

21. DID REACTION REAPPEAR AFTER REINTRODUCTION? ☐ YES ☐ NO ☐ NA

III. CONCOMITANT DRUGS AND HISTORY

22. CONCOMITANT DRUGS AND DATES OF ADMINISTRATION *(Exclude those used to treat reaction)*

23. OTHER RELEVANT HISTORY *(e.g. diagnoses, allergies, pregnancy with LMP etc.)*

IV. ONLY FOR REPORTS SUBMITTED BY MANUFACTURER

24. NAME AND ADDRESS OF MANUFACTURER *(Include Zip Code)*

24a. IND/NDA. NO. FOR SUSPECT DRUG

24b. MFR CONTROL NO.

24c. DATE RECEIVED BY MANUFACTURER

24d. REPORT SOURCE *(Check one)* ☐ FOREIGN ☐ STUDY ☐ LITERATURE ☐ HEALTH PROFESSIONAL ☐ CONSUMER

25. 15 DAY REPORT ☐ YES ☐ NO

25a. REPORT TYPE ☐ INITIAL ☐ FOLLOWUP

V. INITIAL REPORTER *(In confidence)*

26.-26a. NAME AND ADDRESS OF REPORTER *(Include Zip Code)*

26b. TELEPHONE NO. *(Include area code)*

26c. HAVE YOU ALSO REPORTED THIS REACTION TO THE MANUFACTURER? ☐ YES ☐ NO

26d. ARE YOU A HEALTH PROFESSIONAL? ☐ YES ☐ NO

NOTE: Required of manufacturers by 21 CFR 314.80.

FORM FDA 1639 (5/85) PREVIOUS EDITION IS OBSOLETE.

FIG. 21.4. Copy of FDA 1639 form to collect data on adverse reactions. Instructions for completing this form are also shown. This form is completed by investigators for known drugs and by sponsors for serious adverse reactions reported to them.

INSTRUCTIONS FOR COMPLETING FORM FDA - 1639

GENERAL

* Use a separate Form FDA - 1639 for each patient.
* Additional pages may be attached if the space provided on the Form FDA - 1639 is inadequate.
* Non-manufacturers should send forms to Food and Drug Administration, Division of Drug and Biological Product Experience, HFN-730, 5600 Fishers Lane, Rockville, MD 20857.
* For questions call: 301 - 443-4580.
* Patient and initial reporter identification is held in confidence by the FDA and is not subject to release under the Freedom of Information Act.
* Reports of serious, suspect reactions are encouraged.
* Submission of a report does not necessarily constitute an admission that the drug caused the adverse reaction.

SPECIFIC INSTRUCTIONS

I. Reaction Information

Item 2. Age - For children under 5 years of age write in date of birth (DOB) in Item 1. For congenital malformations, give the age and sex of the infant (even though the mother was exposed).

Item 7. Describe reaction - Give signs and/or symptoms, diagnoses, course, etc. Underline the single most important descriptive phrase.

II. Suspect Drug Information

Item 14. Suspect Drug - The trade name is preferred. If a generically produced product is involved, the manufacturer should be identified.

Item 15. Dose - For pediatric patients, also give body weights.

Item 20 and 21. NA - is defined as nonapplicable (e.g. when only one dose given or outcome was irreversible).

V. Initial Reporter

Item 26c. Have you also reported this reaction to the manufacturer? - Your answer facilitates identification of duplicates in the central adverse reaction file. FDA encourages direct reporting even if a report has been submitted to the manufacturer.

NOTE TO MANUFACTURERS *(Refer to 21 CFR 314.80)* Detailed instructions are contained in the "Draft Guideline for Reporting Adverse Drug Reactions" and/or "Draft Guideline for Reporting Adverse Biologics Reactions".

☆ U.S. G.P.O. 1985-461-364/37054

FIG. 21.4. *(Continued)*

The form used to report an adverse drug or biologic reaction to the FDA is the 1639 form (Fig. 21.4). The "yellow card" form (Fig. 21.5) is used for this purpose in the United Kingdom. The speed with which serious adverse reactions must be reported to a regulatory agency vary, depending on the particular situation, but are generally clearly described in the regulations. See 21 CFR 314.80 for details pertaining to FDA requirements.

REGULATORY ISSUES AND PROBLEMS

Different types of deep-seated issues and problems permeate the current regulatory environment. There are usually limited methods available to spon-

IN CONFIDENCE – REPORT ON SUSPECTED ADVERSE REACTIONS

1. Please report all suspected reactions to recently introduced drugs (identified by a black triangle in the British National Formulary), vaccines, dental or surgical materials, IUCD's, absorbable sutures, contact lenses and associated fluids, and serious or unusual reactions to all agents.
2. Record all other drugs etc, including self-medication, taken in the previous 3 months. With congenital abnormalities, record all drugs taken during pregnancy, and date of last menstrual period.
3. Do not be deterred from reporting because some details are not known.
4. Please report suspected drug interactions.

NAME OF PATIENT (To allow for linkage with other reports for same patient. Please give record number for hospital patients.)	Family name Forenames	SEX	AGE or DATE OF BIRTH	WEIGHT (Kg.)

DRUGS, VACCINES (Inc. Batch No.), DEVICES, MATERIALS etc. (Please give Brand Name if known)	ROUTE	DAILY DOSE	DATE STARTED	DATE ENDED	INDICATION
Suspected drug, etc.					
Other drugs, etc. (Please state if no other drug given.)					

SUSPECTED REACTIONS	STARTED	ENDED	OUTCOME (eg. fatal, recovered)

ADDITIONAL NOTES	REPORTING DOCTOR (Block letters please)
	Name:
	Address:
	Tel. No: Specialty:
	Signature: Date:

If you would like information about other reports associated with the suspected drug, please tick box – ☐

AR/20 250,000 2/83 / 52/4266 C.BROS(N/C) Ltd.

FIG. 21.5. Copy of "yellow card" used in the United Kingdom to report adverse reactions.

sors for dealing with these issues in a satisfactory way. These issues are described from a pharmaceutical company perspective, and admittedly do not fully present the viewpoint of the regulatory agency. Most of these issues are particularly involved with the FDA. Issues involving other agencies are not elaborated, although there are many factors that differ between national agencies (see Table 21.14 for some examples).

1. There is in general a continued escalation of regulatory demands over the years for increased quality and amount of data (e.g., number of patients, data tabulations) to be generated by the sponsor for INDs as well as NDAs. One aspect of this issue relates to the tendency by the FDA to require more data at an earlier stage of drug development. Occasionally, manufacturing or control information is requested prior to the NDA to allow ample time for review of those items that have been troublesome for regulators to review in the past. In some instances these data are now being required with the IND. Also, there has been a tendency over the last several years to steadily require more definitive safety and efficacy data on a drug, particularly before women of childbearing potential may be entered in clinical studies. This often creates a "Catch-22" situation when applications are criticized by regulatory personnel for including too large a proportion of male patients.

The FDA has made an effort to decrease the amount of paperwork necessary to be submitted in an NDA by no longer mandating that all data collection forms (case report forms) be sent with the initial application, except for patients who died during a clinical study or who did not complete the study because of an adverse event. But this is often a relatively minor

TABLE 21.14. *Selected regulatory factors that differ between national regulatory agencies*

1. Compulsory licensing of a new drug to nonpatent holders (e.g., Canada)
2. Fees to process regulatory submissions (user fees)
3. "Needs clause," which indicates the basis of why the country has a need for the drug (e.g., Norway)
4. Prices established for new drugs are negotiated with most governments.[a] The United States is an exception
5. Limited period for marketing is implemented (e.g., Japan). At the end of the period the drug may be relicensed and also reevaluated by the regulatory agency
6. Review of promotional material by the regulatory agency prior to complete approval (e.g., Canada)[b]
7. Some countries own manufacturing facilities (e.g., Sweden), which may make a drug that is not being made by a sponsor
8. Specific clinical studies must be performed within the country (e.g., ADME[c] studies in Japan)
9. Specific preclinical studies must be performed within the country

[a] This may be done either before the drug is approved (e.g., Nordic countries) or after the drug is approved (e.g., France).
[b] The "approvable" letter in the United States suggests submission of promotional material to the FDA, but it is not a requirement.
[c] ADME, absorption, distribution, metabolism, and excretion.

point for the sponsor since all of the data have been generated and may be requested at any time by the FDA. In addition, it often requires more time and effort to generate the data tabulations required than it does to supply all data collection forms with the submission.

2. One of the most frustrating of all issues between sponsors and FDA involves the changing criteria by which regulatory submissions are judged. This is often referred to as the sponsor's trying to hit a moving target. Some of the changes may be justified if they relate to major changes in the state-of-the-art within a therapeutic area. Other changes are not justified, especially when they relate to the personal philosophy or views of FDA reviewers and are not a reflection of science, medicine, or regulations. When changes occur as a result of new personnel at the FDA desiring to review an NDA differently than their predecessors, it is difficult to know how to best resolve this question. Most companies merely go along with regulatory requests.

The "moving target" issue concerns virtually all areas of drug testing, manufacture, technical development, and toxicology. Guidelines are often established, such as for toxicology (see Table 21.15), but their implementation and interpretation often depend on the personal views of individuals within regulatory agencies, and it is generally believed that appeals made by sponsors with a strong scientific basis are not usually accepted.

Sponsors would like to reach agreement ahead of time (i.e., prior to the NDA submission) with the FDA on exactly which statistical analyses and stratifications are desired. This would save time and prevent reviewers from stringing out multiple requests for reanalyses of the same data over a long period.

3. There is an adversarial relationship that has built up over the years between regulatory agencies and the pharmaceutical industry. Each side has claimed no fault; however, the relationship between many other industries and agencies of the U.S. Government is often different. There is no *a priori* reason why the relationship cannot be more cooperative, and in some situations this has occurred with mutual benefit.

4. A relatively low priority is usually given by FDA reviewers to evaluating NDAs, even on extremely important NCEs. Procedures require the reviewers to give a higher priority to (1) tasks for Congress, (2) tasks for other government agencies, (3) IND reviews, and (4) other tasks assigned by their supervisors.

5. The FDA sometimes places ongoing clinical studies on hold because of perceived problems of patient safety. This is sometimes done before contacting the company, to determine whether the questions at the FDA may be satisfactorily answered. Occasionally this practice may be justified if the submitted data are unclear or inadequate to allow determination that continued use of the drug is safe. This has created many unnecessary difficulties in some cases, however, because of the complex and time-consuming processes necessary to interrupt a series of clinical studies.

Several of these situations arise because of congressional pressures on

TABLE 21.15. *Suggested guidelines for required toxicology studies for various phases of drug development*[a]

Type of drug	Phase I		Phase II		Phase III	
	Clinical study	Toxicology	Clinical study	Toxicology	Clinical study	Toxicology
Drug for oral or parenteral use	Small single dose to few people	Acute toxicology in minimum of two species Subacute in two species, three doses, 14 days Special tests	1. Single dose 2. 1–2 weeks	1. As Phase I 2. Subacute in two species for 4 weeks	1. Single dose 2. 1–2 weeks	1. As Phase I 2. Chronic two species for 1–3 months
			3. 1–3 months	3. Chronic in two species for 3 months	3. 1–3 months	3. Chronic two species for minimum 3 months
			4. 6 months or more	4. Chronic in two species for 6 months to 2 years Special tests	4. 6 months or more	4. Chronic in two species for 6 months to 2 years Special tests
Inhalation anesthetics	One episode of anesthesia	Acute in four species For subacute, 3-hr exposure for 5 subsequent days	One episode of anesthesia	As Phase I Special tests	One episode of anesthesia	As Phase I Special tests
Drugs for dermal application	Single dose	Acute, oral in two species Dermal exposure for 24 hr and observation for 2 weeks	1. Single dose 2. Short-term (2 weeks)	1. As Phase I 2. Subacute dermal for 3 weeks and observation 2 weeks Sensitivity testing in guinea pigs	1. Brief period 2. Long-term (unlimited)	1. As Phase II 2. 3–6 months, dermal Special tests

Drugs for local ophthalmic application	Single dose	Acute oral and local in two species Rabbit irritation test	Brief period	Subacute in two species for 3 weeks	1. Brief period 2. Long-term	1. As Phase II 2. Chronic for 3–6 months
Drugs for vaginal or rectal application	Single dose	Acute oral and local in one to two species	Brief period	Chronic local in two species for 3 weeks to 3 months	1. Brief period 2. Long-term	1. As Phase II 2. Chronic local for 3 months or more
Combinations, full assay for each single component	Brief period	Acute	Brief period	In rat and dog for 1–3 months	1. Brief period 2. Long-term	1. As Phase II 2. As Phase II
Hormone contraceptives, estrogens and progestagens	Brief period (1 month)	Acute and subacute in rat, dog, and primate for 90 days	3 months	Chronic in rat, dog, and primate for 1 year	3–12 months	Chronic in rat, dog, and primate for 2 years
Contact lenses and lens fluid	Brief period	Acute and subacute tests, locally Oral acute for fluids	Long-term	Chronic in rabbit for 3 weeks or more	Long-term	As Phase II

[a] From *Nordic Guidelines* (Nordic Council on Medicines, 1985).

the FDA and the attitude that has risen at the agency that it is "better to be safe than sorry." For the most part these issues cannot be satisfactorily influenced by the pharmaceutical industry. Nonetheless, dialogue is an important step toward making progress on these issues and improving the relationship between the FDA and the pharmaceutical industry.

SELECTED REGULATIONS AND GUIDELINES

Classification of INDs and NDAs by the FDA

The FDA classifies the clinical type and therapeutic potential of commercially sponsored INDs and NDAs. This system provides a simple means of describing the IND and NDA application. The designation given a specific application may change only until the NDA is approved, at which time it becomes fixed. The classification is used as a basis for priority given to the application's review and also as a factor for determining whether an application should be submitted to an advisory committee for review and whether an end-of-Phase II conference should be held. The end-of-Phase II conference is usually restricted to new drugs that are rated by the FDA as having at least a modest therapeutic gain over current treatments. If a lower rating is given a drug, the sponsor may request that the FDA elevate its rating.

The classification given below is taken from the FDA's Staff Manual Guide.

Chemical Types

Type 1. New molecular entity—i.e., the active moiety is not yet marketed in the United States by any drug manufacturer either as a single entity or as part of a combination product.

Type 2. New salt—i.e., the active moiety is marketed in the United States by the same or another manufacturer, but the particular salt, ester, or derivative is not yet marketed in the United States by any drug manufacturer either as a single entity or as part of a combination product.

Type 3. New formulation—i.e., the compound is marketed in the United States by the same or another manufacturer, but the particular dosage form or formulation is not.

Type 4. New combination—i.e., contains two or more compounds that have not previously been marketed together in a drug product by any manufacturer in the United States.

Type 5. Already marketed drug product—i.e., the product duplicates a drug product (the same active moiety, same salt, same formulation, or same combination) already marketed in the United States by another firm.

Type 6. Already marketed drug product by the same firm—used primarily for new indications for marketed drugs.

These types are not mutually exclusive, since a new formulation (Type 3) or a new combination (Type 4) may also contain a new molecular entity (Type 1) or a new salt (Type 2). In such cases, both numbers should be included in the overall classification number for the drug. For example, a new molecular entity representing an important therapeutic gain would be classified 1A; if the new entity were also in a new combination it would be classified 1,4A.

Therapeutic Potential

Type A. Important therapeutic gain—i.e., drug may provide effective therapy or diagnosis (by virtue of greatly increased effectiveness or safety) for a disease not adequately treated or diagnosed by any marketed drug, or provide improved treatment of a disease through improved effectiveness or safety (including decreased abuse potential).

Type B. Modest gain—i.e., drug has a modest, but real, potential advantage over other available marketed drugs, e.g., greater patient convenience, elimination of an annoying but not dangerous adverse reaction, potential for large cost reduction, less frequent dosage schedule, useful in specific subpopulation of those with disease (e.g., those allergic to other available drugs), etc.

Type C. Little or no therapeutic gain—i.e., drug essentially duplicates in medical importance and therapeutic usage one or more already marketed drugs.

These types are mutually exclusive. Only one of these letters may be included in the overall classification number.

Filing Times and Review Clocks

The two review clocks used by the FDA are illustrated in Fig. 21.6. The FDA has 180 days (by statute) to complete their review of an NDA and to determine whether the application is approved, approvable, or rejected. Sixty days after an NDA is received, a second clock (filing clock) is started. The filing date is established if the NDA's format, content, and administrative details are acceptable.

When a sponsor submits significant new data or information to the NDA, the FDA can restart the 180-day review clock. The FDA is not known for strictly adhering to this clock.

The filing clock (Fig. 21.6) is used when an applicant requests a hearing. This is an administrative appeal which is usually made to plead a case if an

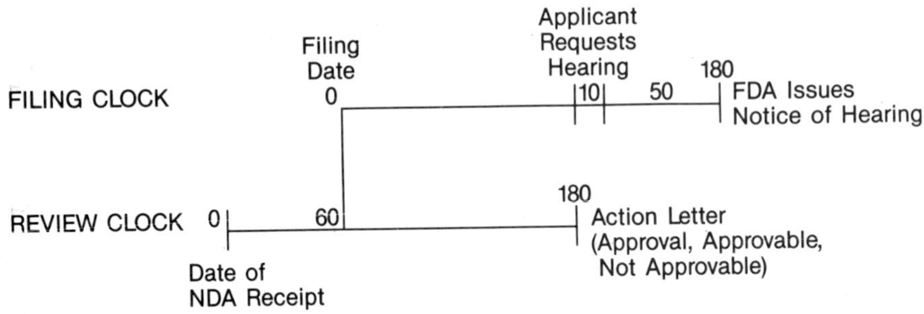

FIG. 21.6. Time frames of the FDA's review clock and filing clock. Numbers refer to days.

application is not approved. The FDA issues a notice of hearing advising the public of a scheduled hearing. This notice is published in the *Federal Register*. The hearing is public, except for any part where discussions involve trade secrets. That part of the meeting may take place in private if a prior request is made by the applicant. See 21CFR.314.200 for more information on this process.

The Drug Master File (DMF)

A drug master file (DMF) is a submission of information to the Food and Drug Administration by a person (the drug master file holder) who intends it to be used for one of the following purposes:

1. To permit the DMF holder to incorporate the information by reference when the holder submits an IND, NDA, or other submission.
2. To permit the DMF holder to authorize other persons or another company to reference the information to support a submission to FDA without the holder having to disclose the specific information to the person or company. For example, a manufacturer of packaging components may submit a DMF and allow all of their customers (companies) to refer to the DMF. Each of the companies which purchase packaging components may have numerous NDAs which refer to the same DMF of the packaging company.

FDA ordinarily neither independently reviews drug master files nor approves or disapproves submissions to a DMF. Instead, the agency customarily reviews the information only in the context of an application.

Much of the information that supports an NDA is similar or identical to that required for multiple regulatory applications. A DMF is submitted once and is then referred to in multiple applications by the sponsor to avoid having to resubmit these data with each application.

Five types of DMFs may be submitted, which relate to:

Type I—Facilities, personnel and general operating procedures.
Type II—Specific drug substances, intermediates, or dosage forms.
Type III—Packaging materials.
Type IV—Colorants, flavors, essences, and other additives used in drug dosage forms.
Type V—Animal and clinical studies. These are usually submitted, however, in a regulatory application and not in a DMF.

Toxicological Guidelines

The FDA does not have strict requirements and standards for number and identity of species and duration of studies for all categories of drugs. There are, however, approximate guidelines that are similar to those of the Nordic countries (Table 21.15). Specific requirements are often discussed with the FDA during meetings or on other occasions.

An important part of the toxicology studies are those involving reproduction. These have become the focus of more attention since the thalidomide disaster and are divided into three segments.

Segment I. Study of fertility and general reproductive performance. The studies provide general data for the effect of the drug on the entire reproductive process (e.g., teratogenesis, late stages of gestation, parturition, lactation) and evaluate the effects on gonadal function, estrous cycles, mating behavior, and conception rates.

Segment II. Study of teratogenesis. Drugs are administered during organogenesis to evaluate whether a drug has a potential for causing toxicity to the embryo or of causing teratogenic effects.

Segment III. Perinatal and postnatal study. The drug is given during the last trimester of pregnancy and during lactation to evaluate the effects of the drug on late fetal development, labor and delivery, lactation, neonatal viability, and growth of the newborn.

Finally, it is worth noting that Federal Guidelines are by definition merely "recommendations." Too often the guidelines are interpreted as legal requirements, both by various companies and by the FDA itself. For more detailed information, see 21CFR 10.90.

22

Interactions of Marketing and Research and Development Departments

Activities Originating in, and Conducted by, Research and Development Departments • Activities Originating in, and Conducted by, Marketing Departments

ACTIVITIES ORIGINATING IN, AND CONDUCTED BY, RESEARCH AND DEVELOPMENT DEPARTMENTS

This chapter deals with interactions of research and development departments with marketing departments. The word "interactions" refers to both joint activities and joint communications. Activities are usually initiated by a specific marketing or research and development department, and are mainly conducted within one of these groups. This section is concerned with those interactions where most activities are performed in, or by, a research and development department.

An important research and development activity which relates to marketing is the conduct of clinical studies to support marketing-related activities. These studies often involve a direct comparison of an investigational drug with a known standard drug. The purpose of such studies is to obtain comparative data on safety, efficacy, and/or pharmacokinetic parameters. These data may eventually be incorporated into promotional materials and publications, and may serve as evidence to support use of the study drug.

Other marketing-related activities in which research and development's clinical staff may participate include (1) review of advertising and other marketing copy to insure that it is accurate and not misleading, (2) participation in the design of scientific exhibits to be used at professional meetings, (3) attendance at scientific exhibits or drug launches, (4) planning and carrying out symposia or other meetings, and (5) preparation of various monographs, materials for a drug's launch, and other scientific documents.

Preclinical staff in research departments also assist marketing efforts in many ways. In addition to providing assistance in many of the clinical activities described above, preclinical staff often assay blood or urine samples from ongoing drug studies in pursuit of new indications, or assist outside laboratories in setting up similar assays. Scientific studies are usually performed to elucidate a drug's mechanism of action, as well as to investigate reasons for purported drug–drug interactions reported in the literature or to the company.

Answering telephone and written requests for routine or emergency information and providing assistance to answer product complaints are additional functions performed by research and development staff. Research staff members also assist in the training programs for sales representatives. Technical departments become involved in the development of new dosage strengths (i.e., size of dose per tablet or unit), dosage forms (e.g., tablet, suppository), and formulations. These products often constitute line extensions for the drug.

ACTIVITIES ORIGINATING IN, AND CONDUCTED BY, MARKETING DEPARTMENTS

Marketing groups provide many important inputs into drug development. At the early stage of drug discovery some companies attempt to concentrate their research in therapeutic areas likely to provide significant commercial returns. If there is a strong influence of marketing views in terms of identifying appropriate therapeutic areas for research and in using marketing criteria to either promote or terminate a project, then the company is said to be "market driven." If marketing influences are not strong at this early stage of drug development and decisions about choosing research areas to search for new drugs are primarily made by research management, by senior research scientists, or by a combination of the two, the company is said to be "research driven." In this situation the marketing division reacts to new drugs developed by research departments. Some companies experience strong internal conflicts and pressures as the nondominant partner attempts to increase its influence in how the company makes decisions and is oriented.

Marketing influences and information are important inputs in choosing directions for drug development once a drug is tested in humans. Information such as capsule or tablet color, size, shape, and dosage strength are obvious examples where marketing input is required. In addition, if a choice of indications to pursue is possible or if there is a choice of dosage forms (e.g., liquid or solid), then it is usually important to obtain input from marketing. As the clinical profile of the drug becomes more clearly established, marketing input is obtained in order to determine which aspects of the profile should be investigated; often, this information is also used to determine which parameters or endpoints should be evaluated. For instance, if a drug has been administered on a three- or four-times-a-day basis in early clinical studies to demonstrate and confirm its activity, but marketing wishes to sell the drug on a once-a-day basis, then studies must be planned and initiated to determine if adequate efficacy and safety will be maintained when the drug is given less frequently. It is often impossible to predict in advance whether a drug will be active for a sufficiently long period when given on a less frequent basis. One reason for this situation is that a drug's biological activity may persist for a period after the drug is excreted from the body or is broken down by the body to inactive metabolites.

Toward the end of the clinical program that is followed for an investigational drug, specialized clinical studies are often initiated specifically for marketing group objectives. These studies usually compare the new drug directly with a standard drug presently used for the same indication or they may evaluate interactions of the new drug with alcohol or other drugs that will be commonly given with the new drug. The drug may also be evaluated in a special type of patient population where results will provide important marketing information.

Marketing Strategies

The marketing strategy may be described as the mix of marketing techniques used by a company to maximize sales and/or profits. These techniques include variables such as (1) which established products are chosen to sell, (2) which new products are chosen to introduce, (3) the price of each product, and (4) the amount of promotion of each product in terms of advertising, detailing, mailings, sampling, and other techniques. Another aspect of strategy relates to the claims made about the drug which attempt to distinguish it from all other products of its class and other competing products. All of

TABLE 22.1. *Clinical questions that should be considered in developing a marketing strategy*

1. What are the best means to demonstrate superiority of a drug over its competitors in clinical studies (e.g., use of special patient populations, comparison of specific efficacy parameters, evaluation of their adverse reaction profile)?
2. What are appropriate means to create an awareness in the medical community of important, but as yet unapproved, indications of a drug (e.g., publications, talks to medical groups, drug studies)?
3. How may a sponsor/inventor obtain the best patent protection possible for the (1) drug, (2) drug uses, (3) dosage forms, and (4) methods of manufacturing?
4. Which clinical studies will provide practitioners with the information needed to effectively treat their patients? This includes the following studies: (1) drug interactions, (2) special populations, and (3) methods to wean patients off other drugs and place them on the new drug
5. Which studies must be conducted to obtain data that will enable undesirable drug labeling to be removed?

TABLE 22.2. *Selected types of marketing strategies to be addressed through conducting clinical studies*

1. Expansion of available dosage forms (e.g., capsules, tablets, caplets, solutions)
2. Expansion of approved indications (e.g., additional diseases, prophylactic use)
3. Reduction of undesirable aspects of drug labeling (e.g., removal of a black box around a warning, reduction of a contraindication to a warning)
4. Conversion of a product from prescription to over-the-counter status[a]
5. License-out a specific drug with a known profile of activity
6. Expansion of number of special patient groups in which the drug may be prescribed (e.g., children, patients with renal failure)
7. Obtain improved labeling about benefits of a drug (e.g., state that the risk of cardiovascular adverse reactions is less than with other standard drugs of the same therapeutic class)
8. Expansion of number of packages available (e.g., ampuls, multidose vials, infusion sets)
9. Comparison with a known standard drug or nondrug treatment
10. Demonstration of a particular point for use in advertising
11. Comparison of drug costs and influence on a patient's quality of life
12. Obtain approval to manufacture a drug at an additional site or by an additional manufacturer through demonstration of bioequivalence

[a] See reference by Hammes and Ciccone (1985) for details.

these techniques have a great impact on the percent of a market (i.e., market share) captured by a drug.

Some relevant questions that may assist in developing a marketing strategy are listed in Table 22.1. Selected types of marketing strategies are listed in Table 22.2. Marketing strategies are described more fully by Slatter (1977) and by Guth (1985).

A company's marketing strategy differs for each product. Each drug is sold in a different therapeutic market, where doctors' prescribing habits and attitudes differ, the nature and intensity of the competition differs, and many of the other factors that may affect a marketing strategy also differ.

Marketing Research

Marketing research attempts to answer questions that assist in developing a marketing strategy and planning relevant clinical studies. The value of a drug from a commercial perspective depends on the (1) amount of sales, (2) cost of goods (manufacturing and distribution costs), and (3) costs of promotion, coupled with the company's overall profit objective.

Some of the types of questions that marketing research attempts to answer are described below.

Before Making New Compounds

1. Which therapeutic areas have a large market size?
2. Which therapeutic areas greatly need medical advances?

TABLE 22.3. *Selected types of marketing advantages sought for a new drug*

A. Improved safety
   1. Less-serious adverse reactions (i.e., lower intensity)
   2. Fewer overall adverse reactions (i.e., lower incidence)
   3. Fewer interactions with other drugs
   4. Greater safety in specific populations (e.g., renal compromised, elderly, cardiovascular compromised)
B. Improved efficacy
   1. Faster onset of activity
   2. Longer duration of action
   3. Increased peak effect
   4. Additional clinical or pharmacological activities
   5. More-predictable response (i.e., less variability)
   6. Decreased need for concomitant therapy
C. Greater patient convenience or acceptability
   1. Less-frequent dosing
   2. Easier to swallow (e.g., film coated, smaller-size capsule)
   3. Easier dosage form to use (e.g., tablet versus aerosol or nasal inhaler)
   4. Easier package to use (e.g., blister pack versus bottle)
   5. Easier storage requirements (e.g., refrigeration no longer necessary)
   6. Improved odor or taste
D. Improved pharmacokinetic profile
   1. More-consistent absorption
   2. More-predictable metabolism
   3. All patients metabolize the drug similarly
   4. Preferred distribution pattern (e.g., does not penetrate into the brain)
   5. Preferred route of excretion
E. Greater economic benefits
   1. Decreased direct cost to patient and/or third-party payers
   2. Decreased length of hospital stay, which saves money for third-party insurers and hospitals
   3. More rapid recovery likely, which allows a more rapid return to work
   4. Decreased costs to institutions for institutionalized patients
   5. Potential savings if traditional concomitant therapies are no longer necessary

3. Which therapeutic areas offer substantial commercial potential for a new drug?
4. What are the characteristics of a new drug that would create a major gain in a given therapeutic area?
5. What drugs are presently competing in a given therapeutic area? What is their share of that market?
6. What are other potentially competitive companies doing about this therapeutic area? Are there new investigational drugs being evaluated that represent major breakthroughs or advances in this therapeutic area?
7. Is this a new therapeutic area for the company or would it be building on an existing franchise?

The types of marketing advantages sought for a new drug include those listed in Table 22.3. Some of the sources of published information of investigational drugs under development are listed in Table 22.4.

TABLE 22.4. *Current sources of published information on pharmaceutical development*[a]

De Haen New Product Survey
Drug Data Report
Inpharma
Investment analyst reports (e.g., Goldman Sacks; Smith, Barney, Harris, Upham, and Co.; Kidder, Peabody, and Co.; Bernstein)
NDA Pipeline
New Drug Commentary
Pharmaprojects
Pharmascope
Pharmaceutical News Capsule
Prospects, Healthcare Forecasting, Inc.
Scrip-World Pharmaceutical News
The Blue Sheet
The Pink Sheet

[a] This is a representative list, not an exhaustive one.

During the Testing of a New Investigational Drug

1. What is the desired clinical profile of the drug (from a marketing perspective) that should be evaluated clinically?
2. How will practitioners use the drug in actual clinical use?
3. Which of the desired clinical characteristics are essential for the drug to be successful commercially?
4. If multiple dosage forms or formulations have been prepared and tested, in which order should they be submitted for approval and marketed?
5. What is the range of the anticipated market size for the new drug? This is based on many factors, including the (1) present market size, (2) market trends, (3) unmet clinical need for an improved drug, (4) clinical characteristics of the drug, and (5) technical characteristics of the drug (e.g., size of pill, taste of drug).

Prior to, During, and After Launch

1. What tactics and strategies should be adopted to introduce the new drug?
2. What strategies should be adopted to follow the use and progress of the drug after it is launched (e.g., use of postmarketing surveillance techniques)?
3. When unanticipated questions arise at any stage of drug discovery or development, panels of physicians or potential purchasers may be assembled to address the issue (e.g., opinion about a controversial ad-

TABLE 22.5. *Factors to consider in designing a marketing interview*

A. Related to physicians interviewed and their practice
   1. Number of physicians to interview
   2. Choice of physician specialty (or specialties) to interview
   3. Geographical distribution of physicians to be interviewed (e.g., East Coast versus West Coast, city versus rural)
   4. Background of physicians (if desired) in terms of age, training, prescribing habits, and other factors
   5. Number of patients with a specified disease which the physician treats each week, month, or year
   6. Type of practice (e.g., hospital based, solo private practice, group practice)
   7. Selection of physicians interviewed may be made on numerous bases (e.g., with structured or unstructured selection criteria)
B. Related to nature of the interview and data generated
   1. Use of telephone interview versus personal visit or mailed questionnaire
   2. Methods to record data
   3. Methods to analyze data collected
   4. Methods to validate the questionnaire
   5. If interviews are used, what training is necessary for the interviewer?
   6. Determine how the response rate of physicians will be estimated
   7. Determine whether payment will be given to respondents. If so, the amount must be determined

ditive; or views about the taste of a syrup among several samples, including those of the competitors).

In order to address these and other questions, market research staff consult a variety of sources. These include published literature, professional organizations that provide marketing data, surveys and interviews of physicians and consumers, and results of preference tests of flavors or other drug characteristics. Marketing surveys require consideration of numerous factors (Table 22.5). A number of questions that physicians may be asked are listed in Table 22.6. Research and development personnel should be consulted in the design of marketing surveys and invited to observe the focus groups or other physician interviews to help improve the acceptance of results within the company. Results of these surveys and marketing research are integrated into the overall drug's development plan through the marketing member on the project team. This individual's role includes participation in those issues listed in Table 22.7.

Market Research Versus Venture Research

Market research primarily involves a retrospective analysis of marketing data and information to establish profiles, trends, and characteristics of drugs and therapeutic areas. Market research utilizes historical data when future projections are made. The projections made are often extrapolations of

TABLE 22.6. *Selected questions that physicians may be asked in a market research interview*[a]

A. Relating to patients presently in their practice
   1. Type(s) of patients seen
   2. Age range of patients seen
   3. Causes of a specified disease in patients they treat
   4. Frequency of seeing the same patients who have a specified disease
   5. Number of patients seen per day
B. Relating to current methods used for diagnosis and treatment of a specific disease or medical problem
   1. Tests commonly used to diagnose patients
   2. Current treatments used
   3. Rationale for using those treatments
   4. Length of treatment with current therapies
   5. Success rate with current therapies
   6. Usual means of monitoring patients
   7. Degree of dissatisfaction with currently available treatments
   8. Problems with current treatments and changes which would be perceived as improvements
C. Relating to a potential new drug
   1. Improvements that are desired in a new drug
   2. Whether a drug with attributes described by the interviewer would be perceived as an important improvement
   3. Whether a drug with the attributes described by the interviewer would be used by the physician. If so, in what proportion of his patients and in which types of patients?

[a] It is assumed that all questions refer to patients with a specific disease in the physician's practice or clinic.

TABLE 22.7. *Role of the marketing representative(s) on the project team*[a]

1. Recommend the desired form(s) of the drug, dose strength (mg), and colors of each dose strength
2. Help determine trade names and provide input into choosing generic names
3. Help determine types of packages (e.g., blister packs, foil samples) and size of packages (i.e., number of tablets per pack or bottle)
4. Coordinate above activities with subsidiaries or parent company in other countries
5. Determine markets to be targeted and in which order
6. Establish needs of physicians through market research
7. Evaluate market sizes; evaluate growth trends of each potential indication
8. Monitor competitive activity
9. Recommend line extensions that are desired
10. Recommend which changes in the package insert would be desirable from a marketing perspective
11. Liaise with other groups in marketing
12. Help instill commercial value in Phase III activities (e.g., recommend quality of life studies, cost-effectiveness studies, and comparisons with standard drugs)

[a] A number of additional roles are listed in Table 13.5.

trends and as such have certain limitations, since probable influences of future events are not generally considered.

Venture research is a future-oriented prospective study of evaluating and prognosticating future trends as well as physician needs and desires. Venture research involves physician interviews to establish what information physicians desire in order to make a choice among different drugs of the same therapeutic class. Their responses often differ by specialty, location of their practice, type of practice, age, and numerous other factors. The information from these interviews help provide, answers to several marketing questions which target a new drug most effectively. Some of these questions are:

1. What information about a new drug could influence a physician's opinion?
2. How do physicians weigh the various types of information they utilize in choosing a drug to use?
3. How do physicians obtain information about drugs, and which sources do they use?
4. Do the physicians interviewed prefer to read studies performed by physicians of the same specialty, or is this not an issue?
5. Is the information presented on the characteristics of a hypothetical drug easily understood by physicians? These characteristics are those of the investigational drug. Would physicians prescribe the new drug?

An important part of a marketing division is their field staff or marketing representatives. Marketing representatives are the sales force of a drug company. They are well trained by their company in the strengths and weaknesses of their products, as well as important selling points. These individuals have become information specialists in recent years and interact with physicians in both private offices and hospitals. Well-trained representatives understand the medical science that underlies their drug and can help educate physicians about new results relating to one or more areas in medicine, as well as the scientific aspects of the drugs they are promoting. See Table 22.8 for specific functions of sales representatives.

Specific marketing activities conducted on a drug depend on whether the drug is established on the market, newly introduced to the market, or investigational. Activities include determining sales strategies for drugs based on the drug's development as a (1) new chemical entity (NCE), (2) line extension (e.g., new dosage form, dose size), (3) conversion from prescription to over-the-counter use, or (4) combination drug. Each of these types of drugs involves specific considerations from a marketing perspective. These considerations plus drug profile and market needs influence the development of the marketing plan developed for each drug.

Role of the Product Champion

The product manager in marketing has an analogous role in many ways to the project leader in research and development. The project leader usually

TABLE 22.8. *Selected functions of pharmaceutical sales representatives*

A. With physicians
   1. Provide information about new products
   2. Provide new information about old products
   3. Provide medical literature and educational materials
   4. Encourage physicians to prescribe certain products
   5. Provide product samples
   6. Help establish and/or monitor clinical studies
   7. Obtain information requested by the physician
   8. Report adverse reactions to the sponsor
B. With pharmacists[a]
   1. Check inventory
   2. Promote over-the-counter drugs
   3. Discuss relevant issues
   4. Encourage pharmacists to dispense the company's products

[a] Most points with part A are also relevant.

shepherds the project from the decision point where it was decided to study the compound in humans until it is approved for marketing, and possibly longer. In some companies a joint research and development plus marketing team is utilized during the transition period. The product manager develops the marketing strategy and approach while the drug is still undergoing investigation. This includes (1) identifying the target audience that will receive most of the promotion, (2) establishing the position of the product so that it stands apart from the competitors, and (3) determining a promotional platform that remains within the drug's labeling. He or she also assists in (1) determining the price that will be charged based on a balance of various factors, (2) forecasting the number of units that will be sold during the first year, (3) placing orders with production personnel to make these units, (4) determining the amount of money to spend on promotion and how it will be spent, and (5) planning many other aspects of the drug's launch and career (see below).

Market Launch

The market launch of a new drug is an important milestone in a drug's life. Planning the various activities involved is important for various reasons, including those listed in Table 22.9. A list of the various activities that may be planned is given in Table 22.10. In addition to all of the activities conducted in various marketing departments that are planning for, and actually launching, a new drug, medical departments also participate. Some of their activities are listed in Table 22.11.

Various plans for launching a drug may be submitted to a decision-making person or group for review and establishment of policy. It is usually im-

TABLE 22.9. *Selected objectives in planning activities that are part of a market launch*

1. Identify milestone dates
2. Identify decision points
3. Identify activities to be conducted by individual departments or groups
4. Identify the shortest route to a product launch
5. Identify activities where liaison with production, research and development, and other areas are required
6. Assist in identifying effects of delay

portant to carefully plan as many launch oriented events as possible to insure that they are handled well and take the minimum amount of time. Certain steps (e.g., drug manufacturing) may be conducted either before or after the final approval letter is received from the regulatory agency. If the company has received an approvable letter, there may be sufficient assurance that the final approval will be received within a reasonable period and a decision may therefore be made to proceed with full-scale manufacturing.

Medical Groups Within Marketing Departments

Several drug companies have allowed their marketing departments to establish and control medical groups that initiate clinical studies. These medical groups are not the company's major medical group or department that investigates new drugs, but are intended to plan, initiate, monitor, analyze, and interpret marketing-oriented clinical studies. These studies include those evaluating (1) a new drug versus established standard drugs, (2) new formulations, (3) line extensions, and possibly (4) new indications. The primary reason why a company would establish a separate medical group within marketing is that marketing studies have traditionally been given a low priority within medical departments. Thus, medical departments often do not initiate and analyze marketing-oriented studies as rapidly as marketing people would like or expect. This often leads to great frustration within marketing, especially when their top priorities for clinical studies are not accorded adequate priority within the medical department and the studies are not performed, or are greatly delayed.

Conversion of Prescription Drugs (Rx) to Over-the-Counter (OTC) Status

When marketing groups have determined that an established prescription product should be converted to OTC status, there is often a significant amount of clinical and technical development work that must be conducted within research and development departments. The strategy of converting

TABLE 22.10. *Factors to schedule and monitor in planning marketing activities to launch a new drug*[a]

A. Projected milestone events
   1. Issue packaging particulars
   2. Finalize market plan completed by marketing representative
   3. Issue package specifications request
   4. Management approves market plan
   5. Issue budget schedule
   6. Issue production order
   7. Develop preliminary launch plan and schedule
   8. Review of NDA by FDA and approvable letter
   9. Final pre-NDA approval of market plans
   10. Receive FDA approval letter

B. Advertising
   1. Determine literature and promotion costs
   2. Determine direct-mail costs
   3. Contact advertising agency
   4. Develop graphic concepts and strategy
   5. Prepare preliminary journal costs
   6. Submit journal schedule
   7. Submit journal advertising proposal
   8. Develop and route direct-mail/ promotion copy
   9. Test and approve journal advertisements
   10. Prepare convention panel (mechanicals)
   11. Develop promotional layout
   12. Prepare advertising film
   13. Review and approve journal schedule
   14. Route and approve promotional material specifications
   15. Prepare and award promotional material bid
   16. Print direct-mail and promotional material
   17. Have advertising agency send insert order to journal(s)
   18. Develop press release
   19. Issue press release to trade journal(s)
   20. Mail promotional material

C. Management committees, coordinating committees, board of directors
   1. Approve market plan
   2. Review progress of marketing activities

D. Marketing services
   1. Collect and analyze marketing data
   2. Prepare initial market plan
   3. Conduct focus group interview(s)
   4. Request works cost analysis
   5. Conduct initial market forecast
   6. Request stability studies
   7. Issue NDA packaging specifications
   8. Determine product and package cost
   9. Focus group data analysis
   10. Issue product and package pricing
   11. Develop final sample package
   12. Develop and route package mechanicals
   13. Issue packaging particulars
   14. Issue packaging specifications request
   15. Issue budget
   16. Issue production order

E. Marketing product planner
   1. Finalize market plan
   2. Submit market plan to management
   3. Contact wholesale services
   4. Contact sales promotion
   5. Contact government services
   6. Contact hospital services
   7. Contact convention department
   8. Contact retail services
   9. Prepare initial market forecast
   10. Prepare preliminary product report
   11. Prepare unit forecast
   12. Propose budget
   13. Request works cost analysis
   14. Finalize forecast

(*Continues on following page*)

TABLE 22.10. *(Continued)*

F. Production
   1. Prepare final packaging specifications
   2. Estimate package plan
   3. Approve bill of materials
   4. Order package components
   5. Write manufacturing plan
   6. Receive package components
   7. Write manufacturing schedule
   8. Order printed labels and inserts
   9. Receive printed labels and inserts
   10. Pass printed labels by quality assurance
   11. Manufacture bulk drug for launch
   12. Pass bulk tablets by quality assurance
   13. Pass package components by quality assurance
   14. Schedule and prepare package order
   15. Package bulk drug
   16. Pass finished product by quality assurance
   17. Ship drug for launch

G. Drug regulatory affairs
   1. Develop label copy

H. Sales administration
   1. Set up market plan
   2. Contact drug distribution data services
   3. Develop slide, tape, and video program(s)
   4. Develop government promotion
   5. Government Service Administration price list addition
   6. Develop hospital promotion
   7. Sales tracking information to drug distribution data
   8. Develop drug distribution report
   9. Develop retail promotion
   10. Drug distribution reports to regional sales managers
   11. Drug distribution reports to district sales managers
   12. Drug distribution reports to staff
   13. Hospital promotion to sales promotion
   14. Medicaid and third-party notification
   15. Notification of General Services Administration
   16. Set automatic ship quantities
   17. Mail launch letter to wholesalers
   18. Addition of products to territory planning system
   19. Develop territory planning system program

I. Sales promotion
   1. Assign detailing positions
   2. Develop selling sheet
   3. Develop preliminary launch plan and schedule
   4. Schedule conventions
   5. Develop convention panels for exhibit
   6. Develop and produce slide, tape, and/or video program(s)
   7. Draft launch and selling plan
   8. Send selling sheet to advertising
   9. Route convention panels
   10. Review launch and selling plan
   11. Produce convention panels
   12. Print launch and selling plan
   13. Send final insert copy to staff
   14. Ship convention panels
   15. Send staff launch and selling plan
   16. Advise staff of final NDA approval
   17. Present slide, tape, and/or video program to staff

J. Sales training
   1. Assessment by training department
   2. Prepare disease and/or product learning unit
   3. Issue disease unit to test staff
   4. Issue product unit to test staff
   5. Send final training unit to staff
   6. Revise training unit with approved label

[a] Each of these activities requires a start and completion date and an indication of whether it is on the critical path. The critical path denotes that (1) other activities cannot be initiated and/or (2) the project will be delayed until this activity is completed.

TABLE 22.11. *Preparations in medical and/or other research and development departments for launch of a new product*

1. Prepare a bibliography of published literature
2. Index the published literature
3. Prepare a list of anticipated questions from physicians and the media
4. Prepare responses to these questions which company personnel may use
5. Train personnel who will provide information to physicians and other health professionals
6. Determine which departments will handle which types of telephone and written questions (e.g., medical questions, marketing questions, orders, complaints)
7. Instruct telephone operators on how to forward calls to the correct departments and individuals

prescription drugs to OTC status has become more important in recent years and will probably continue to grow, at least for the near future.

The group of OTC drugs that were formally prescription drugs has been referred to by some people as "professional OTCs" and are generally seen by the public as being more sophisticated and contemporary than the longtime traditional OTC products. Professional OTCs are believed by the public to have fewer adverse reactions and to be cheaper than prescription drugs. They are increasingly popular as consumers become more sophisticated and more involved in their own treatment.

In conclusion, each sponsor establishes a marketing strategy for each drug. In developing this strategy the possible alternatives should be evaluated by comparing them to corporate and marketing objectives, rather than merely comparing the available alternatives with each other. This latter type of comparison is a common trap that may lead a group into choosing a wrong alternative which may not be consistent with the corporate objectives.

23

Managing Costs of Projects, Clinical Studies, and Drug Development

Types of Costs in Drug Development • Total Cost of a Drug's Development • Monitoring and Budgeting Project Costs • Establishing Fair Market Value for a Single Study • Minimizing Costs of Clinical Studies

TYPES OF COSTS IN DRUG DEVELOPMENT

After a drug is discovered, the costs of new drug development which are perhaps the most visible are those of clinical studies. In addition to costs of clinical studies conducted during Phases I, II, and III there are numerous other types of costs incurred in drug development. Most of these are summarized in a few broad categories.

Nonclinical Studies Conducted After Clinical Studies Are Initiated

This category includes most of the toxicology program. If the drug is to be given chronically, instead of acutely, then there will usually be a need to conduct full 2-year carcinogenicity studies in two species. Advanced studies in pharmacology, biochemistry, metabolism, and other relevant disciplines (e.g., microbiology, immunology) will be conducted during this period, as will most of the technical development activities.

Administrative Costs

Administrative costs are usually quite substantial in the pursuit of a New Drug Application (NDA) on any new drug. In many (if not most) cases, these costs do not differ substantially when comparisons are made between drugs intended for rare diseases and those intended for common diseases. This category includes activities of the Drug Regulatory Affairs Department, which has the task of assembling, checking, and submitting Notice of Claimed Investigational Exemption for a New Drug (IND) and NDA documents to the Food and Drug Administration (FDA). This department remains in contact with the FDA during the review process and even after the drug is approved and marketed. Adverse reactions and other information on the drug must be maintained and reports must be submitted to the FDA. There is also significant time spent on the part of managers and other personnel who directly and/or indirectly supervise and review the progress of the myriad activities necessary to give birth to a new drug.

Patent costs may be considered as part of administrative costs. Most patents require periodic fees to maintain their viability. Also, patents must be filed in many countries, even if it is not certain whether the drug will be eventually registered for sale in any of those countries.

Marketing Costs

Although some drugs are highly profitable, many others are not expected to make a profit for the pharmaceutical company that discovers, develops, and launches them. Several studies have reported that only about one-quarter to one-third of marketed drugs ever repays their costs of development (Grabowski and Vernon, 1982; Drews, 1985; Joglekar and Paterson, 1986). Since marketing resources are limited, a suitable amount of promotion and advertising must be determined. Marketing personnel inform physicians about the new drug, train and educate their own sales force, and provide physicians with promotional materials and information.

Specially trained personnel and/or regular staff in medical and/or marketing departments must answer letters and telephone calls from physicians, pharmacists, nurses, and other professionals about the new product. These costs will arise regardless of the market potential of the drug. A new drug with limited sales potential which receives a great deal of publicity could generate more requests for information than a drug with much greater sales potential.

Manufacturing Costs

Activities involved in the synthesis and manufacture of the drug could raise major issues within a corporation if the manufacturing process required specialized equipment or procedures, or if the needed raw materials are rare and/or expensive. In some situations it is necessary to build a new plant just to make a single drug. A small-volume drug (small in terms of the number of units sold) may tie up manufacturing equipment and production lines required for other products. For example, the cleaning and preparation of large pieces of equipment, for either (1) the next step in the chemical synthesis or manufacturing process or (2) the next drug to be made, may represent a time-intensive process. These steps are often complex and costly, and the magnitude (and expense) of the efforts involved are independent of the drug's eventual use and sales potential.

Other Support Costs

There are many other activities that must be conducted on an ongoing basis for any marketed drug, regardless of whether the drug is for a rare, or for a common, disease. These activities vary in degree and proportion from drug to drug and may also change during the life span of any one drug. Representative activities include: (1) analyzing of blood, urine, or other biological samples for drug levels; (2) analyzing of returned drug samples to evaluate the amount of drug present; (3) providing information to pharmaceutical compendia; (4) monitoring the published literature and adverse reaction reports; (5) presenting of materials to hospital and state formularies; (6) conducting activities to register the drug in other countries; (7) providing various types of technical support for the drug's production; and (8) tracking costs and revenues.

TOTAL COST OF A DRUG'S DEVELOPMENT

It is difficult to generalize about the total costs of all efforts and studies necessary to establish safety and efficacy and to bring a new chemical entity to market. There are many factors involved, and at the initiation of the development process there are many known and unknown hurdles for each drug to overcome. This makes early estimates of total costs for any specific drug only educated guesses.

A number of economists have estimated the costs of developing a new drug. Rather than averaging a number of actual drug development costs, these figures are usually derived by taking the entire research and development budgets of a number of companies over a period of years and dividing that total by the number of new drugs launched. Thus, all money spent on drugs that were therapeutic or toxic failures, and all research on the compounds that went nowhere or were the ancestors of new drugs, are allocated to the few eventually successful drugs. This seems to be a fair method for establishing the cost of developing a single new drug because all of the money attributed to drug failures was actually spent, and at least some of the costs contributed to the discovery of the new drug. It would be generally difficult, if not impossible, to accurately differentiate among those costs spent on activities that did or did not contribute to discovering the new drug.

Using this "fully allocated" technique of summarizing all relevant expenses, the cost of a new drug in 1976 was calculated to be 54 million dollars.

TABLE 23.1. *Selected factors to consider when drug costs are determined by dividing total research costs by number of drugs developed*[a]

A. Total research costs
   1. Should all research costs of the subsidiaries of the parent company be included?
   2. How many years should be included in the analysis, since too short a period may distort the result?
   3. Should some management costs of nonresearch corporate officers be apportioned to research, because of time spent by boards of directors on specific research and drug development issues?
   4. How much computer costs should be allocated to research if they are not part of the research budget?
   5. How much of all the other nonresearch costs involved in operating a facility should be considered if they are not included in the research budget?
   6. How should inflation be considered in adding costs from different years?

B. Number of drugs developed within a defined period
   1. Should only prescription drugs be considered or should over-the-counter drugs be included?
   2. Should each separate dosage form marketed be counted separately or combined and counted as only one drug?
   3. Should only new chemical entities be included?
   4. Should multiple indications for a drug be considered the same as one indication?
   5. Should a drug with sales of less than a million dollars per year be considered and counted the same as a highly successful drug?
   6. Should a drug be counted if it is only introduced into a small country with limited sales and has not yet been approved for sale in an industrialized country?

[a] These questions are intended to illustrate the complexity of the simple ratio and the need to define exactly how the figure is derived. Comparing numbers between companies is fraught with additional difficulties since differences in definitions and accounting practices exist. See Table 23.2 for additional factors.

This figure had climbed to nearly 90 million dollars in 1983 (Hansen, 1983) and is probably close to (or above) 100 million dollars today. The determination of this value for any company should include consideration of a several-year period because most companies do not introduce new drugs each year. The variation in this figure between companies is probably substantial and is a reflection of their research productivity in discovering new drugs and their ability to develop drugs. Both the numerator (total research and development costs) and denominator (number of drugs discovered) are somewhat complex concepts. A number of considerations that enter into each are listed in Table 23.1. This table illustrates that it is not a simple matter to calculate either the numerator or denominator.

The actual ("direct") dollars spent on developing any one specific drug to the market, after it has been "discovered," are always much less than the large totals given by Professor Hansen and others. Actual amounts spent may vary by orders of magnitude from drug to drug and usually range from 2 to 50 million dollars. These costs do not usually include all costs of the research program, which might have been spent while searching for many years before a new drug was discovered.

The money necessary to complete a drug's development may be estimated (usually excluding factors such as inflation and lost financial interest) at the outset of a drug's development. The fair market value of outside clinical and nonclinical studies and in-house costs of various aspects of the drug's development must be established. Knowledge of the number and types of studies required to complete the evaluation of a drug, plus approximate costs of each, will yield a general total figure. "Fudge factors" are sometimes applied to derive a more realistic estimate that allows for unanticipated problems that invariably develop during a drug's development. Actual costs of developing a single drug are often significantly higher than the projected costs established at the initiation of a project. A list of some of the factors to consider in determining costs of a specific drug are listed in Table 23.2.

MONITORING AND BUDGETING PROJECT COSTS

Monitoring Costs of a Project

Costs that are monitored include direct costs for clinical studies paid either to investigators or to institutions on their behalf. There are also direct costs of chemical starting materials and various outside grants for toxicology, data processing, or other activities. These expenses are usually captured and reported as a routine matter in most companies.

Other costs for projects include the time and effort of the staff at the company developing the drug. This topic is rather controversial in many companies because of the varying perspectives of different individuals who participate in these exercises. Financial managers are used to, and generally expect, highly detailed reports and itemizations of time and efforts reports, whereas research managers vary enormously in their interest and desire for specific, as opposed to general, information on project costs. Some managers are clearly not interested in evaluating any cost information.

Clinical staff, scientists, and other workers whose time and effort are being monitored often resent the chore of having to complete the necessary forms to capture such data. The more detailed, frequent, and time-consuming the forms, the more the staff can be expected to resent the activity. Shortcuts are frequently used to circumvent or minimize the activity, such as by submitting duplicate or near-duplicate forms for each reporting period.

Clearly a balance is needed between the needs of all of these groups. A different balance is needed in different companies. A system that requires "too much" information demands large amounts of administrative time of both staff and management and will invariably decrease their productivity. On the other hand, management groups that collect little or no information

TABLE 23.2. *Selected factors to consider in answering the question: How much does a specific drug cost to develop*[a]

1. Should costs of research which directly lead to the drug be included?
2. Should costs of research on the same therapeutic target which did not lead to the drug be included?
3. Should costs be included for other research which was not or has not yet been successful but is conducted each year?
4. Should only direct costs be included or should indirect costs of that drug's development be included?
5. Should relevant overhead costs of management, rent, heat, etc., be included? If not, why?
6. Should costs of all the different dosage forms be included, or only the first one to reach the market?
7. Should costs of developing all line extensions be included regardless of when they were incurred relative to regulatory approval?
8. Should costs of developing line extensions be included if they were being developed while the drug was investigational?
9. Should costs of studies on new clinical indications be included?
10. Should costs of studies on indications be included if the indications failed? What if studies on other indications were completed before the drug was successfully marketed for its major indication?
11. Should development costs be included after the drug was initially launched in the first territory, even though the market size in that territory is extremely small?
12. Should all repetitive costs of drug development in different countries be included if required by several regulatory agencies? What if the studies are only partly repetitive?
13. Should costs of marketing studies be included if they were conducted prior to launching the drug? What if the drug were launched in some countries, but not in all of those where the marketing study results would be used?
14. Should costs of synthesizing additional compounds to protect the patent be included?
15. Should costs of related drugs that were never marketed but assisted in learning about the field and the best investigators, consultants, and other individuals be included?

[a] These questions illustrate the complexity of attempting to determine an accurate figure that simply states the answer to the question. Adding up all of the separate costs is not straightforward, even disregarding inflation and other financial questions.

often do not really know what their staff members are working on and how their resources are being allocated to various projects.

In designing suitable forms to collect these types of data there are several basic questions to address. These include:

1. Whose time and effort will be collected? Is it necessary to collect the time and effort of all clerical staff and service staff (e.g., data entry operators, librarians), or are those of senior (usually scientific) staff who are directly working in the area of drug discovery and development sufficient?
2. How frequently is it necessary to collect these data? Most drug companies that collect these data do so on a monthly or quarterly basis.

3. Who will review these data? Is it strictly for research and development personnel or will it be shared with corporate managers? If so, in what form will it be sent to senior managers?
4. What decisions will be made with these data? These data are usually entered in computers and easily summarized and sorted by variables of interest. These include project(s) studied, departmental and divisional effort, periodic and cumulative costs, and other variables of interest. Since the data are available they may be sorted by variables not originally intended or desired by those who established the system.
5. How much data should be collected? Would the proportion of time spent by each individual on each drug or product be sufficient information? Is it necessary to collect information according to work expended on each major activity on each drug? The amount of time required to accurately complete such forms increases dramatically as the level of detail increases. The reliability of data may decrease as more are collected, unless adequate measures are instituted to insure data accuracy. One means of increasing data accuracy is by requiring certain staff to maintain daily diaries of their activities.
6. Should work performed by outside consultants or others who are operating on a contract basis be captured separately? "Contracts" may be utilized within a company for work requested by different subsidiaries, divisions, or other groups. These data may be collected.
7. What codes could be used to simplify the forms without making them difficult to complete and process?

After these time and effort reports are issued it is possible to conduct various analyses of the results to evaluate changes and trends, or to answer specific questions.

The issue of whether the indirect costs of running a research and development organization should be apportioned in some way to the costs of projects will not be discussed here. This is handled differently within each company. These costs include overhead categories such as rent for space, fringe benefits, management costs (corporate as well as research and development), and support services of both a technical and administrative nature. Unless this administrative and technical infrastructure is in place it will be difficult to discover and develop drugs.

Another issue relates to the means by which staff time is to be converted to dollar terms. An average salary of all workers may be used to multiply by the total time expended to determine the total time and effort costs. Alternative approaches are to use classes of workers (e.g., senior and junior, Grades 1–4, 5–8, 9–12) with an average salary for each class to compute the value of their separate time totals, or to use each individual's exact salary to calculate their precise time and effort costs spent on each project. The total time and effort spent on a specific project would then be the sum of each individual's total time and effort, plus overhead (if relevant).

Budgeting Costs of a Project

This function should be integrated with the process whereby costs of a project are monitored. There may be a separate individual, group, or department charged with the responsibility for maintaining a harmonious balance among activities monitored. Although drug development has a long-term horizon, the project manager's budget usually focuses on a 1- to 3-year horizon. Other managers within the corporation may be concerned about a longer time-frame for monitoring costs. In some organizations each project has a budget and the project manager has the responsibility for spending the money in the most efficient way possible. Part of this manager's performance appraisal is based on how effectively the money was spent. Variations of this approach include having a budget for each project, but assigning the responsibility for its control to an individual other than the project manager.

Many companies have a single sum of money within the research and development function which is allocated to projects according to their requests, priorities, and other considerations. The choice of whether to budget by projects usually depends on the traditions of the company and preferences of the research and development director. The total number of dollars available for each project's activities may be specified at the start of each fiscal year. If it is not, then the total research and development budget minus fixed and committed expenses are in general available to be apportioned to projects according to some criteria. In these situations, the company does not create a budget for each project. If the money needed to advance a project's development is generally used up well before each fiscal year is over, however, there may be pressure to institute a project budget. Another choice is to institute more restraints on spending.

ESTABLISHING A FAIR MARKET VALUE FOR A SINGLE STUDY

An investigator or sponsor may estimate the fair market value of a single study by considering the component parts of the study. An estimate similar to those shown in Fig. 23.1 may be established, although there are many different methods and models for dividing a study into its components (see Figs. 23.2 and 23.3). A standard form may assist in this exercise but is not a necessity, since there are many ways to develop estimates of a study's costs. Many companies do not use standardized forms for establishing a clinical budget.

There are situations when a sponsor intentionally does not carefully compare the total cost per patient for a given study across several potential sites. This may occur if the number of sites that can effectively conduct a particular drug study are limited, or when some sponsors enter a bidding war because

Developing the Costs of a Clinical Study

		Cost Per Patient
A. Examinations		
Initial Patient history and physical examinations		____
Abbreviated physical examinations	(No. of exams × cost per exam = $____)	____
Ophthalmological examinations	(No. of exams × cost per exam = $____)	____
Other examinations ____ ____	(No. of exams × cost per exam = $____)	____
B. Laboratory		
EKG 12 Lead		____
EKG Lead II (No. of tests × cost per test)		____
Clinical Chemistry	(No. of tests × cost per test)	____
Hematology	(No. of tests × cost per test)	____
Urinalysis	(No. of tests × cost per test)	____
Other tests ____ ____	(No. of tests × cost per test)	____
C. Efficacy Examinations		
Test 1	(No. of tests × cost per test)	____
Test 2	(No. of tests × cost per test)	____
Test 3	(No. of tests × cost per test)	____
D. Administration		
Nurse coordinator	(Percent of fulltime × yearly [monthly or other] salary ÷ no. of patients)	____
Telephone, postage, miscellaneous	(Total cost ÷ no. of patients)	____
	Cost per patient =	____
University overhead	(X% × cost per patient)	____
		____ Total cost per patient

Number of patients ____ × Total cost per patient = ____ Total cost of study

FIG. 23.1. Calculating costs of a clinical study.

of limited availability of sophisticated equipment, suitable patients, or qualified and interested investigators. If two or more sponsors are attempting to develop drugs in the same therapeutic area and each requires the services of the few available investigators, most of the "rules" for establishing a fair budget will probably not apply. Some sponsors offer investigators larger

DEVELOPING THE COSTS OF A CLINICAL STUDY

A

Item	Cost Per Item ($)	Per Patient		Total Cost ($)
		Number Of Tests	Cost ($)	

List Each Point of the Protocol for Which There is a Charge.

B

Item	Cost Per Item ($)	Part A of Study Per Patient		Part B of Study				Overall Total Cost
				Screen (n=x)		Study (n=y)		
		Number Of Tests	Total Cost	Number Of Tests	Total Cost	Number Of Tests	Total Cost	

List Each Point of the Protocol for Which There Is a Charge and Total Each Column.

C.

Group of Patients	Number of Patients Per Group	Number of Analyses Per Patient	Cost Per Analysis ($)	Total Cost Per Patient ($)	Total Cost Per Group ($)
1	A				
2	B				
3	C				
4	D				
5	E				
TOTAL					

FIG. 23.2. Calculating costs of a clinical study.

budgets than they might offer otherwise in this situation, to delay their competitor's drug development program.

Some sponsors may conduct a study that is probably not necessary, merely because they were first to contact the investigator and wish to keep the investigator busy with their studies. Investigator's services may also be acquired through (1) bidding wars, (2) long-term contracts, (3) consultancy arrangements, or (4) other negotiations. "Bidding wars" may also be instigated and perpetrated by investigators. Even if an investigator has a monopoly on conducting studies in a certain therapeutic area because of certain equipment, techniques, expertise, or interest, there may not be any need for these types of undesirable negotiations to occur. For example, the investigator may be able to conduct several long-term studies for different sponsors simultaneously or many short-term studies sequentially (or simultaneously). The investigator would thus not have to "choose" between sponsors. These quasi-unethical practices are not believed to be common.

DEVELOPING THE COSTS OF A CLINICAL STUDY

A

	Amount
Microbiology Cultures. Number of Cultures Per Patient Per Week x A Weeks x B $ x C Patients	______
Pharmacy Fees for Dispensing Drugs and Collecting Returns	______
Salaries	
Research Nurse: A Hours at B $ Per Hour x C Patients	______
Secretarial Support:	______
Professional Support:	______
Data Analysis	______
SUBTOTAL	______
OVERHEAD (X%)	______
TOTAL	______
COST PER PATIENT	______

B

Equipment	______
Individual Patient Costs	______
Patient Recruitment (Includes Advertising Costs)	______
Patient Stipend (Includes Meals)	______
Electrocardiograms	______
Ophthalmological Examinations	______
Technical Support (Includes Computer Fees)	______
Medical Support	______
Physical Examinations	______
Clerical Support	______
TOTAL COST PER PATIENT	______
TOTAL STUDY COST	______

C

	Salary	**Benefits**	**Total Cost**
Dr. A. at 25% of Time	______	______	______
Dr. B. at 10% of Time	______	______	______
Office Supplies (Copying, Phone, Typing, etc.)	______	______	______
Professional Travel to One Meeting Each for Drs. A & B			______
TOTAL			______

D

Personnel		
Anesthesiologists (n=A)	X Days at Y $ Per Day	______
Recovery Room Nurses (n=B)	X Days at Z $ Per Day	______
EEG Technician (n=C)	X Days at E $ Per Day	______
Research Coordinator	H Days at F $ Per Day	______
Secretarial Assistance	J Days at G $ Per Day	______
Operating Room Use of Space and Equipment X Days at K $ Per Day		______
Operating Room: Supplies and Drugs		______
Pharmacy Supplies		______
Laboratory Procedures		______
Each Listed, Plus Number of Times Performed Times Cost, Times Number of Patients		______
TOTAL COST PER STUDY		______
TOTAL COST PER PATIENT		______

FIG. 23.3. Calculating costs of a clinical study.

E

	Total Cost
Laboratory Assessments	
Itemize—Number Done Per Patient at Cost in $	________
Clinical Assessments	
Itemize—Cost Per Patient	________
Personnel Costs	
Research Coordinator Cost Per Patient	________
Secretary and Clerical Cost Per Patient	________
Estimated Costs Per Patients Prematurely Discontinued	________
TOTAL	________

F

Personnel Costs (% Effort of Each Worker Listed)	________
Study Administration Costs (Each Aspect Listed)	________
Patient Management	
Laboratory Examinations	________
ECG Evaluations	________
Psychiatric Consultations	________
Other Aspects Listed	________
TOTAL	________
TOTAL COST PER PATIENT	________

G

	Cost Per Volunteer
Hospitalization	
Beds and Food	________
Volunteer Payment	________
Test Procedures (List Each)	________
Personnel Fees	________
Overhead (X%)	________
TOTAL COST PER VOLUNTEER	________
TOTAL COST FOR STUDY	________

H

	Cost Per Patient	**Total Study Cost**
Screening (X Patients)		
Clinic Visit	________	________
History and Physical Examination	________	________
Laboratory Tests (Specify)	________	________
Special Tests (Specify)	________	________
Baseline Period (Y Patients)		
Clinic Visit	________	________
Laboratory Tests (Specify)	________	________
Special Tests (Specify)	________	________
Treatment Period (Y Patients)		
Clinic Visit	________	________
Physical Examination	________	________
Laboratory Tests (Specify)	________	________
Special Tests (Specify)	________	________
Posttreatment Period (Y Patients)		
Clinic Visit	________	________
Physical Examination	________	________
Laboratory Tests (Specify)	________	________
Special Tests (Specify)	________	________
Personnel		
List Each	________	________
Institution Overhead	________	________
Total Cost Per Patient	________	
Total Study Cost		________

FIG. 23.3 (*Continued*)

Sponsors rarely require an academic investigator to work exclusively on their products or new drugs. Indeed, it would not be in keeping with the spirit of academic freedom or integrity to do so. An exception to this principle sometimes occurs in drug evaluation units established in academic centers or hospitals, which are funded and sometimes staffed by a single sponsor.

MINIMIZING COSTS OF CLINICAL STUDIES

The major technique for an investigator or sponsor to minimize the costs of a clinical study is to break down the total financial cost into its components and to analyze each component for potential savings. A number of questions to pose for different parts of a study are:

Overall Questions for a Sponsor

1. Would the study be less expensive if it were conducted in a different country? If the answer is yes, then many other types of costs must be considered to determine whether this is a viable option. This issue is discussed further in Chapter 13 and at the end of this chapter. Also, would the foreign data be accepted by the FDA and/or other regulatory agencies?
2. Would the study be less expensive if it were conducted in a small city or less well-known hospital? Expenses in large cities are often greater than in smaller ones. One must be extremely cautious about the approach to this question because of differences in quality of the investigators, conduct of the study, diagnosis of patients, and many other factors.

Laboratory Evaluations

1. Could the number of different laboratory tests listed in the protocol be decreased without affecting patient safety?
2. Could the number of times each test is requested be reduced without affecting patient safety?
3. Could the tests be conducted at lower cost by an outside laboratory rather than the hospital laboratory, or by a *different* outside laboratory if one is already being used?
4. Could assays for blood or urine levels of the study drug be conducted by a central facility rather than at each study site? If so, is this a less costly method after including shipping and other costs brought about by this approach?
5. Could a better price be obtained for a study where several specialized

laboratory studies are to be performed at a single laboratory (e.g., assays of various hormones)? Even if only a single test is being performed, it may be performed on many patients or on many samples of a few patients and negotiations might lead to decreased laboratory costs.

6. Could samples be frozen to analyze for blood levels of the study drug at a later date, when specific criteria about the drug's safety and efficacy are met? If these criteria are not met, then the samples never need to be analyzed.

Safety Evaluations

1. Could an abbreviated electrocardiogram (i.e., Lead II) be used rather than a complete 12-lead electrocardiogram for some or all recordings?
2. Could an abbreviated physical examination be conducted at different points in the study, rather than a complete physical each time a physical is requested? The same question applies for neurological, ophthalmological, and other examinations.
3. Could a trained nurse or other professional conduct certain examinations, rather than the principal investigator or a physician?
4. Could some parts of an examination or test be modified or deleted to save money (e.g., deleting the sleep, photic stimulation, and/or hyperventilation parts of the electroencephalogram)?

Efficacy Evaluations

Questions similar to those for safety evaluations and laboratory evaluations apply.

Study Design

1. Could the study be conducted at two or more sites at a lower total cost than at one site (or vice versa)? The decision to use two or more sites for a clinical study raises many issues, and financial cost is often one of the least important issues. From the point of view of the statistical analyses of data obtained, it is generally preferable to conduct a study at one site.
2. Could the study be conducted in outpatients instead of inpatients?
3. Could inpatients be discharged when improved, and continue to receive treatment as outpatients?

Monitoring

1. Could monitors who are based near the study site (rather than at a central location) oversee the study?
2. Could data be transmitted electronically in a cost-effective manner?

Study Conduct

1. Would it be cost effective to have the sponsor pay for a full-time research coordinator in terms of (1) having improved rate of patient enrollment because of more efforts expended on this task, (2) increased patient compliance because of greater attention to patient reminders and other details, (3) decreased patient dropouts due to more personal involvement, and (4) more-accurate and complete data, because of time to devote to this effort? In certain cases the answer is clearly yes.

Overhead

1. More and more organizations (e.g., hospitals, academic centers, clinics) are including overhead as a separate line item in their budget. The percent used to calculate this value varies enormously and may often be negotiated.
2. Avoid paying overhead on items where overhead is already built into the price. It is important to determine whether overhead is already included in a charge prior to the application of a general overhead factor.

In addition to financial costs, several other types of costs are associated with many clinical studies. These costs should be considered when the "real" price of a study is being determined and evaluated.

1. *Lost opportunity costs*. For each study conducted, there are usually a number of other studies that could have been conducted in its place on the same (or different) drug. If the study actually conducted has little inherent value or fails to answer its objectives, then there is a cost of lost opportunity. This occurs even though the preferable study may still be able to be conducted at a later date.
2. *Costs of slow development*. For investigational drugs that are being developed there is a cost associated with the time that the drug is not available on the market. An actual figure may be determined, based on the time delay and anticipated sales, which in turn is affected by patient need and by competitive advantages of a drug. If the development process of a drug is slowed, then costs associated with that

TABLE 23.3. *Various means of paying investigators to conduct clinical studies*

1. A lump sum for a clinical study, regardless of what data are eventually collected
2. Payment only for precisely those tests and procedures actually performed
3. Payment that specifies some or all of the following amounts to be paid for each patient who:
   a. Is screened
   b. Passes the screen
   c. Is enrolled
   d. Completes baseline period
   e. Begins treatment
   f. Completes part of treatment (payments may be prorated based on length of treatment completed)
   g. Completes entire treatment (this period is usually defined as at least a specific proportion of the study)
   h. Completes follow-up
4. Payment for patients who drop out because of adverse reactions is sometimes given as if they were completed patients
5. Payment for patients who either drop out without reason or are discontinued for lack of cooperation or inadequate compliance is often given on a prorated basis

drug will be markedly increased. Another aspect of this issue relates to delays in regulatory reviews.

3. *Costs of additional resources.* There are finite resources available for each project within a sponsoring institution. When these are allocated to one project they are unavailable elsewhere, and if new resources are not obtained the development of other projects would be slowed. To prevent this occurrence, new resources of equipment and staff are sometimes obtained.

Pharmaceutical corporations differ in their approach to the question of who negotiates budgets for clinical studies. Whereas monitors play the leading role in certain companies, others give this authority to regional representatives. Although there is no special prerequisite background necessary to conduct this negotiation, it is important for the individual in charge to have experience or training in the approaches and attitudes of the company toward the various financial issues relating to drug development.

After the budget for a study is established various means of disbursing funds must be considered (Table 23.3). Early payment or receipt of funds may have various consequences vis-à-vis inclusion or exclusion of the money in a particular fiscal year or source of funding, which in turn may have other implications for both payer and payee. Dividing the funds into three or more fractional payments allows the sponsor to encourage continued conduct of the study, retain necessary leverage in cases of failure to adhere to protocol requirements, and to collect interest on the balance of the grant during the remaining period. In general, it is important to pay for work completed rather than work promised. One exception is for the initial partial payment, which

TABLE 23.4. *Sample table headings to track financial expenses for clinical studies on a project*[a]

A

Project no. and name	Study no.	Name of investigator and city	Title of study	Total no. of patients to be enrolled	Grants budgeted ($)	Grants spent to date ($)	Grants remaining ($)

B

Project and study no.	Name of investigator	Patient no.	Check after completed						Additional charges	Total cost per patient	Cumulative cost of study
			Screen	Baseline	First third of treatment	Second third of treatment	Total treatment	Follow-up			

[a] Figure 19.5 contains a form that may be used to monitor grant payments on a single study.

should be sufficient for the study to start on a high note, yet not so high as to stunt the investigator's motivation to proceed. In all negotiations, a fair settlement and equitable arrangement should be sought, since no investigator will participate enthusiastically in a study in which he/she believes the agreement or contract is unfair. Many circumstances change during the course of a study, and these sometimes present a need to alter a contract during a study to bring it in line with the changed circumstances. Two sample forms that may be used to track financial costs for clinical studies are illustrated in Table 23.4.

Other Issues

Numerous other financial issues arise in drug development. These include the following.

1. A progressively important parameter in drug marketing relates to the cost of a drug. This issue is more realistically noted in terms of cost of treatment. A drug that costs twice as much as another on a per tablet basis, but is only taken one-third as often (e.g., because of a long half-life), would actually cost less per week or per treatment. Various means of comparing drug costs are illustrated in Table 23.5.
2. Diagnosis-Related Groups (DRGs) and other cost-containment measures are placing more emphasis on the cost associated with new drugs. This can often lead to difficult situations where it is not easy to assign a cash value. For example, if a new drug improves the quality of life for patients by allowing them an additional half hour of sleep every night, or reduces nausea by 15%, how much more can be allowed in

TABLE 23.5. *Types of cost comparisons that may be made between treatments*[a]

1. Cost per tablet or other dosage form
2. Cost per dose of medication (e.g., two tablets may constitute one dose)
3. Cost per day or week for single-drug treatment. This allows for an equitable comparison between a drug taken twice a day and another taken four times a day
4. Cost per day for all drugs taken. Some drugs may require concomitant drugs (e.g., diuretics that require potassium supplements)
5. Cost per day for all necessary treatments. This figure may also factor in other direct costs, primarily for inpatient studies
6. Cost per patient per year per episode. Includes all ancillary direct costs of treatment (e.g., laboratory monitoring, medical care, nursing care)
7. Comparison of average total treatment costs of two groups of patients[b]

[a] This table describes comparisons of direct medical costs. Indirect costs (e.g., administrative costs, transportation, babysitters) and intangible costs (e.g., pain, suffering, inconvenience) may also be considered.

[b] This comparison should generally include costs of all patients who failed treatment and thus it would be a comparison of costs per successful treatment.

the cost of a new drug? If another drug has an improved safety profile compared with standard drugs, but is slightly less efficacious, how would the new drug's price be established and viewed by formulary committees?

3. Various issues of cost-benefit and cost-effectiveness are discussed in Chapter 27 of *Guide to Clinical Interpretation of Data* (Spilker, 1986).

24

Terminating a Project

Value in Terminating a Project • When to Terminate a Study or Project • Alternatives to Terminating a Project

VALUE IN TERMINATING A PROJECT

Drug projects are eventually terminated for one of three reasons. The first and best reason is when a project has successfully achieved its objectives [usually New Drug Application (NDA) approval] and the reasons for its existence no longer exist. The second reason is when the drug may have failed to meet its objectives, usually because of toxicity or lack of efficacy and the project is terminated. In this case the project itself may be viewed successfully in that it efficiently learned about the drug's negative characteristics in a timely fashion. The third and least frequent reason is that the project itself may have failed to meet its objectives, but the drug may still be viable and may be taken over by a new project group or it may be licensed to another company for development.

In the case of the drug industry, the successful end of a project may be viewed as the time of (1) submission of an NDA to the Food and Drug Administration (FDA), (2) approval of the NDA by the FDA (and subsequent launch), or (3) sales of a drug that pay back the money invested. There are pros and cons to each of these three definitions and no clear reason why only one definition should be used as a yardstick for measuring success of all drugs. It is the author's view that approval of the NDA by the FDA and launch of the drug should usually be considered as the point at which the project may be stated to have attained success. In addition, the timely termination of an unsuccessful project, for whatever reason, is also a successful end to a project. Some of the benefits that accrue in this situation are discussed in Chapter 32 of *Guide to Clinical Interpretation of Data* (Spilker, 1986).

It is important to view projects objectively, because it assists in the process of reaching a dispassionate decision to terminate them at the appropriate time. When one or more senior managers have vested their reputations on a drug's success, they sometimes exert pressures to keep the project alive past its realistic time of demise. Sponsors are sometimes unwilling to accept the obvious truth about a drug's likelihood of success, and often resort to progressively less probable scenarios of how the drug can be shown to be active and worth marketing.

There are numerous benefits that accrue to a sponsor when an unsuccessful project is terminated expeditiously. These include: (1) resources become available to use on other projects, (2) staff morale generally improves as new challenges emerge and problems from what may be an albatross around the corporate neck are shed, and (3) the terminated project is disassembled and future costs are saved. If there is a back-up drug or medical device candidate to study, then most or all of the experiences plus contacts with investigators and consultants will be useful for investigating and developing the new drug or device. Lessons learned from the terminated project may often be applied to ongoing or new projects, especially to those in the same therapeutic area.

WHEN TO TERMINATE A STUDY OR PROJECT

Early Termination of a Study with a Positive Outcome

Terminating a study early because of statistically significant beneficial differences between two treatment groups may be a major mistake if the data are not sufficient to convince most physicians of their clinical importance. Rules may be established to terminate a study prematurely, if it achieves certain criteria. A study may be terminated early when there are provisions written in a study protocol to discontinue it when a preset statistically significant benefit is observed. This approach has been used to terminate certain large multicenter studies early [(e.g., Beta-Blocker Heart Attack Trial (BHAT)].

Major reasons to establish rules are (1) because of potential ethical problems if the study is continued or (2) to save valuable resources. If a study is discontinued for ethical reasons it will generally make it difficult or impossible to conduct a similar study in the future. If the clinical importance of the data at the time of discontinuing the study is obvious to most physicians and they will alter their medical practice as a result of the new information from the study, then the decision to discontinue the study was correct. If, however, many physicians are either skeptical or unconvinced about the clinical importance of the data, then discontinuing the study was an error. This mistake may also decrease the likelihood that a real change in physicians' attitudes and medical practice will occur as a result of data from a subsequent study.

When an investigator terminates a study, careful consideration must be given as to how to best phase patients back to their prestudy care and treatment. In many situations this will be a simple issue to address, but when patients have benefited greatly from being in a study, the transition from frequent contact with the investigator and staff, plus benefits of treatment, may present a challenge.

Ware et al. (1985) stated that protocols of clinical studies usually do not consider the possibility arising where a positive result is unlikely to occur and that the study should therefore be prematurely terminated. They proposed a new measure termed "The Futility Index" which would deal with this situation, so that more studies could be prematurely terminated.

Terminating a Project

Although the major reasons for project termination usually relate to safety and efficacy, there are numerous other reasons. An unacceptable pharmacokinetic profile may be sufficient grounds for termination (e.g., inadequate drug absorption, inadequate drug half-life), as would the inability to solve problems of technical development (e.g., inadequate formulation in terms of dissolution). Patent or regulatory difficulties that cannot be resolved are additional reasons for project termination. Nonetheless, agreements between two or more companies on patent issues may sometimes resolve what would otherwise be difficult or impossible issues to circumvent. Two other reasons for terminating a project include (1) changes in medical practice that make the project drug or device obsolete and (2) new products on the market which make the project drug or device noncompetitive.

The least controversial reason for terminating a project usually relates to safety considerations. If unexpected (or even expected) toxicological findings of a significant nature occur in animal studies which are not acceptable to patients and physicians from a benefit-to-risk consideration, and there is a reasonable possibility of these occurring in humans, there may be great pressure to terminate the project. Even when no human cases have been reported and the possibility of observing a severe toxic effect in humans is totally unknown, the project is usually terminated.

Projects may also be terminated for occurrence of toxic events (adverse reactions) in humans. Many severe adverse reactions are not acceptable, if observed in humans. The major criteria used to judge the implications of a severe adverse reaction that occurs in humans are: (1) How severe is the reaction? (2) What are the clinical repercussions? (3) What is the incidence of the event? (4) What are the risk factors? (5) Can it be predicted? (6) How safe are alternative treatments? (7) How severe is the disease being treated? (8) What is the therapeutic index (dose at which a toxic effect is noted, divided by the minimal therapeutic dose)? Overall, how is the benefit-to-risk ratio affected by the adverse reaction?

Another reason for terminating projects involving new drugs is for a lack of efficacy determined in well-controlled studies. One difficulty with terminating a project as a result of inadequate efficacy is that there are usually individuals who claim that if the drug were tested under other conditions there is a likelihood that it would be active. Such situations are rarely totally clear to predict. In addition, some patients may benefit from treatment, but they may represent a small proportion of the total patient population and cannot be readily identified with objective measures prior to treatment. Setting minimal standards in advance for the project to reach will assist the decision to terminate, and avoid the "what if" game that is sometimes used to keep projects alive long after their effective demise. These projects are sometimes referred to as "Lazarus" or "Phoenix" projects, because of the hopes of their champions for the project's eventual resurrection.

Prentis and Walker (1986) reported that seven United Kingdom drug companies tested 197 new chemical entities in humans for the first time during a 17-year period (January 1, 1964 to January 1, 1981). Of these compounds 35 (18%) were marketed by early 1984, and 25 (13%) were still in development. The balance (137 compounds) were terminated. The reasons for termination were adverse reactions (7%), toxicity in animals (6%), lack of efficacy (16%), pharmacokinetic reasons (34%), and miscellaneous reasons (6%). The percents given are calculated based on the total number (197) of compounds studied. Prentis and Walker point out that the high percentage of failures attributable to pharmacokinetic reasons reflects the specific therapeutic areas of the drugs in the sample. Antiinfective drugs accounted for 42% of the data base. When all of the values were recalculated excluding antiinfectives, the category of pharmacokinetic reasons decreased to 25%.

There are some techniques that facilitate the termination of projects. One of the most important is to establish minimum requirements at the outset of a project to continue development of a project. If these standards are not met then there are grounds for terminating the project. Unfortunately, life is rarely that simple and all of a project's goals are seldom totally met or unmet. Some goals will probably be achieved or at least partially achieved, and others will not be met. As the medical characteristics of an investigational drug change, so too does the marketing assessment of where the drug may be successfully positioned in the market and how well it is expected to do financially. If the therapeutic value of a drug is diminishing, at a certain point it will become unreasonable to pursue the drug's development because of the minimal commercial potential in comparison with actual and projected costs to develop and market the drug. An important technique to facilitate the termination of a project is to involve the people in the decision-making process who will be affected by the project's demise. By discussing the rationale and benefits of termination, the group is more likely to agree with and support the decision.

What to Do With a Drug with a Marginal Efficacy or Safety Profile

There are many cases when it is not obvious if a project should be terminated or continued. It is important to guard against too rapid a termination

TABLE 24.1. *Selected considerations that could increase the therapeutic ratio of a drug*

1. Decrease the dosage to find the minimal effective dose
2. Modify the schedule of dose administration (e.g., use b.i.d. instead of q.d. dosing to reduce peak concentrations of the drug in blood)[a]
3. Change the route of administration (e.g., use a slow-release depot)
4. Have patients use another drug concomitantly (e.g., to potentiate effects, reduce adverse reactions)
5. Use a more relevant patient population to evaluate the drug (e.g., drug naive, mildly ill rather than severely ill patients, severely ill rather than mildly ill patients)
6. Pursue a different indication where efficacy may be demonstrated at a lower dose
7. Determine whether an adverse reaction that is commonly observed may be used as a therapeutic goal for a new indication (e.g., sedation that is undesirable for one drug may be used as a goal to develop the drug as a sleep-inducing agent, emesis could be used as a goal to develop a new emetic agent)
8. Have patients take the drug with or after meals to decrease the rate of drug absorption

[a] b.i.d., twice a day; q.d., once a day.

of a project when the consensus of opinion is starting to turn against a drug's potential for success, when some important questions have not been answered. It is possible to reduce the resources and efforts expended while the last remaining questions are addressed.

A drug with a marginal efficacy or safety profile may or may not be able to be converted into a worthwhile drug from medical and commercial points of view. A number of considerations that potentially may increase the therapeutic ratio of a drug are given in Table 24.1. Some of these are intended to improve either efficacy or safety.

ALTERNATIVES TO TERMINATING A PROJECT

In certain situations when it is not clear that a project should be terminated but the original expectations are not being met, there is usually a desire to do "something." That "something" may be:

1. Convene a panel of internal and/or external consultants who review the data and perhaps suggest alternative development paths, study designs, formulations, indications, and so on.
2. Deemphasize the project in terms of priority and resources, while allowing it to proceed at a slower pace.
3. Redefine the objectives and redirect the project in a new direction. At some point, however, it is not fruitful to continue developing a drug that is "looking for a disease."
4. Put in a new leader on the project and possibly several new members as well.

5. Reassess the feasibility of the project and the indication(s) being pursued.
6. Have an independent audit performed of specific questions relating to the project.
7. Solicit ideas for revitalizing the project.
8. Attempt to increase the therapeutic ratio (see Table 24.1) if that ratio is low.

In seeking to perform some of these steps it may become apparent that saving the project would be unwise and a more confident decision may then be reached to terminate it. It is often more palatable for a team to recommend termination than for one person to do so. Reasons for termination are usually based on failure to meet established criteria. At that point it is usually valuable to extract the lessons learned and to make them part of the institutional memory by writing them in a formal report. Collections of such lessons may provide valuable education for relevant new individuals who join the institution.

Appendix

TABLES

FIGURES

OTHER

COMMENTS

The tables and figures in this appendix provide copies of forms used to submit an IND or NDA, plus outlines of information included in various regulatory submissions. The Declaration of Helsinki presents the guidelines promulgated by the World Medical Association for the ethical conduct of clinical studies.

TABLE A.1. *Summary of contents of a new drug application (NDA)*

- I. Overall summary (see Table 21.1 for contents)
- II. Technical sections
  - A. Chemistry, manufacturing, and controls
    - 1. Drug substance
      - a. Physical characteristics
      - b. Chemical characteristics
      - c. Stability
      - d. Name/address of manufacturer
      - e. Method of synthesis/purification
      - f. Process controls in manufacturing and packaging
      - g. Specifications and analytical methods as necessary to assure identity, strength, quality, purity, and bioavailability of the drug substance
      - h. Alternate suppliers, process controls, etc.
    - 2. Drug product
      - a. List of all components used in manufacture
      - b. Composition of drug product
      - c. Specifications/analytical methods for each component
      - d. Name/address of each manufacturer
      - e. Manufacturing/packaging procedure
      - f. In-process controls
      - g. Specifications/analytical methods
      - h. Stability with expiration dating
      - i. Alternative components, suppliers, methods, etc.
    - 3. Environmental impact analysis report
  - B. Nonclinical pharmacology and toxicology
    - 1. Pharmacology studies in relation to
      - a. Proposed therapeutic indication
      - b. Studies that otherwise define the pharmacologic properties of the drug
      - c. Studies pertinent to adverse effects
    - 2. Toxicology studies relating to clinical use, including:
      - a. Acute studies
      - b. Subacute studies
      - c. Chronic studies
      - d. Carcinogenicity studies
      - e. Special studies relating to route of administration or conditions of use
      - f. Reproduction studies
      - g. Studies on the developing fetus
    - 3. Studies of the absorption, distribution, metabolism, and excretion of the drug in animals
    - 4. For each nonclinical laboratory study, a statement that it complies with Good Laboratory Practices (GLP) regulations or a brief statement of the reason for the noncompliance
  - C. Human pharmacokinetics and bioavailability
    - 1. A description of each bioavailability and pharmacokinetic study performed in humans, including:
      - a. Analytical methods
      - b. Statistical methods
      - c. Statement that study was conducted in compliance with Institutional Review Board (IRB) regulations
      - d. Statement that study was conducted in compliance with informed consent regulations
    - 2. A rationale for establishing a specification or analytical method necessary to assure bioavailability
    - 3. A summary and analysis of the pharmacokinetics and metabolism of the active ingredients and the bioavailability/bioequivalence of the drug product
  - D. Microbiology section (for antiinfective and antiviral drugs)
    - 1. Description of the drug's biochemical basis of action on microbial physiology
    - 2. Description of the antimicrobial spectra of the drug (include *in vitro* preclinical studies demonstrating concentrations of drug required for effective use)
    - 3. Descriptions of any known mechanisms of resistance to the drug
    - 4. Description of clinical microbiology laboratory methods needed for effective use of the drug

TABLE A.1. *(Continued)*

- E. Clinical data
  - 1. Clinical pharmacology, including:
    - a. Study description
    - b. Study analysis description
    - c. Comparison with animal pharmacology/toxicology
  - 2. Controlled clinical studies pertinent to a proposed use of the drug, including:
    - a. Protocol
    - b. Description of statistical analysis
    - c. Include unanalyzed, controlled studies along with a brief description of the results and status of the study
  - 3. Uncontrolled clinical studies, including:
    - a. Description
    - b. Summary of results
    - c. Statement explaining why the study is classified as uncontrolled
  - 4. Additional information received by applicant from any source, including:
    - a. Foreign studies
    - b. Clinical studies on additional indications
    - c. Commercial marketing experience
    - d. Published scientific papers
    - e. Unpublished scientific papers
  - 5. An integrated efficacy summary, including:
    - a. Evidence to support dosage and administration in labeling
    - b. Evidence to support dosage and dose interval recommended
    - c. Evidence to support dosage modifications for specific subgroups:
      - i. Pediatrics
      - ii. Geriatrics
      - iii. Etc.
  - 6. An integrated summary of all available safety information including:
    - a. At initial NDA filing:
      - i. Pertinent animal data
      - ii. Demonstrated or potential adverse drug reactions
      - iii. Clinically significant drug–drug interactions
      - iv. Additional information, such as from epidemiological studies
      - v. Description of statistical analysis used, unless submitted in II.E.2.b (above)
    - b. Periodic updates:
      - i. Content and format as in II.E.6.a (above)
      - ii. Case report forms for each patient who died or did not complete the study due to an adverse drug reaction
      - iii. Timing of safety updates
        - α. Four (4) months following initial submission
        - β. Upon receipt of approvable letter
        - γ. At other times, as requested by Food and Drug Administration (FDA)
    - c. For controlled substances only: analysis of studies or information related to the abuse of the drug, proposal for scheduling under the controlled substances act and overdosage information (dialysis, antidotes, etc.)
  - 7. Risk/benefits summary
    - a. Discussion of why the benefits exceed the risks under the conditions stated in the labeling
  - 8. Statement that each human study was conducted in compliance with Part 50 (informed consent regulations) and Part 56 (IRB regulations) of the Code of Federal Regulations (CFR).
- F. Statistical section
  - 1. Describe the statistical evaluation of clinical data, including:
    - a. Copy of information submitted in II.E.2 (above) concerning (for controlled clinical studies):
      - i. Description
      - ii. Analysis
  - 2. Additionally, for controlled clinical studies, submit:

TABLE A.1. *(Continued)*

- a. Documentation
- b. Supporting statistical analysis used in evaluation
3. Describe statistical evaluation of safety data, including:
   - a. Copy of information submitted in II.E.6.a (above)
   - b. Documentation and supporting statistical analysis used in evaluating the safety information

III. Samples and labeling
- A. Samples
  1. Four samples of the following (submit upon FDA request):
     - a. Drug product
     - b. Drug substance used in manufacture of drug product (above)
     - c. Reference standards and blanks
  2. Samples of finished market package (if requested)
  3. In the archival copy of the application, submit
     - a. Three copies of the analytical methods and related descriptive information contained in the manufacturing/controls section (II.A.1 and 2 above)
- B. Labeling (in archival copy of application)
  1. Copies of the label and all labeling, as follows:
     - a. If draft, four copies
     - b. If final, 12 copies

IV. Case report forms and tabulations
- A. Case report tabulations (in archival copy)
  1. Tabulations of all data from:
     - a. All clinical pharmacology studies (Phase I)
     - b. Each adequate and well-controlled study (Phases II and III) for indication(s) sought
  2. Tabulations of safety data from:
     - a. Uncontrolled clinical studies
     - b. Other clinical studies
- B. Case report forms (in archival copy)
  1. Required for:
     - a. Each patient who died during a clinical study
     - b. Each patient who did not complete a clinical study because of an adverse reaction, whether drug-related or not, including patients receiving reference drugs or placebo
- C. Additional data
  1. Submit additional case report forms/tabulations as requested by FDA

TABLE A.2. *Summary of contents of a registration dossier for the European Economic Community (EEC)*

A. Flyleaf
   1. Name or business name of applicant for marketing authorization
   2. Full address of applicant
   3. a. Name and address of manufacturer
      b. Name and address of importer
   4. Name of the proprietary medicinal product
   5. Pharmaceutical form
   6. Method and route of administration
   7. Number of annexes supplied in support of the application
B. Annex I: General information
   1. Name of the proprietary medicinal product
   2. Pharmaceutical form
   3. Qualitative and quantitative composition in terms of active principles
   4. Therapeutic indications
   5. Dosage
   6. Contraindications
   7. Warnings and precautions (including during pregnancy)
   8. Side effects
   9. Directions for use (where applicable)
   10. Shelf life and storage precautions
C. Annex II: Information and documents concerning physicochemical, biological, or microbiological tests
D. Annex II.A: Complete qualitative and quantitative composition
   1. Name of product
   2. Composition
   3. Container (brief description)
E. Annex II.B: Method of preparation
   1. Manufacturing formula
   2. Manufacturing process including in-process control and the pharmaceutical assembly process
F. Annex II.C: Control of starting materials
   1. Active principles
      a. Active principles described in a pharmacopeia
      b. Active principles not described in a pharmacopeia
   2. Other constituents
      a. Constituents described in a pharmacopeia
      b. Constituents not described in a pharmacopeia
G. Annex II.D: Control tests on intermediate products (if necessary)
H. Annex II.E: Control tests on the finished product
   1. General characteristics; other quality control tests required by the nature of the products (appearance, dimension, shape, color, odor, distinguishing features, etc.)
   2. Identification and quantitative determination of the active principle or principles; other quality control tests, with a description of the methods employed [including (if necessary) and depending on the nature of the product; biological and microbiological methods]
   3. Identification and quantitative determination of the other constituents (if necessary)
I. Annex II.F: Stability tests
   1. Proposed shelf life (depending on the type of container)
   2. Information concerning stability, including physical stability:
      a. Number of batches tested
      b. Storage conditions
      c. Methods employed
      d. Description of containers
   3. Results and interpretations
J. Annex II.G: Conclusions
   Certificate by the expert analyst on the application of the methods and justification of the control methods to be used by the manufacturer
K. Annex III: Toxicological and pharmacological tests (summary of the tasks performed by the expert pharmacologist)
   The following information must be provided in respect of each test:
   1. Animals used (species, strain, sex, etc.)
   2. Experimental conditions, including diet
   3. Results
L. Annex III.A: Acute toxicity
M. Annex III.B: Toxicity with repeated administration
   1. Subacute toxicity trials
   2. Chronic toxicity trials

TABLE A.2. *(Continued)*

N. Annex III.C: Fetal toxicity
   1. Tests for teratogenicity (dosing during period of organogenesis)
   2. Pre- and postnatal dosing of the mother to demonstrate effects on late pregnancy, parturition, and lactation

O. Annex III.D: Fertility studies

P. Annex III.E: Carcinogenicity and mutagenicity

Q. Annex III.F: Pharmacodynamics
   1. Actions relevant to the proposed therapeutic uses
   2. Other actions investigated
   3. Interactions

R. Annex III.G: Pharmacokinetics
   1. Absorption (serum levels of the medicinal product)
   2. Distribution of the medicinal product
   3. Biotransformation
   4. Excretion of the medicinal product and metabolites

S. Annex IV: Clinical trials (summary of the tasks performed by the expert clinician)

T. Annex IV.A: Human pharmacology

U. Annex IV.B: Clinical data
   1. Individual data-clinical reports
   2. Summary
   3. Conclusions

V. Annex IV.C: Side effects and interactions
   Information on side effects and interactions observed when used in other countries (the extent of usage in terms of number of prescriptions and duration of use is useful in assessing the frequency of the adverse reaction)

W. Annex V: Special particulars

X. Annex V.A: Dosage forms
   1. Packaging
   2. Label
   3. Package insert

Y. Annex V.B.: Samples

Z. Annex V.C.: Manufacturer's authorization

AA. Annex V.D.: Marketing authorization

TABLE A.3. *Contents of a notice of claimed investigational exemption for a new drug (IND)*[a]

Item 1:	Name, chemical structures, dosage form, and route(s) of administration of the new drug
Item 2:	List of all components of the drug entity, including reasonable alternates for inactive components
Item 3:	Quantitative composition of the drug entity, including reasonable variations that may be expected during the investigational stage
Item 4:	Source and preparation of new drug substances used as components; this includes (1) manufacturing processes for new drug substances(s) and (2) dosage form
Item 5:	Methods, facilities, and controls used for the manufacturing, processing, and packing of the new drug; the establishment and maintenance of appropriate standards of identity, strength, quality, and purity
Item 6:	Preclinical pharmacology, toxicology, and drug metabolism data; available clinical data if drug was used previously (e.g., in another country) or is a combination of previously investigated or marketed drugs
Item 7:	Informational material to be provided to investigators; this includes (1) a copy of the labels to be on the drug containers identifying the drug as investigational and (2) a clinical monograph describing the drug, possible utility, prior investigations, and known hazards, contraindications, side effects, and precautions
Item 8:	A statement of the training and experience required of investigators
Item 9:	The names and credentials of the monitors and investigators. A statement that the sponsor has received from the investigator a signed form that the investigator understands and accepts his responsibilities regarding record keeping, informed consent, and supervision of subjects
Item 10:	Outline of the clinical investigation, including specification of phase involved: Phases I and II (clinical pharmacology) or Phase III (broad clinical trial)
Item 11:	Agreement to notify Food and Drug Administration (FDA) if investigation is discontinued, with explanation
Item 12:	Agreement to notify investigators if investigation is discontinued or a New Drug Application (NDA) for the investigational drug is approved
Item 13:	Completed only if sponsor wishes to sell, rather than distribute, test drug free to investigators; the reason for the need to sell must be explained
Item 14:	Agreement not to ship drug or use in humans until 30 days after receipt of IND by FDA
Item 15:	An environmental impact statement when requested
Item 16:	Statement that all nonclinical laboratory studies comply with Good Laboratory Practices (GLPs)

[a] The forms used to file an IND are shown in Figs. A.1–A.3. These items refer to a synopsis of requirements listed in Form FDA 1571 (Fig. A.1).

DEPARTMENT OF HEALTH AND HUMAN SERVICES PUBLIC HEALTH SERVICE FOOD AND DRUG ADMINISTRATION **NOTICE OF CLAIMED INVESTIGATIONAL EXEMPTION FOR A NEW DRUG**	*Form Approved; OMB No. 0910-0014* *Expiration Date: December 31, 1984* **NOTE:** No drug may be shipped or study initiated unless a complete statement has been received. *(21 CFR 312.1(a)(2)).*

Name of Sponsor ______________________ Date ____________

Address ______________________ Telephone (   ) ____________

Name of Investigational Drug ______________________

FOR A DRUG:

Food And Drug Administration
Office of New Drug Evaluation *(HFN-106)*
5600 Fishers Lane
Rockville, Maryland 20857

FOR A BIOLOGIC:

Food and Drug Administration
Office of Biologics *(HFN-823)*
8800 Rockville Pike
Bethesda, Maryland 20205

Dear Sir:

The sponsor, ______________________, submits this notice of claimed investigational exemption for a new drug under the provisions of section 505(i) of the Federal Food, Drug, and Cosmetic Act and § 312.1 of Title 21 of the Code of Federal Regulations.

Attached hereto in triplicate are:

1. The best available descriptive name of the drug, including to the extent known the chemical name and structure of any new-drug substance, and a statement of how it is to be administered. (If the drug has only a code name, enough information should be supplied to identify the drug.)

2. Complete list of components of the drug, including any reasonable alternates for inactive components.

3. Complete statement of quantitative composition of drug, including reasonable variations that may be expected during the investigational stage.

4. Description of source and preparation of, any new-drug substances used as components, including the name and address of each supplier or processor, other than the sponsor, or each new-drug substance.

5. A statement of the methods, facilities, and controls used for the manufacturing, processing, and packing of the new drug to establish and maintain appropriate standards of identity, strength, quality, and purity as needed for safety and to give significance to clinical investigations made with the drug.

6. A statement covering all information available to the sponsor derived from preclinical investigations and any clinical studies and experience with the drug as follows:

a. Adequate information about the preclinical investigations, including studies made on laboratory animals, on the basis of which the sponsor has concluded that it is reasonably safe to initiate clinical investigations with the drug: Such information should include identification of the person who conducted each investigation; identification and qualifications of the individuals who evaluated the results and concluded that it is reasonably safe to initiate clinical investigations with the drug and a statement of where the investigations were conducted and where the records are available for inspection; and enough details about the investigations to permit scientific review. The preclinical investigations shall not be considered adequate to justify clinical testing unless they give proper attention to the conditions of the proposed clinical testing. When this information, the outline of the plan of clinical pharmacology, or any progress report on the clinical pharmacology, indicates a need for full review of the preclinical data before a clinical trial is undertaken, the Department will notify the sponsor to submit the complete preclinical data and to withhold clinical trials until the review is completed and the sponsor notified. The Food and Drug Administration will be prepared to confer with the sponsor concerning this action.

b. If the drug has been marketed commercially or investigated (e.g. outside the United States), complete information about such distribution or investigation shall be submitted, along with a complete bibliography of any publications about the drug.

c. If the drug is a combination of previously investigated or marketed drugs, an adequate summary of preexisting information from preclinical and clinical investigations and experience with its components, including all reports available to the sponsor suggesting side-effects, contraindications, and ineffectiveness in use of such components: Such summary should include an adequate bibliography of publications about the components and may incorporate by reference any information concerning such components previously submitted by the sponsor to the Food and Drug Administration. Include a statement of the expected pharmacological effects of the combination.

d. If the drug is a radioactive drug, sufficient data must be available from animal studies or previous human studies to allow a reasonable calculation of radiation absorbed dose upon administration to a human being.

7. A total (one in each of the three copies of the notice) of all informational material, including label and labeling, which is to be supplied to each investigator: This shall include an accurate description of the prior investigations and experience and their results pertinent to the safety and possible usefulness of the drug under the conditions of the investigation. It shall not represent that the safety or usefulness of the drug has been established for the purposes to be investigated. It shall describe all relevant hazards, contraindications, side-effects, and precautions suggested by prior investigations and experience with the drug under investigation and related drugs for the information of clinical investigators.

8. The scientific training and experience considered appropriate by the sponsor to qualify the investigators as suitable experts to investigate the safety of the drug, bearing in mind what is known about the pharmacological action of the drug and the phase of the investigational program that is to be undertaken.

9. The names and a summary of the training and experience of each investigator and of the individual charged with monitoring the progress of the investigation and evaluating the evidence of safety and effectiveness of the drug as it is received from the investigators, together with a statement that the sponsor has obtained from each investigator a completed and signed form, as provided in subparagraph (12) or (13) of this paragraph, and that the investigator is qualified by scientific training and experience as an appropriate expert to under-

FORM FDA 1571 (9/84) PREVIOUS EDITION ARE OBSOLETE.

FIG. A.1. Form used to file an IND (FDA 1571).

take the phase of the investigation outlined in section 10 of the "Notice of Claimed Investigational Exemption for a New Drug." (In crucial situations, phase 3 investigators may be added and this form supplemented by rapid communication methods, and the signed Form FD-1573 shall be obtained promptly thereafter.)

10. An outline of any phase or phases of the planned investigations and a description of the institutional review committee, as follows:

a. Clinical pharmacology. This is ordinarily divided into two phases: Phase I starts when the new drug is first introduced into man - only animal and in vitro data are available - with the purpose of determining human toxicity, metabolism, absorption, elimination, and other pharmacological action, preferred route of administration, and safe dosage range; phase 2 covers the initial trials on a limited number of patients for specific disease control or prophylaxis purposes. A general outline of these phases shall be submitted, identifying the investigator or investigators, the hospitals or research facilities where the clinical pharmacology will be undertaken, any expert committees or panels to be utilized, the maximum number of subjects to be involved, and the estimated duration of these early phases of investigation. Modification of the experimental design on the basis of experience gained need be reported only in the progress reports on these early phases, or in the development of the plan for the clinical trial, phase 3. The first two phases may overlap and, when indicated, may require additional animal data before these phases can be completed or phase can be undertaken. Such animal tests shall be designed to take into account the expected duration of administration of the drug to human beings, the age groups and physical status, as for example, infants, pregnant women, premenopausal women, of those human beings to whom the drug may be administered, unless this has already been done in the original animal studies. If a drug is a radioactive drug, the clinical pharmacology phase must include studies which will obtain sufficient data for dosimetry calculations. These studies should evaluate the excretion, whole body retention, and organ distribution of the radioactive material.

b. Clinical trial. This phase 3 provides the assessment of the drug's safety and effectiveness and optimum dosage schedules in the diagnosis, treatment, or prophylaxis of groups of subjects involving a given disease or condition. A reasonable protocol is developed on the basis of the facts accumulated in the earlier phases, including completed and submitted animal studies. This phase is conducted by separate groups following the same protocol (with reasonable variations and alternatives permitted by the plan) to produce well-controlled clinical data. For this phase, the following data shall be submitted:

i. The names and addresses of the investigators. (Additional investigators may be added.)

ii. The specific nature of the investigations to be conducted, together with information or case report forms to show the scope and detail of the planned clinical observations and the clinical laboratory tests to be made and reported.

iii. The approximate number of subjects (a reasonable range of subjects is permissible and additions may be made), and criteria proposed for subject selection by age, sex, and condition.

iv. The estimated duration of the clinical trial and the intervals, not exceeding 1 year, at which progress reports showing the results of the investigations will be submitted to the Food and Drug Administration.

c. Institutional review board (IRB). The sponsor must give assurance that an IRB that complies with the requirements set forth in Part 56 of this chapter will be responsible for the initial and continuing review and approval of the proposed clinical study. The sponsor must also provide assurance that the investigators will report to the IRB all changes in the research activity and all unanticipated problems involving risks to human subjects or others, and that the investigators will not make any changes in the research without IRB approval, except where necessary to eliminate apparent immediate hazard to the human subjects. FDA will regard the signing of the Form FDA-1571 as providing the necessary assurances above.

(The notice of claimed investigational exemption may be limited to any one or more phases, provided the outline of the additional phase or phases is submitted before such additional phases begin. A limitation on an exemption does not preclude continuing a subject on the drug from phase 2 to phase 3 without interruption while the plan for phase 3 is being developed.)

Ordinarily, a plan for clinical trial will not be regarded as reasonable unless, among other things, it provides for more than one independent competent investigator to maintain adequate case histories of an adequate number of subjects, designed to record observations and permit evaluation of any and all discernible effects attributable to the drug in each individual treated, and comparable records on any individuals employed as controls. These records shall be individual records for each subject maintained to include adequate information pertaining to each, including age, sex, conditions treated, dosage, frequency of administration of the drug, results of all relevant clinical observations and laboratory examinations made, adequate information concerning any other treatment given and a full statement of any adverse effects and useful results observed, together with an opinion as to whether such effects or results are attributable to the drug under investigation.

11. A statement that the sponsor will notify the Food and Drug Administration if the investigation is discontinued, and the reason therefor.

12. A statement that the sponsor will notify each investigator if a new-drug application is approved, or if the investigation is discontinued.

13. If the drug is to be sold, a full explanation why sale is required and should not be regarded as the commercialization of a new drug for which an application is not approved.

14. A statement that the sponsor assures that clinical studies in humans will not be initiated prior to 30 days after the date of receipt of the notice by the Food and Drug Administration and that he will continue to withhold or to restrict clinical studies if requested to do so by the Food and Drug Administration prior to the expiration of such 30 days. If such request is made, the sponsor will be provided specific information as to the deficiencies and will be afforded a conference on request. The 30-day delay may be waived by the Food and Drug Administration upon a showing of good reason for such waiver; and for investigations subject to institutional review committee approval as described in item 10c above, and additional statement assuring that the investigation will not be initiated prior to approval of the study by such committee.

15. When requested by the agency, an environmental impact analysis report pursuant to § 25.1 of this chapter.

16. A statement that all nonclinical laboratory studies have been, or will be, conducted in compliance with the good laboratory practice regulations set forth in Part 58 of this chapter, or, if such studies have not been conducted in compliance with such regulations, a statement that describes in detail all differences between the practices used in conducting the study and those required in the regulations.

Very truly yours,

SPONSOR	PER
	INDICATE AUTHORITY

(This notice may be amended or supplemented from time to time on the basis of the experience gained with the new drug. Progress reports may be used to update the notice.)

ALL NOTICES AND CORRESPONDENCE SHOULD BE SUBMITTED IN TRIPLICATE.

★ U.S.GPO:1984-0-454-393/18778

FIG. A.1. *(Continued)*

DEPARTMENT OF HEALTH AND HUMAN SERVICES
PUBLIC HEALTH SERVICE
FOOD AND DRUG ADMINISTRATION

STATEMENT OF INVESTIGATOR
(Clinical Pharmacology)

Form Approved; OMB No. 0910-0015
Expiration Date: December 31, 1984.

NOTE: No drug may be shipped or study initiated unless a completed statement has been received *(21 CFR 312.1(a)(12)).*

TO: SUPPLIER OF THE DRUG *(Name and address, include ZIP Code)*	NAME OF INVESTIGATOR *(Print or Type)*
	DATE
	NAME OF DRUG

Dear Sir:

The undersigned, ______________________________

submits this statement as required by section 505(i) of the Federal Food, Drug, and Cosmetic Act and § 312.1 of Title 21 of the Code of Federal Regulations as a condition for receiving and conducting clinical pharmacology with a new drug limited by Federal (or United States) law to investigational use.

1. A STATEMENT OF THE EDUCATION AND TRAINING THAT QUALIFIES ME FOR CLINICAL PHARMACOLOGY

2. THE NAME AND ADDRESS OF THE MEDICAL SCHOOL, HOSPITAL, OR OTHER RESEARCH FACILITY WHERE THE CLINICAL PHARMACOLOGY WILL BE CONDUCTED

3. The investigator assures that an IRB that complies with the requirements set forth in Part 56 of this chapter will be responsible for the initial and continuing review and approval of the proposed clinical study. The investigator also assures that he/she will report to the IRB all changes in the research activity and all unanticipated problems involving risks to human subjects or others, and that he/she will not make any changes in the research that would increase the risks to human subjects without IRB approval. FDA will regard the signing of the Form FD 1572 as providing the necessary assurances stated above.

4. THE ESTIMATED DURATION OF THE PROJECT AND THE MAXIMUM NUMBER OF SUBJECTS THAT WILL BE INVOLVED

FORM FDA 1572 (10/83) PREVIOUS EDITIONS ARE OBSOLETE.

FIG. A.2. Form used with the IND application (FDA 1572).

5. GENERAL OUTLINE OF THE PROJECT TO BE UNDERTAKEN *(Modification is permitted on the basis of experience gained without advance submission of amendments to the general outline, but with the approval of the review committee and upon notification of the sponsor.)*

6. THE UNDERSIGNED UNDERSTANDS THAT THE FOLLOWING CONDITIONS GENERALLY APPLICABLE TO NEW DRUGS FOR INVESTIGATIONAL USE GOVERN HIS RECEIPT AND USE OF THIS INVESTIGATIONAL DRUG

a. The sponsor is required to supply the investigator with full information concerning the preclinical investigation that justifies clinical pharmacology.

b. The investigator is required to maintain adequate records of the disposition of all receipts of the drug, including dates, quantity, and use by subjects, and if the clinical pharmacology is suspended, terminated, discontinued, or completed, to return to the sponsor any unused supply of the drug. If the investigational drug is subject to the Comprehensive Drug Abuse Prevention and Control Act of 1970, adequate precautions must be taken, including storage of the investigational drug in a securely locked, substantially constructed cabinet, or other securely locked, substantially constructed enclosure access to which is limited, to prevent theft or diversion of the substance into illegal channels of distribution.

c. The investigator is required to prepare and maintain adequate case histories designed to record all observations and other data pertinent to the clinical pharmacology.

d. The investigator is required to furnish his reports to the sponsor who is responsible for collecting and evaluating the results, and presenting progress reports to the Food and Drug Administration at appropriate intervals, not exceeding 1 year. Any adverse effect which may reasonably be regarded as caused by, or is probably caused by, the new-drug shall be reported to the sponsor promptly; and if the adverse effect is alarming it shall be reported immediately. An adequate report of the clinical pharmacology should be furnished to the sponsor shortly after completion.

e. The investigator shall maintain the records of disposition of the drug and the case reports described above for a period of 2 years following the date the new-drug application is approved for the drug; or if no application is to be filed or is approved until 2 years after the investigation is discontinued and the Food and Drug Administration so notified. Upon the request of a scientifically trained and specifically authorized employee of the Department, at reasonable times, the investigator will made such records available for inspection and copying. The names of the subjects need not be divulged unless the records of the particular subjects require a more detailed study of the cases, or unless there is reason to believe that the records do not represent actual studies or do not represent actual results obtained.

f. The investigator certifies that the drug will be administered only to subjects under his personal supervision or under the supervision of the following investigators responsible to him,

____

____

____

____

and that the drug will not be supplied to any other investigator or to any clinic for administration to subjects.

g. The investigator certifies that he will inform any patients or any persons used as controls, or their representatives, that drugs are being used for investigational purposes, and will obtain the consent of the subjects, or their representatives, except where this is not feasible or, in the investigator's professional judgment, is contrary to the best interests of the subjects.

h. The investigator is required to assure the sponsor that for investigations subject to an institutional review requirement under Part 56 of this chapter the studies will not be initiated until the institutional review board has reviewed and approved the study. (The organization and procedure requirements for such a board as set forth in Part 56 should be explained to the investigator by the sponsor.)

Very truly yours,

Name of Investigator ________________________

Address ________________________ Telephone (   ) ____________

FIG. A.2. *(Continued)*

DEPARTMENT OF HEALTH AND HUMAN SERVICES PUBLIC HEALTH SERVICE FOOD AND DRUG ADMINISTRATION **STATEMENT OF INVESTIGATOR**	*Form approved; OMB No. 0910-0013* *Expiration Date: December 31, 1984.* **Note:** No drug may be shipped or study initiated unless a completed statement has been received *(21 CFR 312.1(a)(12)).*
TO: SUPPLIER OF DRUG *(Name, address, and Zip Code)*	NAME OF INVESTIGATOR *(Print or Type)* DATE NAME OF DRUG

Dear Sir:

The undersigned, ______________________________
submits this statement as required by section 505(i) of the Federal Food, Drug, and Cosmetic Act and §312.1 of Title 21 of the Code of **Federal Regulations as a condition for receiving** and conducting clinical investigations with a new drug limited by Federal *(or United States)* **law to investigational use.**

1. THE FOLLOWING IS A STATEMENT OF MY EDUCATION AND EXPERIENCE:

a. COLLEGES, UNIVERSITIES, AND MEDICAL OR OTHER PROFESSIONAL SCHOOLS ATTENDED, WITH DATES OF ATTENDANCE, DEGREES, AND DATES DEGREES WERE AWARDED

b. POSTGRADUATE MEDICAL OR OTHER PROFESSIONAL TRAINING. GIVE DATES, NAMES OF INSTITUTIONS, AND NATURE OF TRAINING.

c. TEACHING OR RESEARCH EXPERIENCE. GIVE DATES, INSTITUTIONS, AND BRIEF DESCRIPTION OF EXPERIENCE.

d. EXPERIENCE IN MEDICAL PRACTICE OR OTHER PROFESSIONAL EXPERIENCE. GIVE DATES, INSTITUTIONAL AFFILIATIONS, NATURE OF PRACTICE, OR OTHER PROFESSIONAL EXPERIENCE.

e. REPRESENTATIVE LIST OF PERTINENT MEDICAL OR OTHER SCIENTIFIC PUBLICATIONS. GIVE TITLES OF ARTICLES, NAME OF PUBLICATIONS AND VOLUME, PAGE NUMBER, AND DATE.

IF THIS INFORMATION HAS PREVIOUSLY BEEN SUBMITTED TO THE SPONSOR, IT MAY BE REFERRED TO AND ANY ADDITIONS MADE TO BRING IT UP-TO-DATE.

FORM FDA 1573 (10/83) PREVIOUS EDITIONS ARE OBSOLETE.

FIG. A.3. Form used with the IND application (FDA 1573).

2a. The investigator assures that an IRB that complies with the requirements set forth in Part 56 of this chapter will be responsible for the initial and continuing review and approval of the proposed clinical study. The investigator also assures that he/she will report to the IRB all changes in the research activity and all unanticipated problems involving risks to human subjects or others, and that he/she will not make any changes in the research that would increase the risks to human subjects without IRB approval. FDA will regard the signing of the Form FDA 1573 as providing the necessary assurances stated above.

b. A description of any clinical laboratory facilities that will be used. (If this information has been submitted to the sponsor and reported by him on Form FDA 1571, reference to the previous submission will be adequate).

3. *The investigational drug will be used by the undersigned or under his supervision in accordance with the plan of investigation described as follows: (Outline the plan of investigation including approximation of the number of subjects to be treated with the drug and the number to be employed as controls, if any; clinical uses to be investigated; characteristics of subjects by age, sex and condition; the kind of clinical observations and laboratory tests to be undertaken prior to, during, and after administration of the drug; the estimated duration of the investigation; and a description or copies of report forms to be used to maintain an adequate record of the observations and test results obtained. This plan may include reasonable alternates and variations and should be supplemented or amended when any significant change in direction or scope of the investigation is undertaken.)*

4. **THE UNDERSIGNED UNDERSTANDS THAT THE FOLLOWING CONDITIONS, GENERALLY APPLICABLE TO NEW DRUGS FOR INVESTIGATIONAL USE, GOVERN HIS RECEIPTS AND USE OF THIS INVESTIGATIONAL DRUG:**

a. The sponsor is required to supply the investigator with full information concerning the preclinical investigations that justify clinical trials, together with fully informative material describing any prior investigations and experience and any possible hazards, contraindications, side-effects, and precautions to be taken into account in the course of the investigation.

b. The investigator is required to maintain adequate records of the disposition of all receipts of the drug, including dates, quantities, and use by subjects, and if the investigation is terminated, suspended, discontinued, or completed, to return to the sponsor any unused supply of the drug. If the investigational drug is subject to the Comprehensive Drug Abuse Prevention and Control Act of 1970, adequate precautions must be taken including storage of the investigational drug in a securely locked, substantially constructed cabinet, or other securely locked substantially constructed enclosure, access to which is limited, to prevent theft or diversion of the substance into illegal channels of distribution.

c. The investigator is required to prepare and maintain adequate and accurate case histories designed to record all observations and other data pertinent to the investigation on each individual treated with the drug or employed as a control in the investigation.

d. The investigator is required to furnish his reports to the sponsor of the drug who is responsible for collecting and evaluating the results obtained by various investigators. The sponsor is required to present progress reports to the Food and Drug Administration at appropriate intervals not exceeding 1 year. Any adverse effect that may reasonably be regarded as caused by, or probably caused by, the new drug shall be reported to the sponsor promptly, and if the adverse effect is alarming, it shall be reported immediately. An adequate report of the investigation should be furnished to the sponsor shortly after completion of the investigation.

e. The investigator shall maintain the records of disposition of the drug and the case histories described above for a period of 2 years following the date a new-drug application is approved for the drug; or if the application is not approved, until 2 years after the investigation is discontinued. Upon the request of a scientifically trained and properly authorized employee of the Department, at reasonable times, the investigator will make such records available for inspection and copying. The subjects' names need not be divulged unless the records of particular individuals require a more detailed study of the cases, or unless there is reason to believe that the records do not represent actual cases studied, or do not represent actual results obtained.

f. The investigator certifies that the drug will be administered only to subjects under his personal supervision or under the supervision of the following investigators responsible to him,

____

____

____

and that the drug will not be supplied to any other investigator or to any clinic for administration to subjects.

g. The investigator certifies that he will inform any subjects including subjects used as controls, or their representatives, that drugs are being used for investigational purposes, and will obtain the consent of the subjects, or their representatives, except where this is not feasible or, in the investigator's professional judgment, is contrary to the best interests of the subjects.

h. The investigator is required to assure the sponsor that for investigations subject to an institutional review requirement under Part 56 of this chapter the studies will not be initiated until the institutional review board has reviewed and approved the study. (The organization and procedure requirements for such a board as set forth in Part 56 should be explained to the investigator by the sponsor.)

Very truly yours,

Name of Investigator ________________________________

Address ____________________ Telephone (   ) __________

____

(This form should be supplemented or amended from time to time if new subjects are added or if significant changes are made in the plan of investigation.)

FIG. A.3. (*Continued*)

DEPARTMENT OF HEALTH AND HUMAN SERVICES PUBLIC HEALTH SEVICE FOOD AND DRUG ADMINISTRATION **APPLICATION TO MARKET A NEW DRUG FOR HUMAN USE OR AN ANTIBIOTIC DRUG FOR HUMAN USE** *(Title 21, Code of Federal Regulations, 314)*	*Form Approved: OMB No. 0910-0001* *Expiration Date; May 31, 1986.*	
	FOR FDA USE ONLY	
	DATE RECEIVED	DATE FILED
	DIVISION ASSIGNED	NDA/ANDA NO. ASS.

NOTE: No application may be filed unless a completed application form has been received *(21 C.F.R. Part 314).*

NAME OF APPLICANT	DATE OF SUBMISSION
ADDRESS *(Number, Street, City, State and Zip Code)*	TELEPHONE NO. *(Include Area Code)*

NEW DRUG OR ANTIBIOTIC APPLICATION NUMBER *(If previously issued)*

DRUG PRODUCT

ESTABLISHED NAME *(e.g., USP/USAN)*	PROPRIETARY NAME *(If any)*	
CODE NAME *(If any)*	CHEMICAL NAME	
DOSAGE FORM	ROUTE OF ADMINISTRATION	STRENGTH(S)

PROPOSED INDICATIONS FOR USE

LIST NUMBERS OF ALL INVESTIGATIONAL NEW DRUG APPLICATIONS *(21 CFR Part 312)*, NEW DRUG OR ANTIBIOTIC APPLICATIONS *(21 CFR Part 314)*, AND DRUG MASTER FILES *(21 CFR 314.420)* REFERRED TO IN THIS APPLICATION:

INFORMATION ON APPLICATION

TYPE OF APPLICATION *(Check one)*

☐ THIS SUBMISSION IS A FULL APPLICATION *(21 CFR 314.50)*

☐ THIS SUBMISSION IS AN ABBREVIATED APPLICATION *(ANDA) (21 CFR 314.55)*

IF AN ANDA, IDENTIFY THE APPROVED DRUG PRODUCT THAT IS THE BASIS FOR THE SUBMISSION

NAME OF DRUG	HOLDER OF APPROVED APPLICATION

STATUS OF APPLICATION *(Check one)*

☐ ORIGINAL APPLICATION

☐ AN AMENDMENT TO A PENDING APPLICATION

☐ RESUBMISSION

☐ SUPPLEMENTAL APPLICATION

PROPOSED MARKETING STATUS *(Check one)*

☐ APPLICATION FOR A PRESCRIPTION DRUG PRODUCT*(Rx)*

☐ APPLICATION FOR AN OVER - THE - COUNTER PRODUCT *(OTC)*

FORM FDA 356h (5/85) PREVIOUS EDITION IS OBSOLETE.

FIG. A.4. Form used with the NDA application (FDA 356h).

CONTENTS OF APPLICATION	
This application contains the following items: *(Check all that apply)*	
1. Index	
2. Summary *(21 CFR 350.50(c))*	
3. Chemistry, manufacturing, and control section *(21 CFR 314.50 (d) (1))*	
4. Nonclinical pharmacology and toxicology section *(21 CFR 314.50 (d)(2))*	
5. Human pharmacokinetics and bioavailability section *(21 CFR 314.5 (d) (3))*	
6. Microbiology section *(21 CFR 314.50 (d) (4))*	
7. Clinical data section *(21 CFR 314.50 (d) (5))*	
8. Statistical section *(21 CFR 314.50 (d) (6))*	
9. Safety update report *(21 CFR 314.50 (d) (5) (vi) (b))*	
10. a. Samples *(21 CFR 314.50 (e) (1)) (Submit only upon FDA's request)*	
b. Methods Validation Package *(21 CFR 314.50 (e) (2) (i))*	
c. Labeling *(21 CFR 314.50 (e) (2) (ii))*	
i. draft labeling *(4 copies)*	
ii. final printed labeling *(12 copies)*	
11. Case report tabulations *(21 CFR 314.50 (f) (1))*	
12. Case reports forms (21 CFR 314.50 (f) (1))	
13. Patent information on any patent which claims the drug *(21 U.S.C. 355 (b) or (c))*	
14. A patent certification with respect to any patent which claims the drug *(21 U.S.C. 355 (b) (2) or (j) (2) (A))*	
15. OTHER *(Specify)*	

I agree to update this application with new safety information about the drug that may reasonably affect the statement of contraindications, warnings, precautions, or adverse reactions in the draft labeling. I agree to submit these safety update reports as follows: (1) 4 months after the initial submission, (2) following receipt of an approvable letter and (3) at other times as requested by FDA. If this application is approved, I agree to comply with all laws and regulations that apply to approved applications, including the following:

1. Good manufacturing practice regulations in 21 CFR 210 and 211.
2. Labeling regulations in 21 CFR 201.
3. In the case of a prescription drug product, prescription drug advertising regulations in 21 CFR 202.
4. Regulations on making changes in application in 21 CFR 314.70, 314.71, and 314.72.
5. Regulations on reports in 21 CFR 314.80 and 314.81.
6. Local, state and Federal environmental impact laws.

If this application applies to a drug product that FDA has proposed for scheduling under the controlled substances Act I agree not to market the product until the Drug Enforcement Administration makes a final scheduling decision.

NAME OF RESPONSIBLE OFFICIAL OR AGENT	SIGNATURE OF RESPONSIBLE OFFICIAL OR AGENT	DATE
ADDRESS *(Street, City, State, Zip Code)*	TELEPHONE NO. *(Include Area Code)*	
(**WARNING:** A willfully false statement is a criminal offense. U.S.C. Title 18, Sec. 1001.)		

*U.S. GOVERMENT PRINTING OFFICE 1985 461-364/37052

FIG. A.4. (*Continued*)

DECLARATION OF HELSINKI

Recommendations guiding medical doctors in biomedical research involving human subjects.

Adopted by the 18th World Medical Assembly, Helsinki, Finland, 1964, and as revised by the 29th World Medical Assembly, Tokyo, Japan, 1975, and by the 35th World Medical Assembly, Venice, Italy, 1983.

Introduction

It is the mission of the medical doctor to safeguard the health of the people. His or her knowledge and conscience are dedicated to the fulfillment of this mission.

The Declaration of Geneva of The World Medical Association binds the physician with the words, "The health of my patient will be my first consideration," and the International Code of Medical Ethics declares that "A physician shall act only in the patient's interest when providing medical care which might have the effect of weakening the physical and mental condition of the patient."

The purpose of biomedical research involving human subjects must be to improve diagnostic, therapeutic and prophylactic procedures and the understanding of the etiology and pathogenesis of disease.

In current medical practice most diagnostic, therapeutic or prophylactic procedures involve hazards. This applies especially to biomedical research.

Medical progress is based on research which ultimately must rest in part on experimentation involving human subjects.

In the field of biomedical research a fundamental distinction must be recognized between medical research in which the aim is essentially diagnostic or therapeutic for a patient, and medical research, the essential object of which is purely scientific and without implying direct diagnostic or therapeutic value to the person subjected to the research.

Special caution must be exercised in the conduct of research which may affect the environment, and the welfare of animals used for research must be respected.

Because it is essential that the results of laboratory experiments be applied to human beings to further scientific knowledge and to help suffering humanity, The World Medical Association has prepared the following recommendations as a guide to every physician in biomedical research involving human subjects. They should be kept under review in the future. It must be stressed that the standards as drafted are only a guide to physicians all over the world. Physicians are not relieved from criminal, civil and ethical responsibilities under the laws of their own countries.

I. Basic principles

1. Biomedical research involving human subjects must conform to generally accepted scientific principles and should be based on adequately performed laboratory and animal experimentation and on a thorough knowledge of the scientific literature.

2. The design and performance of each experimental procedure involving human subjects should be clearly formulated in an experimental protocol which should be transmitted to a specially appointed independent committee for consideration, comment and guidance.
3. Biomedical research involving human subjects should be conducted only by scientifically qualified persons and under the supervision of a clinically competent medical person. The responsibility for the human subject must always rest with a medically qualified person and never rest on the subject of the research, even though the subject has given his or her consent.
4. Biomedical research involving human subjects cannot legitimately be carried out unless the importance of the objective is in proportion to the inherent risk to the subject.
5. Every biomedical research project involving human subjects should be preceded by careful assessment of predictable risks in comparison with foreseeable benefits to the subject or to others. Concern for the interests of the subject must always prevail over the interests of science and society.
6. The right of the research subject to safeguard his or her integrity must always be respected. Every precaution should be taken to respect the privacy of the subject and to minimize the impact of the study on the subject's physical and mental integrity and on the personality of the subject.
7. Physicians should abstain from engaging in research projects involving human subjects unless they are satisfied that the hazards involved are believed to be predictable. Physicians should cease any investigation if the hazards are found to outweigh the potential benefits.
8. In publication of the results of his or her research, the physician is obliged to preserve the accuracy of the results. Reports of experimentation not in accordance with the principles laid down in this Declaration should not be accepted for publication.
9. In any research on human beings, each potential subject must be adequately informed of the aims, methods, anticipated benefits and potential hazards of the study and the discomfort it may entail. He or she should be informed that he or she is at liberty to abstain from participation in the study and that he or she is free to withdraw his or her consent to participation at any time. The physician should then obtain the subject's freely-given informed consent, preferably in writing.
10. When obtaining informed consent for the research project the physician should be particularly cautious if the subject is in a dependent relationship to him or her or may consent under duress. In that case the informed consent should be obtained by a physician who is not engaged in the investigation and who is completely independent of this official relationship.
11. In case of legal incompetence, informed consent should be obtained from the legal guardian in accordance with national legislation. Where physical or mental incapacity makes it impossible to obtain informed consent, or when the subject is a minor, permission from the responsible relative replaces that of the subject in accordance with national legislation. Whenever the minor child is in fact able to give a consent, the minor's consent must be obtained in addition to the consent of the minor's legal guardian.

12. The research protocol should always contain a statement of the ethical considerations involved and should indicate that the principles enunciated in the present Declaration are complied with.

II. Medical research combined with professional care (clinical research)

1. In the treatment of the sick person, the physician must be free to use a new diagnostic and therapeutic measure, if in his or her judgment it offers hope of saving life, reestablishing health or alleviating suffering.
2. The potential benefits, hazards and discomfort of a new method should be weighed against the advantages of the best current diagnostic and therapeutic methods.
3. In any medical study, every patient-including those of a control group, if any-should be assured of the best proven diagnostic and therapeutic method.
4. The refusal of the patient to participate in a study must never interfere with the physician-patient relationship.
5. If the physician considers it essential not to obtain informed consent, the specific reasons for this proposal should be stated in the experimental protocol for transmission to the independent committee. (I.2)
6. The physician can combine medical research with professional care, the objective being the acquisition of new medical knowledge, only to the extent that medical research is justified by its potential diagnostic or therapeutic value for the patient.

III. Nontherapeutic biomedical research involving human subjects (Nonclinical biomedical research)

1. In the purely scientific application of medical research carried out on a human being, it is the duty of the physician to remain the protector of the life and health of that person on whom biomedical research is being carried out.
2. The subjects should be volunteers—either healthy persons or patients for whom the experimental design is not related to the patient's illness.
3. The investigator or the investigating team should discontinue the research if in his/her or their judgment it may, if continued, be harmful to the individual.
4. In research on man, the interest of science and society should never take precedence over considerations related to the well-being of the subject.

References

Abt, K., and Krupp, P. (1986): Pooling of laboratory safety data in multicenter studies. *Drug Inf. J.*, 20:311–313.

Asbury, C. H. (1985): *Orphan Drugs—Medical Versus Market Value*. Lexington Books, Lexington, MA.

Association of the British Pharmaceutical Industry (1983): Compensation and drug trials. Guidelines: Clinical trials—compensation for medicine induced injury. *Br. Med. J.*, 287:675.

Baum, M. (1983): The practical and ethical defects of surgical randomised prospective trials. Commentary. *J. Med. Ethics*, 9:92–93.

Beecher, H. K. (1961): Surgery as placebo. *J.A.M.A.*, 176:1102–1107.

Begg, C. B., Carbone, P. P., Elson, P. J., and Zelen, M. (1982): Participation of community hospitals in clinical trials: Analysis of five years of experience in the eastern cooperative oncology group. *N. Engl. J. Med.*, 306:1076–1080.

Bell, G. D. (1973): *The Achievers: Six Styles of Personality and Leadership*. Preston-Hill, Chapel Hill, North Carolina.

Bettis, J. W. (1985): Manufacture of clinical supplies. *Drug Dev. Ind. Pharm.*, 11:1685–1702.

Bleich, H. L., Beckley, R. F., Horowitz, G. L., Jackson, J. D., Moody, E. S., et al. (1985): Clinical computing in a teaching hospital. *N. Engl. J. Med.*, 312:756–764.

Bonchek, L. I. (1979): Are randomized trials appropriate for evaluating new operations? *N. Engl. J. Med.*, 301:44–45.

Bonchek, L. I. (1982): The role of the randomized clinical trial in the evaluation of new operations. *Surg. Clin. North Am.*, 62:761–769.

Breuning, S. E., Ferguson, D. G., and Cullari, S. (1980): Analysis of single–double blind procedures, maintenance of placebo effects, and drug-induced dyskinesia with mentally retarded persons. *Appl. Res. Ment. Retard.*, 1:175–192.

Byer, A. (1983): The practical and ethical defects of surgical randomised prospective trials. *J. Med. Ethics*, 9:90–93.

Cardon, P. V., Dommel, F. W., and Trumble, R. R. (1976): Injuries to research subjects—a survey of investigators. *New Engl. J. Med.*, 295:650–654.

Challah, S., and Mays, N. B. (1986): The randomised controlled trial in the evaluation of new technology: A case study. *Br. Med. J.*, 292:877–879.

Chalmers, T. C., and Sacks, H. (1979): Letter to the editor. *N. Engl. J. Med.*, 301:1182.

Cleland, D. I. and King, W. R., eds. (1983): *Project Management Handbook*. Van Nostrand Reinhold Co., New York.

Cobb, L. A., Thomas, G. I., Dillard, D. H., Merendino, K. A., and Bruce, R. A. (1959): An evaluation of internal-mammary-artery ligation by a double-blind technic. *N. Engl. J. Med.*, 260:1115–1118.

Cocchetto, D. M. (1986): An orientation program for new clinical trial monitors. *Clin. Res. Practices Drug Reg. Affairs*, 4:235–250.

Committee for the Protection of Human Participants in Research (1982): *Ethical Principles in the Conduct of Research with Human Participants*. American Psychological Association, Washington, D.C.

Cori, K. A. (1985): Fundamentals of master scheduling for the project manager. *Project Manage. J.*, 16:78–89.

Côté, R. A., and Robboy, S. (1980): Progress in medical information management: Systematized nomenclature of medicine (SNOMED). *J.A.M.A.*, 243:756–762.

Crawley, R., Belsey, R., Brock, D., and Baer, D. M. (1986): Regulation of physicians' office laboratories: The Idaho experience. *J.A.M.A.*, 255:374–382.

Darragh, A., Kenny, M., Lambe, R., and Brick, I. (1985): Sudden death of a volunteer. *Lancet*, I:93–94.

DeCosse, J. J., Donegan, W. L., Sedransk, N., Jones, N. F., and Claudon, D. B. (1980):

Operative procedures: Is standardization feasible or necessary? *Cancer Treat. Rep.*, 64:419–423.

de Maar, E. W. J. (1986): The global core clinical protocol and its rational adaptations. *Drug Inf. J.*, 20:257–261

Dimond, E. G., Kittle, C. F., and Crockett, J. E. (1960): Comparison of internal mammary artery ligation and sham operation for angina pectoris. *Am. J. Cardiol.*, 5:483–486.

Dinnerstein, A. J., and Halm, J. (1970): Modification of placebo effects by means of drugs: Effects of aspirin and placebos on self-rated moods. *J. Abnorm. Psychol.*, 75:308–314.

Drews, J. (1985): Judging pharmaceutical research and development from a financial point of view. *Swiss Pharm.*, 7:21–23.

Drury, M., and Hull, F. M. (1981): Prospective monitoring for adverse reactions to drugs in general practice. *Br. Med. J.*, 283:1305–1307.

Dubey, S. D. (1986): Current thoughts on crossover designs. *Clin. Res. Practices Drug Reg. Affairs*, 4:127–142.

Faust, R. E. (1982): Project selection factors in pharmaceutical R & D. In: *Drug Development*, edited by C. E. Hamner. CRC Press, Boca Raton, FL.

Folland, E., Hammermeister, K. E., Khuri, S., Rahimtoola, S. H., Sethi, G., et al. (1979): Letter to the editor. *N. Engl. J. Med.*, 301:1182–1183.

Forbes, M. B., Perez, A. E., and Gelberg, A. (1986): FDA's adverse drug reaction drug dictionary and its role in post-marketing surveillance. *Drug Inf. J.*, 20:135–145.

Fowler, N. O. (1979): Randomized clinical trials in surgery. *N. Engl. J. Med.*, 301:1181.

Frelick, R. W., and Kyle, A. (1984): Cancer clinical trial records: Physician responsibility. *Prog. Clin. Biol. Res.*, 156:369–378.

Gilbert, J. P., McPeek, B., and Mosteller, F. (1977): Progress in surgery and anesthesia: Benefits and risks of innovative therapy. In: *Costs, Risks and Benefits of Surgery*, edited by J. Bunker, B. Barnes, and F. Mosteller, pp. 124–169. Oxford University Press, New York.

Glicksman, A. S., Reinstein, L. E., Brotman, R., and McShan, D. (1980): Quality assurance programs in clinical trials. *Cancer Treat. Rep.*, 64:425–433.

Grabowski, H., and Vernon, J. (1982): A sensitivity analysis of expected profitability of pharmaceutical research and development. *Managerial and Decision Economics*, 3:36–40.

Graham, R. J. (1985): *Project Management: Combined Technical and Behavioral Approaches for Effective Implementation.* Van Nostrand Reinhold Co., New York.

Griffin, J. P., and Weber, J. C. P. (1985): Voluntary systems of adverse reaction reporting—Part I. *Adv. Drug React. Ac. Pois. Rev.*, 4:213–230.

Griffin, J. P., and Weber, J. C. P. (1986): Voluntary systems of adverse reaction reporting—Part II. *Adv. Drug React. Ac. Pois. Rev.*, 1:23–55.

Guth, W. D. (1985): *Handbook of Business Strategy.* Warren, Gorham and Lamont, Boston.

Guy, W. (1979): Documentation of early phase II trials. In: *Coordinating Clinical Trials in Psychopharmacology: Planning, Documentation, and Analysis*, DHEW Publication No. (ADM) 79-803, edited by J. Levine. U.S. Government Printing Office, Washington.

Guyatt, G., Sackett, D., Taylor, D. W., Chong, J., Roberts, R., et al. (1986): Determining optimal therapy: Randomized trials in individual patients. *N. Engl. J. Med.*, 314:889–892.

Haines, S. J. (1983): Randomized clinical trials in neurosurgery. *Neurosurgery*, 12:259–264.

Hammes, C. E., and Ciccone, P. E., eds. (1985): The impact of the Rx-to-OTC switch process: Present and future. *Drug Inf. J.*, 19(2), Special Issue:85–203.

Hansen, H. J., Caudill, S. P., and Boone, J. (1985): Crisis in drug testing: Results of CDC blind study. *J.A.M.A.*, 253:2382–2387.

Hansen, R. W. (1983): International Issues of Drug Regulation. *Zeitschrift fur die gesamte Staatswissenschaft* (*J. Inst. Theoret. Econ.*), 139:568–577.

Hayes, R. H. (1985): Strategic planning—forward in reverse? *Harv. Bus. Rev.*, 63(6):111–119.

Hopkins, J. A., Shoemaker, W. C., Greenfield, S., Chang, P. C., McAuliffe, T., et al. (1980): Treatment of surgical emergencies with and without an algorithm. *Arch. Surg.*, 115:745–750.

Inman, W. H. W., ed. (1986): *Monitoring for Drug Safety.* MTP Press, Lancaster, UK.

Jay, A. (1976): How to run a meeting. *Harv. Bus. Rev.*, 54(2):43–57.

Joglekar, P., and Paterson, M. L. (1986): A closer look at the returns and risks of pharmaceutical R & D. *J. Health Econ.*, 5:153–177.

Johnsson, G., Åblad, B., and Hansson, E. (1984): Prediction of adverse drug reactions in clinical practice from animal experiments and phase I–III studies. In: *Detection and Prevention of Adverse Drug Reactions* (*Skandia International Symposia*), edited by H. Boström, and N. Ljungstedt, pp. 190–199. Almqvist and Wiksell International, Stockholm.

Jones, J. K. ed. (1985): International adverse reaction surveillance. *Drug Inf. J.*, 19:205–393.

Kent, D. L., Shortliffe, E. H., Carlson, R. W., Bischoff, M. B., and Jacobs, C. D. (1985): Improvements in data collection through physician use of a computer-based chemotherapy treatment consultant. *J. Clin. Oncol.*, 3:1409–1417.

Landauer, A. A., and Pocock, D. A. (1984): Stress reduction by oxprenolol and placebo: Controlled investigation of the pharmacological and non-specific effects. *Br. Med. J.*, 289:592.

Lasagna, L. ed. (1975): *Combination Drugs: Their Use and Regulation*. Stratton Intercontinental Medical Book Corp., New York.

Lasagna, L. (1986): On reducing waste in foreign clinical trials and postregulation experience. *Clin. Pharm. Ther.*, 40:369–372.

Loh, I. K. (1979): Letter to the editor. *N. Engl. J. Med.*, 301:1182.

Mazzoni, D. J. (1972): Rx for the pharmaceutical marketer: Preventive marketing. *Med. Mark. Media*, 7:16–28.

McLeod, R. S., Taylor, D. W., Cohen, Z., and Cullen, J. B. (1986): Single-patient randomised clinical trial: Use in determining optimum treatment for patient with inflammation of Kock continent ileostomy reservoir. *Lancet*, I:726–728.

Mezey, K. C., ed. (1980): *Fixed Drug Combinations—Rationale and Limitations*. International Congress and Symposium Series, No. 22. Royal Society of Medicine, London; Academic Press, London: Grune and Stratton, New York.

Moses, L. E. (1984): The series of consecutive cases as a device for assessing outcomes of intervention. *N. Engl. J. Med.*, 311:705–710.

Murray, G. D. (1986): Use of an international data bank to compare outcome following severe head injury in different centres. *Stat. Med.*, 5:103–112.

Nordic Council on Medicines. (1983): *Clinical Trials of Drugs: Nordic Guidelines*. NLN publication, No. 11. Nordiska Läkemedelsnämnden, Uppsala, Sweden.

Pocock, S. J. (1985): Current issues in the design and interpretation of clinical trials. *Br. Med. J.*, 290:39–42.

Prentis, R. A., and Walker, S. R. (1986): Trends in the development of new medicines by UK-owned pharmaceutical companies (1964–1980). *Br. J. Clin. Pharmacol.*, 21:437–443.

Revill, J. P., ed. (1978): *Drug Information Sources: A World-wide Annotated Survey*. Gothard House Publications, Oxon, U.K.

Ruffin, J. M., Grizzle, J. E., Hightower, N. C., McHardy, G., Shull, H., et al. (1969): A cooperative double-blind evaluation of gastric "freezing" in the treatment of duodenal ulcer. *N. Engl. J. Med.*, 281:16–19.

Sackett, D. L., Haynes, R. B., and Tugwell, P. (1985): *Clinical Epidemiology: A Basic Science for Clinical Medicine*. Little, Brown and Company, Boston.

Saltzman, A. (1985): Adverse reaction terminology standardization: A report on Schering-Plough's use of the WHO dictionary and the formation of the WHO adverse reaction terminology users group (WUG) consortium. *Drug Inf. J.*, 19:35–41.

Sheiner, L. B., and Benet, L. Z. (1985): Premarketing observational studies of population pharmacokinetics of new drugs. *Clin. Pharmacol. Ther.*, 38:481–487.

Sills, J. M., Faich, G. A., Milstien, J. B., and Turner, W. M. (1986): Postmarketing reporting of adverse drug reactions to the FDA: An overview of the 1985 FDA guideline. *Drug. Inf. J.*, 20:151–156.

Slatter, S. St. P. (1977): Competition and Marketing Strategies in the Pharmaceutical Industry. Holmes and Meier Publishers, New York.

Sloboda, W., and Currier, C. (1985): FDA's monitoring of clinical trials. *Psychopharmacol. Bull.*, 21:105–106.

Snoddy, C. S., Jr., Michalak, R. A., and Kaufman, L. S. (1985): The pyramid concept. *Drug Inf. J.*, 19:27–33.

Sogliero-Gilbert, G., Mosher, K., and Zubkoff, L. (1986): A procedure for the simplification and assessment of lab parameters in clinical trials. *Drug Inf. J.*, 20:279–296.

Spilker, B. (1984): *Guide to Clinical Studies and Developing Protocols*. Raven Press, New York.

Spilker, B. (1985): Development of orphan drugs. *Trends Pharmacol. Sci.*, 6:185–188.

Spilker, B. (1986): *Guide to Clinical Interpretation of Data*. Raven Press, New York.

Spodick, D. H. (1973): The surgical mystique and the double standard. Controlled trials of medical and surgical therapy for cardiac diseases: Analysis, hypothesis, proposal. *Am. Heart J.*, 85:579–583.

Stephens, M. D. B. (1985): *The Detection of New Adverse Drug Reactions*. Stockton Press, New York.

Teal, T. W., and Dimmig, A. L. (1985): Adverse drug experience management: A brief review of the McNeil pharmaceutical system. *Drug Inf. J.*, 19:17–25.

Trombitas, I. D., and Simpson, R. L., Jr. (1986): Monitoring the world's published literature for adverse drug experiences. *Drug Inf. J.*, 20:57–62.

Turner, W. M., Milstien, J. B., Faich, G. A., and Armstrong, G. D. (1986): The processing of adverse reaction reports at FDA. *Drug Inf. J.*, 20:147–150.

van der Linden, W. (1980*a*): Pitfalls in randomized surgical trials. *Surgery*, 87:258–262.

van der Linden, W. (1980*b*): On the generalization of surgical trial results. *Acta Chir. Scand.*, 146:229–234.

Ware, J. H., Muller, J. E., and Braunwald, E. (1985): The futility index: An approach to the cost-effective termination of randomized clinical trials. *Am. J. Med.*, 78:635–643.

Williams, M. E. (1985): Electronic databases. *Science*, 228:445–456.

Yu, G. C. S. (1986): Remote data entry and retrieval: The human and administrative aspects. *Drug Inf. J.*, 20:103–107.

Zarafonetes, C. J. D., Riley, P. A. Jr., Willis, P. W. III, Power, L. H., et al. (1978): Clinically significant adverse events in a Phase 1 testing program. *Clin. Pharmacol. Ther.*, 24:127–132.

Subject Index

F